Volume Replacement

Monographs of the Physiological Society

Members of the Editorial Board

Corticospinal Function
and
Voluntary Movement

Robert Porter

Monash University
Melbourne, Australia

and

Roger Lemon

University of Cambridge

CLARENDON PRESS · OXFORD

Oxford University Press, Walton Street, Oxford OX2 6DP

Oxford   New York
Athens   Auckland   Bangkok   Bombay
Calcutta   Cape Town   Dar es Salaam   Delhi
Florence   Hong Kong   Istanbul   Karachi
Kuala Lumpur   Madras   Madrid   Melbourne
Mexico City   Nairobi   Paris   Singapore
Taipei   Tokyo   Toronto

and associated companies in
Berlin   Ibadan

Oxford is a trade mark of Oxford University Press

Published in the United States
by Oxford University Press Inc., New York

A catalogue record for this book is available from the British Library

Library of Congress Cataloging in Publication Data
Porter, Robert, 1932–
Corticospinal function and voluntary movement / Robert Porter and
Roger Lemon.
p.   cm. – (Monographs of the Physiological Society ; no. 45)
Includes bibliographical references and index.
1. Pyramidal tract.   2. Motor neurons.   3. Kinesiology.
I. Lemon, Roger.   II. Title.   III. Series.
QP370.5.P67   1993   612.8'252 – dc20   93-14881
ISBN   0 19 852375 0

Printed in Great Britain by St Edmundsbury Press Ltd, Bury St Edmunds, Suffolk

Preface

Our aim is to illustrate the way in which experimental observations, especially those which provide descriptions of anatomical connectivity within the primate brain and those which test the physiological correlation, with aspects of movement performance, of given neural elements within such connected systems, have delineated functional anatomical substrates for the management of movement in human primates. In recent years, measurements of regional brain activities in normal human subjects and in persons with brain disorders have provided for increasing comparisons between results obtained in monkeys and those obtained in man. Neurologists and psychologists are now able, more directly than ever before, to relate the findings of the experimental neuroanatomist and neurophysiologist to the human problems which they are studying. It therefore seems to be an appropriate time to summarize our knowledge of these anatomical and physiological observations and to relate such facts to our understanding of the significance of the observations being made in man, at least as they concern the performance of voluntary movement.

As is usual for these publications by The Physiological Society, this monograph will develop its theme by drawing heavily on the personal observations and experience of the authors and their associates. We shall not attempt to be comprehensive in our coverage of all the relevant literature or experiments. Our scientific colleagues are already aware of the respect with which we regard them and their work. Our original publications in the scientific literature refer directly to the contributions of others to the development of our ideas. It is rather to provide a personal, general commentary on the overall state of knowledge relevant to understanding of the control of voluntary movement that this book is addressed. We shall include descriptions of the major scientific observations which have contributed to our present understanding and we hope we have identified sufficient references to the multitude of contributions of the host of other significant workers in this field, to allow the interested reader to be led to the detailed original reports which contain full descriptions of the scientific findings from which we have made our selections.

Because this book was conceived, in some measure, as a sequel to an earlier monograph of The Physiological Society entitled *Corticospinal neurones: their role in movement* (Phillips and Porter 1977), the historical background to more recent work and the experimental observations covered in that book will be dealt with in much less detail in the present volume. Nevertheless, we have tried, without repeating extensive descriptions, to provide sufficient historical context, within which the most recent observations may be interpreted, to allow this book to stand alone and to pursue its own thematic development. We identify, in Chapter 1, the evolution of concepts of localization of motor function largely within the precentral convolution of the cerebral cortex and its immediately adjacent regions. We have given special attention to early histological and electrical studies which examined the human brain because these provide the descriptions of functional geography in man. Against this background it is possible to analyse the interpretations of modern observations in both monkeys and human subjects. Also, in this chapter, we introduce the study of the organization of the spinal cord and the analysis of synaptic connectivities within the spinal cord. These provide a substrate for corticospinal actions to be enabled to influence movement. They also elucidate the details of synaptic mechanisms themselves and provide the rules which must operate in the interactions between connected cells within the cerebral cortex itself or in other parts of the brain. Microphysiological principles have been established through experiments on spinal synaptic mechanisms.

We then proceed to deal with the detailed cellular anatomy of the principal motor region of the cerebral cortex and with the experimental information which is concerned with development of the corticospinal tract both phylogenetically and in some primate species. Our title indicates that we continue to ascribe to corticospinal connections a major significant role in the execution of voluntary movement, and it is principally with corticospinal structure and functions that this book will be concerned. Therefore we need to understand the details of the anatomy of these fibres and of the intracortical connections that will allow them to be selected and engaged in motor outputs. Study of corticospinal anatomy must extend to the divergence of its influences to subcortical structures and, in particular, to its impact on the complex, organized spinal machinery for ordered activation of muscles via the final common path from motoneurones to motor units in selected muscles. This task of concentrating on the experimental study of corticospinal involvement in voluntary movement precludes the comprehensive review of such complex issues as the detailed delineation of boundaries for the motor cortex.

Our descriptions provide the anatomical substrate for the examination of output functions as they can be revealed by direct recordings from neuronal elements in the cerebral cortex during movement performance and by the indirect identification of regional changes in neural activation by studies of blood flow and metabolism in the human brain. Here again it is possible to identify that the parallel results obtained by sampling the discharges of individual neurones in conscious monkeys are consistent with measurements made in human subjects performing appropriate motor tasks. Moreover, the general indications of regional specialization in connection with some aspects of human behaviour can direct attention to the need to re-examine these regions using electrophysiological methods in subhuman primates to analyse the neuroanatomical and neurophysiological basis of such regional specialization.

From the very earliest experimental studies of voluntary movement and from analysis of the acquisition of human skills, it is clear that there is a major involvement in movement performance of those parts of the nervous system which are concerned with sensory experience. Before the turn of the century, Mott and Sherrington (1895) had stated that the 'whole sensory path is in action during voluntary movement'. Against this background, our account examines the anatomy and physiology of some of the inputs to the brain which relate to the performance of voluntary movement. We also address other 'circuits' which must be examined to define their involvement in the management of movement. Some of these connect more or less directly to the cells of origin of the corticospinal system and could influence the outputs through this system. Intracortical circuits involve regions such as the premotor cortex and supplementary motor area which are closely associated with the precentral motor cortex. Others involve deep brain structures known to influence movement performance. It will be essential to understand the regional and cellular connectivities which provide the basis for the functional role of these circuits.

Dynamic changes occur in the brain during the establishment of behaviours, during the acquisition of motor skills, in attention, in learning new performances, and following perturbations in some parts of the brain's movement control systems. It is now becoming possible to examine some of this plasticity in identified regions of the human brain. Renewed efforts are being made in animal experiments to elucidate the nature of the plastic transformation and its underlying anatomical and physiological basis. For our purposes, we need to ask whether the techniques that are at present available to the neurophysiologist allow us to interpret the dynamic changes in the regional maps of motor functional anatomy and to explain them on a micro-anatomical and microphysiological basis.

Our final task has been to attempt a synthesis which gives our impressions of the operations of the brain, the co-operative and continuous interactions within its many connected regions, and especially of the activation of the corticospinal tract in the management of voluntary movement. We are aware that much of the material which we have reviewed here will have been enriched and modified by new observations even before this book is published. In the light of new findings, our identification of those observations which we regard as most important and our interpretations of the significance of the experimental results obtained will also need re-evaluation. Our purpose will have been served, however, if the young people interested in this subject because they are embarked on a career in basic neuroscience, in human movement studies, in neurology, in psychology, in physiotherapy, or in education or rehabilitation can be stimulated to challenge our conclusions and to become personally involved in extending the knowledge base which we have attempted to encompass.

Cambridge   R. P.
June 1992   R. N. L.

Acknowledgements

The opportunity for the development of the approach of this book, and for the preparation of first drafts of a good part of the text, was generously provided by support from the British Council and the award of a Commonwealth Senior Medical Fellowship to Bob Porter. This allowed two separate periods of collaboration between the authors while Porter was given the privilege of taking up residence in New Hall, Cambridge and having membership of the Senior Common Room. Excellent facilities for collaborative work were provided by the Anatomy Department in Cambridge and access to that Department's library and to the Cambridge University library was very valuable. The support of the Vice Chancellor of Monash University (Professor Mal Logan) in allowing two short periods of leave to undertake outside studies programs is acknowledged.

The material in the book is based on our work and is particularly dependent on the contributions of our many scientific colleagues to both the literature and to fruitful intellectual interactions. Special acknowledgement is required for the important influences of Charles Phillips of Oxford and the late Hans Kuypers on our work and on the development of our ideas. Also contributing in a major way have been the large number of close colleagues whose association with us over the years has contributed so much to the background and also to the detail of this book. Principal among these immediate colleagues have been Jean Armand, Parveen Bawa, Keree Bennett, Cobie Brinkman, Brian Bush, Steve Edgley, Janet Eyre, Didier Flament, Soumya Ghosh, Mosjé Godschalk, Marie-Claude Hepp-Reymond, Jonathan Hore, Malcolm Horne, Robert Iansek, Julian Jack, Ted Jones, Donald Lawrence, Murray Lewis, Geert Mantel, Simon Miller, Ray Muir, Peter Rack, John Rawson, Stephen Redman, Ed Schmidt, Tom G. Smith Jnr, David Tracey, Bruce Walmsley, and Wilfried Werner.

We acknowledge that many of the most important new ideas referred to in this book have come from the work of scientists working in other laboratories round the world. Reference to the dependence of what we have done or what we have written on their contributions is included in the text.

All the original material from our own scientific observations has been made possible through continuous support for this work, since the 1960s, by the Wellcome Trust, by the National Health and Medical Research Council in Australia, the Australian Research Grants Committee, the Medical Research Council (UK), Action Research, and the East Anglian Regional Health Authority. A special acknowledgement is needed for the support of Action Research, then called the National Fund for Research into Crippling Diseases, for the provision of a postdoctoral Research Fellowship to Roger Lemon to enable him to travel to Australia in 1974 to join Bob Porter and to commence the scientific associations and collaboration in this field of endeavour. His introduction to the experimental approaches which were then in progress in the Department of Physiology at Monash University provided the basis for much of the scientific work described in this book.

At Monash, Canberra, Sheffield, Rotterdam, and Cambridge the contributions of a large number of technical staff and other have been involved in facilitating our work. Julie Norman cared for the monkeys at Monash, and Garry Rodda assisted with experiments at The John Curtin School of Medical Research. Hans van der Burg and Eddie Dalm provide excellent support in Rotterdam as did Rosalyn Cummings in Cambridge.

The preparation of the book itself has also involved the devoted efforts of many of our associates. Rosalyn Cummings in Cambridge undertook the mammoth task of compiling and checking the reference list. Typing, corrections, and reorganization of computer readable discs was done by Ruby Watson and Angela Lester at the Australian end. Preparation of the illustrations was handled by Stuart Butterworth at The John Curtin School of Medical Research in Canberra and by John Bashford and his staff, Rosalyn Cummings, and Rachel Chesterton in Cambridge.

Opportunities for continuing use of the excellent facilities of The John Curtin School and its unsurpassed biomedical science library were provided to Bob Porter by the Director of that School, Professor David Curtis, who arranged for a Visiting Fellowship to be available after Porter's return to Monash.

We should also like to thank Alan Brown, Chairman of the Physiological Society's Editorial Board for Monographs, for his continued advice, patience, and encouragement. The cooperation, advice, and assistance of the staff of Oxford University Press is gratefully acknowledged.

Contents

Contents

Previous Volumes in this Series

Volumes marked with an asterisk are now out of print.

1

The background: relationships between structure and function

1.1 LOCALIZATION

Nineteenth century considerations of the relationships between brain structure and motor function explored key issues which are still relevant as we approach the end of the twentieth century. The tools that were available for use by all the early workers in the field were quite inadequate for the demanding task of examining relationships between structure and function in the mammalian brain. Yet, using the then available histological techniques, crude electrical stimulation and the earliest forms of mechanical registration of muscle contractions, important indications were obtained of the background for present-day evaluation of modern studies of the human brain in health and disease, using positron emission tomography and other forms of imaging, as well as modern methods of microneurography and magnetic brain stimulation in conscious human subjects. We shall endeavour to build on this background, and incorporate the results of detailed observations from experimental interventions in laboratory primates, in order to provide for a more confident approach to descriptions of the relationships between structure and function in the brain's machinery for voluntary movement performance.

A major desire to understand the mechanisms for initiation and control of voluntary movement performance in man and to account for the disturbances of motor function which accompany human disease, clearly motivated many medical scientists and continues to be a major stimulus for investigation of brain function. In addition to the scientific challenge itself, major theoretical and philosophical questions, which go far beyond the issue of defining the chains of nervous connections that are essential for the production of movement, have been raised and seriously debated throughout the last century. These include: the relationship between anatomical development of nervous connectivity and the learning of motor skills as behaviour becomes established from infancy to adulthood; the precise nature of the association between morphological structures in the brain and defined minute or global functions; the fixity or flexibility of these associations; the capacity for inducing new functions within a given structure, with potential implications for recovery of function; and the very concept of dependence on particular brain structures and defined connections of such concepts as 'free will' (in the context of deciding to move, planning a voluntary movement or deciding not to move).

Following the examples set by Broca (1861) and Hughlings Jackson (1874), examination of human subjects whose disorders had been documented at the bedside provided increasing evidence for localization of function in the human cerebral cortex and of the status of corticospinal connections as a substrate for aspects of the control exerted by the cerebral cortex on spinal motor nuclei. This background is described in detail and commented upon in Phillips and Porter (1977, Chapter 2). Goldstein (1953) summarized Broca's historic presentation in the following words:

It was a memorable day in 1861 when Broca demonstrated before the *Société d'anthropologie* in Paris — with his venerable father looking on in silent admiration — the lesion in the left frontal lobe of his patient who had suffered from *aphémie* (renamed 'aphasia' by Trousseau in 1861). From this and subsequent observations he concluded that the integrity of the posterior part of the third frontal convolution was indispensable to articulate speech, and therefore termed this region the *circonvolution du langage*. (Later Ferrier referred to it as 'Broca's convolution'.)

The theory of circumscribed localisation was considered to be established beyond doubt. His views took on even more importance when, in 1874, Wernicke localised the corresponding disturbance in the sensory part of language, sensory aphasia, and elaborated his psycho-physical theory of brain function. However, Broca was not infallible: Pierre Marie, in the early 1900's sought out Broca's brain specimens in the old Musée Dupuytren and found that the very brain Broca described had parieto-temporal as well as frontal lesions.

Efforts to develop experimental approaches that, in modern terminology, might yield 'animal models' of human disorder led, towards the end of the nineteenth century, to fierce controversy, even about the fact of localization of motor function within the cerebral cortex. Hence, in 1881, 'a battle of the giants, Goltz and Ferrier, on the question of localization of motor control in the cortex of the brain' was clearly the most significant debate of the day (Liddell 1960). So contentious was the issue that, at the Seventh International Medical Congress in London in 1881, it was decided that the brain from one of Goltz's experimental dogs, which exhibited no evidence in favour of localization, and the brain of one of the hemiplegic monkeys of Yeo and Ferrier, in which localized lesions had been followed by localized effects in the limbs, should be subjected to independent detailed morphological examination.

1.2 FUNCTIONAL SIGNIFICANCE OF LOCALIZATION

This was the event which provided the introduction of the young Sherrington, still an undergraduate medical student, to physiology. Langley was given the task of examining the cerebral hemisphere of Goltz's dog and he was joined in this endeavour by Sherrington, whose name appears with Langley's on the paper describing the degeneration in the brain which followed the long established cortical lesion (Langley and Sherrington 1884). Another paper under Sherrington's sole authorship appeared in 1885, although he was clearly assisted by, and had access to material from, the experiments of Goltz. This work is expertly summarized by Liddell (1960). Some important observations were made. Consistent with the earlier evidence of others, Sherrington confirmed that 'voluntary power was maintained in the dog after large destruction of both pyramidal tracts', that 'the knee jerk was found to be depressed after removal of the 'cord area', but was later exaggerated', and that 'the defect of motion is observable only as clumsiness in the execution of fine movements'. These were Sherrington's 'first recorded contributions to the study of function during life' (quotations from Liddell 1960, p. 107).

It became clear to Sherrington, as it is clear to us, that in the search for a structural basis for the function of voluntary motor performance, he should follow the example of Ferrier (1876) and examine brain–cord connections in the monkey. He was also persuaded that 'anatomy had to come before physiology' (Liddell 1960, p. 131) and that it was essential to develop descriptions of the structural basis of the functional outcomes in which he was interested. He therefore turned to the monkey for experiments which examined the sensory and motor innervation of the limbs and the detailed anatomical basis for sensory and motor function in primates (Sherrington 1893; 1898). His first paper on 'brain–cord connections' in the monkey (Sherrington 1889) indicated that, following shallow lesions of the precentral gyrus, there were

no neat bundles of degenerated fibres in the pyramidal tracts, but a wide scatter of degenerated fibres all through the pyramid. Further, after lesions in the 'arm area' there were degenerated fibres all the way down the spinal cord as far as the sacral region, which was remarkable. Similarly, lesions of the 'leg area' produced degeneration in fibres which ended in the cervical enlargement of the cord (Liddell 1960).

1.3 SENSATION AND MOVEMENT

Because of the impact which this early work of Sherrington had on the progress of our understanding, and because of the influence which Sherrington exerted on his pupils and his associates, who then extended the experimental study of motor functions of the cerebral cortex into human subjects, as well as other experimental mammals, it is worthwhile documenting a few other elements of the background to modern investigations which were provided by his work. Mott and Sherrington (1895) observed monkeys for a period of months after section of the dorsal roots of the spinal cord. They reported that voluntary movement was more impaired by dorsal root section than by cortical ablation. The 'apaesthetic' limb was rendered useless and pendular by section of its dorsal roots. They concluded that their experiments implied an 'influence of sensation upon voluntary movement, in as much as they indicate not only the cortex but the whole sensory path from the periphery to the cortex cerebri is in action during voluntary movement.' In spite of the removal of afferent signals, and of this paralysis of voluntary movement, electrical stimulation of the cortex in these animals produced the usual movements of thumb, hallux, and digits. The implication was that the connections necessary for the production of movement were intact. However, without sensory input from the limb these connections could not be utilized to generate movement voluntarily.

Consistent with his emerging theories that implicated the distance receptors of an animal organism in guiding and directing purposive motor performance ('movement as an outcome of the working of the brain', as it is styled in *The integrative action of the nervous system*) Sherrington (1906) concentrated part of his commentary on the special features and 'refined duties of sensation and motor action' of the apex of the limb: 'That which the delicate yellow spot is to the sentifacient sheet of the retina, may the thumb and the index be said to constitute in the great sentifacient field of the limb'.

1.4 MAPS: THE SEQUENCE AND SIGNIFICANCE OF MOVEMENT RESPONSES

Just before the turn of the century, and following his move from Cambridge to Liverpool, Sherrington began to examine the 'maps' of cortical localization of motor responses which could be revealed by electrical stimulation of the surface of the brain in anaesthetized apes. This work provides one of the starting points for the examination of the anatomical substrates of the functions with which this book will be concerned. It sets the scene for the histological descriptions of identifiable and separable structural zones within the cerebral cortex of both apes and man, especially revealed in the work of Campbell (1905), on which foundations the results of the electrical stimulation experiments in human subjects performed by Penfield, Foerster, and others were to be interpreted. In this chapter we shall provide a very brief introduction to this line of study. It will set the scene for the later description, in Chapters 2, 3, and 4, of more recent contributions to these anatomical substrates for movement performance, whether these have been revealed by conventional microscopic observations or by electro-anatomical methods (Phillips and Porter 1977).

1.5 THE FINAL COMMON PATH

In addition, we shall have to be concerned with a second field of investigation, as central to the understanding of mechanisms for movement and functional outcomes of neuronal activity as is the detailed study of the nature of cerebral representation. This is the machinery for movement which resides in the spinal cord and its associated connections. Liddell (1960) quotes Sherrington as saying: 'My own work began by chance at the wrong end — the cortex, pyramidal degenerations, etc.'. And it is certain that the lifelong pursuit of the detailed study of function by Sherrington and his many students and collaborators was so enormously successful because the anatomical facts of spinal innervation could be established by experiment. These facts could be used appropriately to ask realistic questions about function in decerebrate and spinal animals. The rules which applied to the connectivities underlying a number of reflex functions could be established, and the role of the synapse in conferring a single direction on the propagation of nervous impulses through a chain of nerve cells could be defined.

Sherrington's work, characterized by persistence in the exploration of the multiplicity of details of functional organization and by immense insight which gave weight to his interpretations of experimental observations, led on to the modern analysis of spinal cord organization and reflexes, which will be summarized in later chapters. This complex machinery does not deal only with the mechanisms of reflex function, however. It provides the essential basis for, and details the synaptic processes involved in, the understanding of functional connectivity which will have to be explored within the cerebral cortex itself. It also exists as the inbuilt machinery for functional influences exerted by the brain on the spinal cord, where similar or the same, common synaptic machinery provides the substrate for the brain's own functional impact on the spinal systems.

1.6 PRIMATE MOTOR MAPS

To return to the systematic mapping of motor output responses of the primate cerebral cortex and the correlation of these maps with histologically defined zones or regions, we need to examine the observations of Grünbaum and Sherrington (dealt with *in extenso* by Leyton (previously Grünbaum) and Sherrington 1917) which were reported first in 1901. The major paper reports the results of faradization with just threshold stimuli, of the cerebral cortex of twenty two chimpanzees, three gorillas, and three orang-utans. Others (Mott, Schuster, and Graham Brown among them) contributed to the experiments which are here documented. The studies addressed particularly the question of localization of motor function and concluded that the representation of motor responses was limited, in these anthropoids, to the precentral gyrus. This contrasted with the results obtained by Beevor and Horsley (1890) who elicited motor responses from both precentral and postcentral cortex. Leyton and Sherrington (1917) reported that

a very considerable number of different movements are obtainable from the motor cortex of the anthropoid, far more than can be obtained from the dog or macaque.

. . . the individual movements, elicited by somewhat minutely localised stimulations, are, broadly speaking, fractional, in the sense that each, though co-ordinately executed, forms, so to say, but a unitary part of some more complex act, that would, to attain its purpose, involve combination of that unitary movement with others to make up a useful whole. . . .

It is the isolated and restricted character of the primary movements elicited by punctate stimulation of the cortex, or, to repeat the term introduced above, their fractional character, which makes so equivocal any purpose that an observer, who would interpret their purpose, can assign to them. Such a movement as the extension of the index finger can serve many purposes. . . .

The motor cortex appears to be par excellence a synthetic organ for motor acts. . . . The motor cortex seems to possess, or to be in touch with, the small localized movements as separable units, and to supply great numbers of connecting processes between these, so as to associate them together in extremely varied combinations. The acquirement of skilled movements, though certainly a process involving far wider areas (cf. V. Monakow) of the cortex than the excitable zone itself, may be presumed to find in the motor cortex an organ whose synthetic properties are part of the physiological basis that renders that acquirement possible.

This paper also describes, in minute detail, with meticulous recording of the precise observations made in each individual experiment, the effects of ablation of circumscribed areas of anthropoid motor cortex, defined by the responses produced in them by electrical stimuli. Temporary, localised paresis of a contralateral limb was produced and its characteristics documented. The recovery of function was said not to depend on surrounding precentral or postcentral regions of cerebral cortex taking over functions of the zone removed. Degeneration of the corticospinal fibres was traced through the pyramidal tracts and into the spinal cord and it is stated that

the pyramidal tract in the anthropoid (chimpanzee) more closely resembles the human than does that of any other animal so far examined: . . . there is a well marked uncrossed ventral column bundle belonging to the tract. The uncrossed ventral column bundle shows degeneration after arm area lesions as well as after leg area lesions, but in the latter case its degeneration is traceable into the lumbar region, whereas in the former it ceases much higher up the cord, although there it may be large.

The pyramidal tract degeneration after the arm area lesion was traceable [in the contralateral dorsolateral segment of the cord] to much below the brachial enlarge-

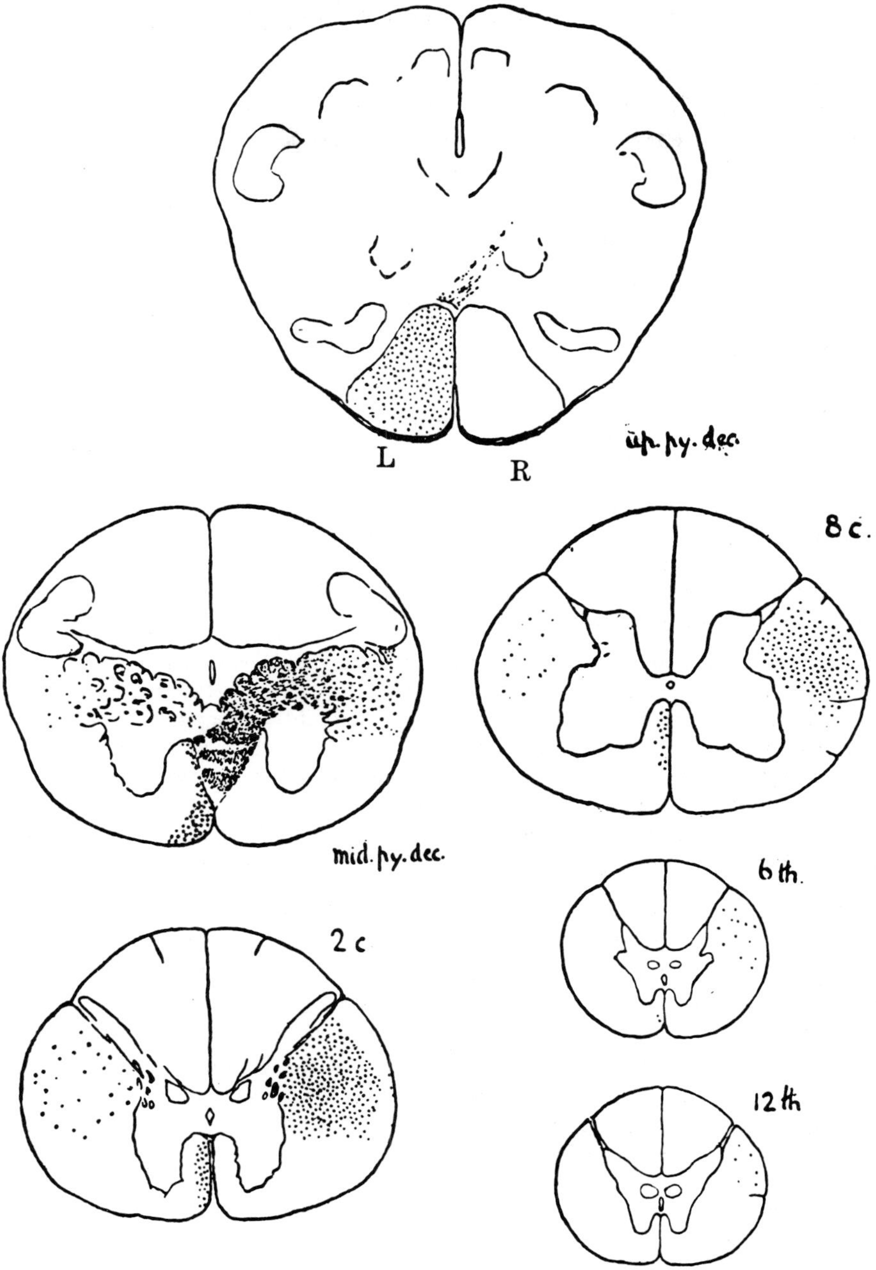

FIG 1.1 Spinal cord degeneration after a unilateral lesion in the arm area of the motor cortex of a chimpanzee. This figure reproduces Fig. 20 of Leyton and Sherrington (1917). The longitudinal distribution of corticospinal fibres is more restricted in the higher apes than it is in the monkey and this diagram illustrates that the corticospinal innervation is for the most part limited to cervical (c) segments of the spinal cord.

ment, . . . but did not reach the lumbosacral. In the grey matter of the ventral gray horn of the side contralateral to the cortical lesion a heavy degeneration in the minute fibres was evident, in the brachial segments after arm area lesion, in the lumbosacral enlargement after leg area lesion [see Fig. 1.1].

It is clear from these studies that the longitudinal distribution of corticospinal fibres from the arm representation in the cerebral cortex is more restricted in the higher apes than it is in the monkey: it appears to be more limited to innervation of the cervical segments of the spinal cord.

The paper by Leyton and Sherrington (1917) contains a large number of detailed diagrams of the closely-spaced points stimulated and the movements elicited in a large number of individual hemispheres. Only for the brain of the gorilla is a more diagrammatic summary provided which illus-

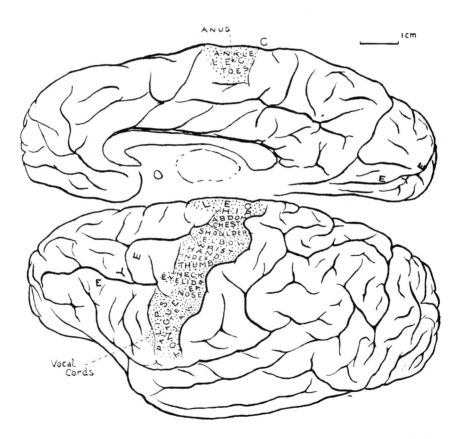

FIG 1.2   A diagram of the sequence of representation of movements revealed by electrical stimulation of the brain of a gorilla. This reproduces Fig. 10 of Leyton and Sherrington (1917).

trates the generalized arrangement of the sequence elicited for the localization of motor responses (Fig. 1.2)

The most schematic summary of the arrangement of the responses obtained
from stimulation of the precentral cortex seems to be the one used by
Sherrington in the second Silliman Memorial Lecture at Yale and published
in 1906 as '*The integrative action of the nervous system*'. This is a diagram
of the brain of a chimpanzee and a redrawn and relabelled version of it
is reproduced here as Fig. 1.3.

An extensive discussion of the discovery of localized outflow from the
cerebral cortex by the use of electrical stimulation of its surface in a large
number of animal species has been provided in Chapter 2 of Phillips and
Porter (1977). The foregoing observations by Sherrington and his colleagues
are there analysed in the context of the contributions those reports made
to emerging ideas about the corticospinal outflow and its functional significance. They are also evaluated in terms of their relevance to major questions about the nature and meaning of cortical representations. Many of
the earliest workers considered that they were, indeed, revealing, by electrical stimulation of the cortex, the representation of movement itself,
rather as the phrenologists, Gall and Spurzheim (1810), had imputed a

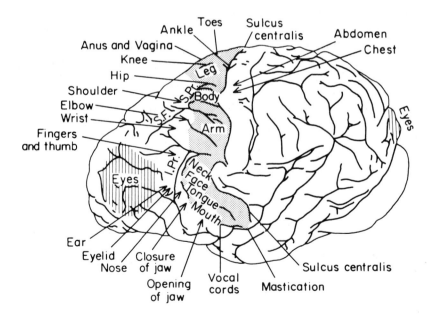

Fig 1.3   A diagram of the motor responses obtained by stimulation of the brain
of a chimpanzee. This is a redrawn and relabelled version of the diagram which
was presented as Fig. 72 of Sherrington (1906).

'representation' to sensations, emotions, ideas, and thought processes within particular localized regions of the brain. Here we wish to link those findings on motor responses obtained by brain stimulation to anatomical, structural elements, as far as that is possible.

1.7 HISTOLOGICAL FEATURES OF THE CEREBRAL CORTEX

A number of cerebral hemispheres from two chimpanzees and one orang-utan which had been subjected to electrical stimulation experiments by Sherrington and Grünbaum were made available to Dr A. W. Campbell for histological study. Campbell (Fig. 1.4) was working at the Rainhill Asylum and he had set out to examine regional differences in the histological structure of parts of the human brain which could be identified as having particular functions localized within them. Until Campbell undertook his laborious and detailed work, only piecemeal observations on structural differences in different parts of the cerebral cortex existed.

At the most two functional areas, the motor and visuo-sensory, can be pointed to as having their boundaries accurately delineated by cytological methods, and it is plain that observers have previously baulked an attempt to explore the whole surface in a comprehensive and complete manner on account of the magnitude of the task. To the accomplishment of this undertaking I now lay claim; and its independent value is materially enhanced by the fact that it has enabled me to make a collateral comparison of cell lamination and fibre arrangement in section after section and millimetre by millimetre over the entire surface of the human cerebrum.

A footnote to this statement indicates:

In more than one case, I have converted an entire cerebral hemisphere into serial sections and alternately stained these for the display of nerve cells and nerve fibres. (Campbell 1905, p. xvii).

Figure 1.5 summarizes Campbell's diagram of the human cerebrum. The legend to his diagram explains that

the figures are especially misleading in regard to some of the most important areas: thus the floor not the lip of the fissure of Rolando is the boundary between precentral and postcentral fields, and accordingly the concealed portion of these areas is almost equivalent to that exposed.

Campbell subjected the hemispheres of the chimpanzees and the orang-utan to the same careful detailed study that had enabled him confidently to describe the principal, histologically separable areas of the cerebral cortex of man. Moreover, since these brains had been 'mapped' by electrical stimulation, the correlation between the motor area of the cerebral cortex, as so revealed, and its histological organization could be established with

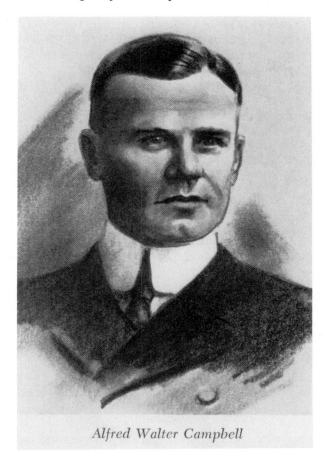

Alfred Walter Campbell

Fig 1.4   A. W. Campbell. We learn from pp 16–18 of *The founders of neurology* (1953) (ed. Webb Haymaker) that Alfred Walter Campbell (1868–1937) was born on his father's station at Cunningham Plains, near Harden, in the hills of New South Wales. He studied medicine in Edinburgh, graduating in 1889. He was captain of cricket and soccer teams. He studied in Vienna and Prague and obtained his doctorate in 1892, 'On the pathology of alcoholic insanity', and his thesis won him the gold medal at the University of Edinburgh. He then spent 13 years as resident medical officer and director of pathology at the Rainhill Asylum near Liverpool. He returned to Sydney in 1905 where he took up the practice of neurology and psychiatry in which he continued with great distinction until he retired in 1937. This portrait is reproduced from *The founders of Neurology*; the original appeared in *The Medical Journal of Australia* (1938), Volume 1, p. 1820.

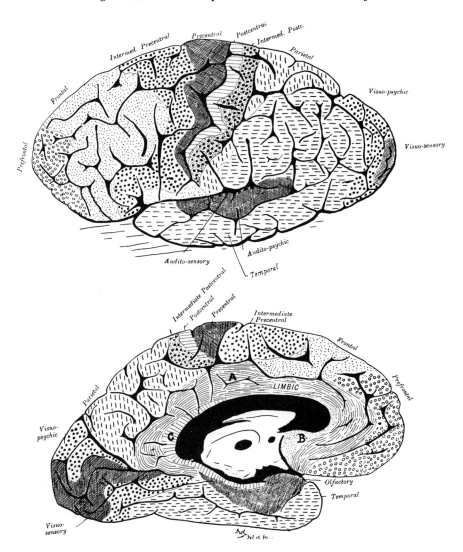

FIG 1.5 Diagrams which are reproduced from Plate I of Campbell's (1905) treatise. The original legend described the diagrams as 'orthogonal tracings of the lateral and mesial surfaces (the former somewhat tilted to show the convexity) of the left cerebral hemisphere'. This brain was obtained from a 41-year-old male. 'In a surface diagram it is impossible to give a true idea of the extent of many of these fields, because cortex concealed within fissures cannot be indicated'.

some confidence. The main conclusion was that motor responses were essentially limited to the precentral region in the apes.

Campbell reported that

it has been satisfactory to find that the delicate methods of electrical excitation employed in stimulating the cortex in those researches has not in any way damaged the brain for histological purposes.

This histological investigation I undertook with the object of ascertaining whether the cortex of parts which responded to electrical excitation could be differentiated from the 'silent' parts, by the possession of any distinctive histological structure; and, leaving details for later reference, I may here mention that no small measure of success attended the effort, for I think I was able to prove to Professor Sherrington and Dr. Grünbaum's satisfaction, that it is just as possible to define the motor area on the histological bench, as on the operating table.

Of course it was also possible for Campbell to make direct extrapolation from his histological findings in the apes (in this case the orang-utan) to his descriptions of the histological structure of the normal human brain (Fig. 1.6) giving confidence to his delineation of the precentral area as the motor cortex in humans.

In addition, Campbell provided detailed accounts of the appearances of the cerebral cortex in two patients who had suffered amyotrophic lateral sclerosis. He also described the 'reactive alterations' in the cortex in seven patients who had been subjected to amputation of one or another limb. These findings have as much importance today, when the results of brain stimulation and cerebral blood flow studies in such patients must be interpreted in the light of structural and functional changes which may have occurred, as they did at the turn of the century when correlations between histological organization and functional capacity were being sought. From Campbell's examination of these clinical cases, the sequence of representation of the limbs along the precentral motor area which was so evident in the results of electrical stimulation of the ape's brains, was confirmed for the human brain, because the changes in cortical cellular structure which followed amputation of the leg, for example were limited to the upper extremity of the precentral gyrus. Campbell (1905, p. 64) noted that

In two cases of amputation of the arm through the humerus, degenerated cells were found over an extended area corresponding very closely with Professors Sherrington and Grünbaum's experimentally located areas for finger, wrist, and elbow movements.

Campbell's classification of cell lamination was based on his identification of seven layers in the cortex. Most subsequent work (Brodmann 1906; Vogt and Vogt 1919) and modern accounts recognize only six laminae because they include both of Campbell's adjacent 'layer of medium sized pyramidal cells (3)' and 'external layer of large pyramidal cells (4)' within

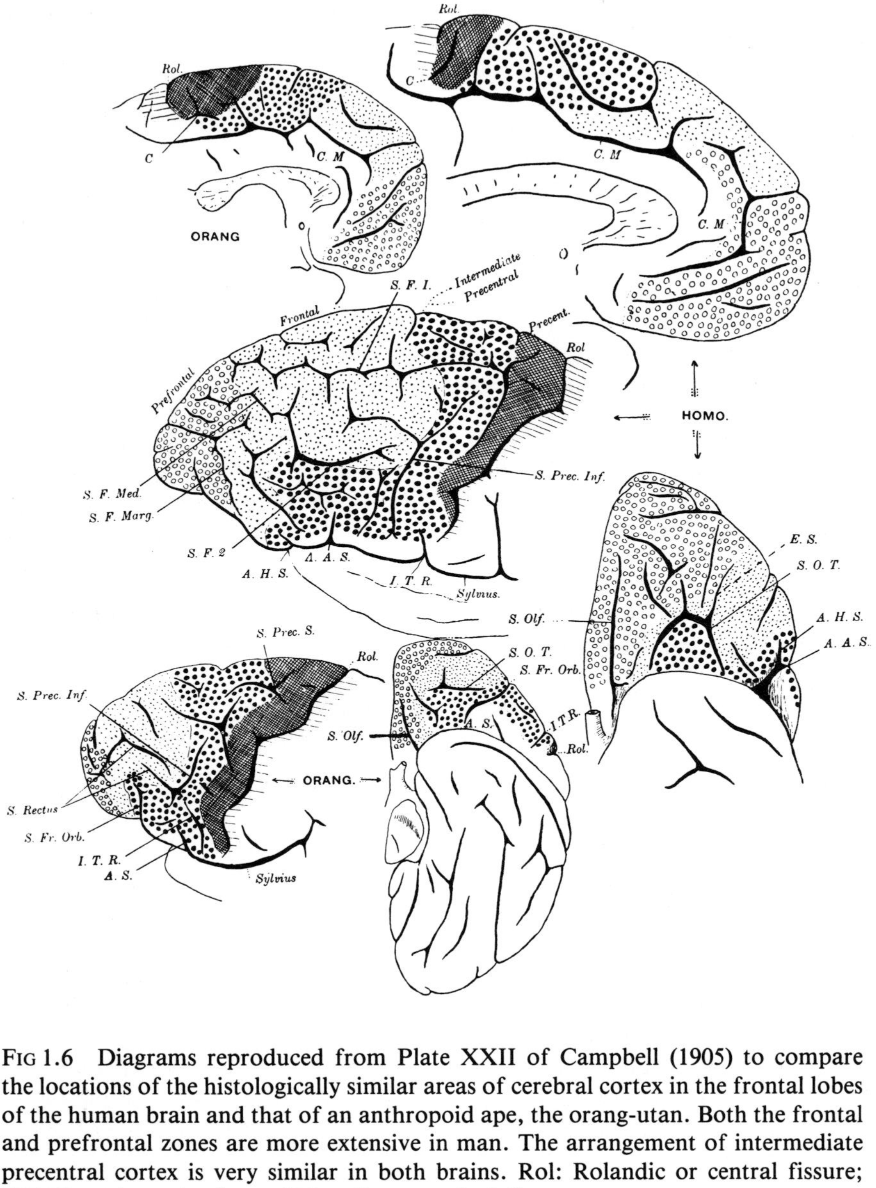

FIG 1.6   Diagrams reproduced from Plate XXII of Campbell (1905) to compare the locations of the histologically similar areas of cerebral cortex in the frontal lobes of the human brain and that of an anthropoid ape, the orang-utan. Both the frontal and prefrontal zones are more extensive in man. The arrangement of intermediate precentral cortex is very similar in both brains. Rol: Rolandic or central fissure; SFI: Sup. frontal sulcus; CM: callosomarginal fissure.

lamina III. The fibre and cellular arrangements in the precentral motor areas of the human cerebral cortex are illustrated in Fig. 1.7 (taken from Campbell's book).

We should note before concluding this account of Campbell's pioneering studies that he identified a zone of cerebral cortex which he styled the 'intermediate precentral area' (Fig. 1.5). He described his anatomical observations concerning the organization of this region and presented a discussion of Hughlings Jackson's concepts of several levels of cortical representation (re-representation). According to Penfield and Welch (1951), Munk (1881) had already suggested that Jackson's highest level of representation of movement resided in this region. Because of the inclusion of Broca's area within the intermediate precentral zone and from the descriptions of clinical cases of motor aphasia and agraphia with which he had had personal experience at the Rainhill Asylum, Campbell drew a number of conclusions about the physiological links between this zone and the 'primary' motor cortex. He concluded that the intermediate precentral area must have an association with higher order aspects of motor function. He speculated about the 'possible share taken by this cortex in the execution of what we understand by skilled movements.' Then he went on:

I am of the opinion that this particular stretch of cortex is specially designed for the execution of complex movements of an associated kind, of skilled movements, of movements in which consciousness or volition takes an active part, as opposed to automatic movements.

1.8 MOTOR RESPONSES FROM THE CEREBRAL CORTEX OF MAN

Among those who worked with Sherrington after he was elevated to the Waynflete Chair in Oxford was an American Rhodes Scholar, Wilder Penfield, who would have become familiar with all the background to electrical stimulation of the cerebral cortex in subhuman primates and the speculations about the relationship of the results of such studies to the natural function of purposive movement. Later, he also leaned heavily on the descriptions of the histology of the human cerebral cortex which had been provided by Campbell and extended by Brodmann (1906) and the Vogts (1919). He would have been familiar with Campbell's speculations concerning functional associations of the several histological zones which had been delineated.

In Canada, where he soon became established as the leading neurosurgeon, he set about the task of making direct observations by stimulating the human brain with weak electrical shocks in conscious patients undergoing surgery, under local anaesthesia, for the removal of cerebral tumours, vascular malformations or epileptic foci. In 1937, Penfield and Boldrey summarized their observations on the localization of motor responses

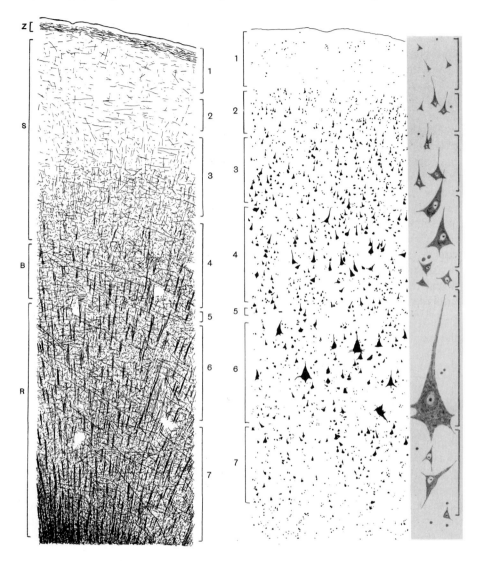

FIG 1.7   This is a reproduction of Plate III from Campbell (1905). On the left is shown the fibre arrangement in the precentral motor area from a section through the precentral gyrus 15 mm from the upper border of the hemisphere. The cell lamination in precentral cortex as seen in a section through the paracentral lobule is shown on the right. Campbell described the arrangement of fibres as having zonary (Z) supraradiary (S) and radiary (R) layers; B indicates the line of Baillarger. The numbering of the cortical laminae is different from the modern convention.

collected from the study of 163 patients examined between 1928 and 1937. They reported that often they found it impossible to ascribe the representation of function to a strict cytoarchitectonic region. In many of the patients the operation was performed for the relief of epilepsy and it is possible that the cortex stimulated could have exhibited increased excitability, expanding the zone within which a particular response could be obtained through activation of cortico-cortical systems.

Finger movements were among the best localized of the responses that could be observed and of such responses, 77 were obtained from precentral sites compared with 25 postcentral. Penfield and Boldrey (1937) found that 'flexion and extension responses' [of the digits] 'were often separable in an individual case, and points for one digit were sometimes found separated rather widely as though these members had a comparatively large amount of cortex devoted to them'. While recognizing the problems inherent in the superimpositions on a schematic brain of the observations derived from a very large number of partial maps from different individuals, Penfield and Boldrey summarized their general conclusions as shown in Fig. 1.8. This reveals that 'movement has a proportionately larger representation anterior to the central fissure and sensation a larger representation posteriorly, and the two areas, motor and sensory, overlap each other consistently and

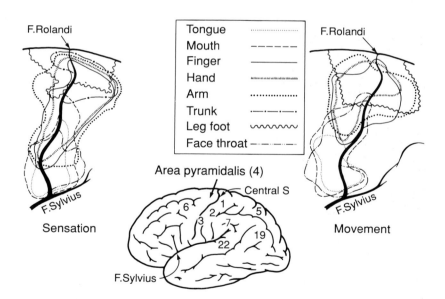

FIG 1.8 Originally presented as Fig. 25 of Penfield and Boldrey (1937), this diagram has been redrawn to illustrate the cortical territories within which motor or sensory responses were obtained by stimulation of the brain of conscious patients undergoing neurosurgical procedures.

correspond to each other horizontally'. The areas defined within these boundaries encompassed all the points from which a given response had been obtained. However, the individual motor points were densely clustered in the vicinity of the central sulcus and very close to it anteriorly. So the elements involved in the production of the evoked movements were not uniformly spread through these zones.

The sequence of motor representation from above downwards was 'almost invariable'. While the purpose of Fig. 1.9 was to illustrate this sequence (from toes through to tongue and swallow) it is presented as a series of lines whose length is related to the *number of responsive points* in front of and behind the Rolandic fissure (the length of the line is not proportional to the extent or magnitude of the responsive zone, as is often implied).

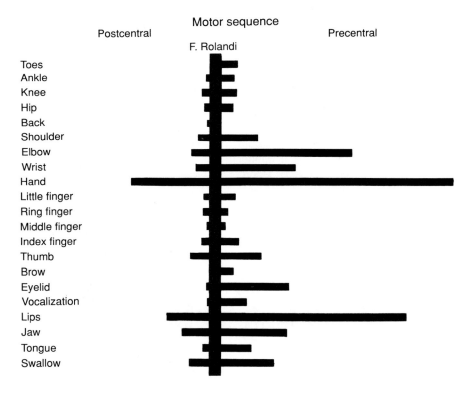

FIG 1.9   This diagram, redrawn from Penfield and Boldrey (1937), in which it appeared as the left-hand half of Fig. 26, illustrates the sequence of motor representation on the human cerebral cortex (from above downwards) with lines whose length is related to the number of points from which movement responses of that body part were obtained.

The extent of the cortical region over which a response could be obtained was judged by the vertical disposition along the standardized Rolandic fissure of the points from which this response was obtained in a large number of subjects when all the results were superimposed. This could be justified by the dense clustering of such points along the fissure. In spite of the major problems inherent in this approach, which is subject to considerable potential error, the conclusion reached was that the largest representations were devoted to the tongue, mouth, thumb, index and little finger, and the great toe, roughly in that order. Using this impression, Penfield and Boldrey constructed a caricature of the human form with body parts drawn in sizes proportional to the presumed extent of their representations. A modified version of this cartoon was later published as an homunculus in the book by Penfield and Rasmussen (1952), which summarized the results now accumulated from some 400 patients, and this diagram appears in most neurological textbooks (Fig. 1.10).

Penfield and Boldrey recognized the difficulties which surrounded the

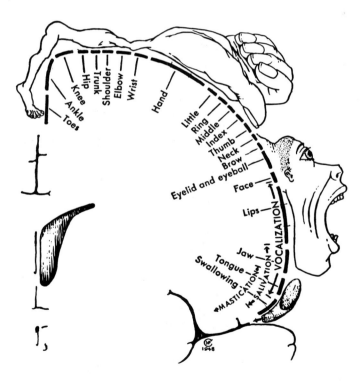

FIG 1.10 The representation as a caricature (homunculus) of movements of the human body which result from stimulation of the contralateral cerebral cortex as depicted in Fig. 22 of Penfield and Rasmussen (1952). Reproduced with permission.

interpretation of the responses which they observed. They accepted that the apparently wide dispersion of the points from which a given response could be obtained could have resulted from abnormal excitability of the epileptic cortex (even in the absence of seizures), from the instability (facilitation, reversal, or deviation) of the response as analysed by Brown and Sherrington (1912), and from the artefact of superimposition of observations from a large number of studies. They concluded that the results from stimulation of the human brain resembled most those obtained by Grünbaum and Sherrington in the chimpanzee and suggested that their own findings of motor responses from the postcentral gyrus (one of the key areas of debate at that time) was revealed because their experiments were conducted without the suppression of excitability which would have been caused by light anaesthesia in the animal studies. Further, they acknowledged the possibility that their finding of responses from area 6a alpha, further forward on the precentral gyrus, could result from activation of neural connections of this region with area 4, even using a minimal stimulus.

According to Penfield and Boldrey (1937, p.441), 'The responses of the cerebral cortex to punctate stimulation are crude'. In his book with Rasmussen (Penfield and Rasmussen 1952, p. 13), Penfield states:

It is a far cry from the gross movement produced by cortical stimulation to the skilled voluntary performance of the hand of man or monkey. Our problem is to discover, if we can, how this cortical mechanism is utilized in the composition of such performance.'

Again, in the same publication (p. 47),

the movements produced by cortical stimulation are never skilled, acquired movements but instead consist of either flexion or extension of one or more joints, movements which are not more complicated than those the newborn infant is able to perform.

All movements of the extremities were contralateral to the site of stimulation. The patients reported that these movements had been imposed upon them by the surgeon: they were not willed responses and the subjects did not experience a desire to perform the motor act.

1.9 SUPPLEMENTARY MOTOR AREA

In addition to the descriptions of the motor responses obtained from stimulation near the central sulcus, Penfield and Rasmussen (1952, p. 62)) reported

an area from which bilaterally *synergic movements* may be produced. For lack of a more descriptive name we have called it the supplementary motor area to distin-

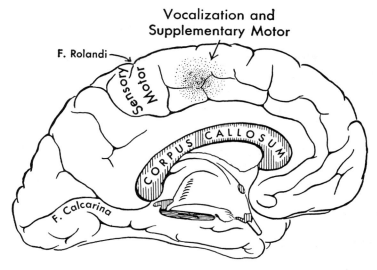

FIG 1.11 The location of the supplementary motor area is indicated in this diagram which originally appeared as Fig. 26 of Penfield and Rasmussen (1952). Reproduced with permission.

guish it from the classical sensorimotor area and the second sensory and motor representation [in or close to the bank of the Sylvian fissure]. This supplementary area is comparatively small and is situated within the superior intermediate frontal region within the longitudinal fissure [see Fig. 1.11].

Penfield and Welch (1951) provided a full account of the observations on which the existence of the supplementary motor area in the human brain was based, and, in addition, and quite unusually for Penfield, included a series of experimental studies on electrical stimulation of an analogous area of the cortex of the monkey.

Electrical excitation of the mesial and superior surfaces of the cortex anterior to the precentral gyrus in man produced an unexpected variety of responses — vocalization; movements of the head, face, arms, trunk and legs; inhibition of voluntary activity [in which the test situation was frequently speech]; aphasia; eye movements; cardiac acceleration, and arrest of breathing.

The threshold stimuli needed to produce these responses were sometimes higher than those needed for movements to be elicited from the pre-Rolandic cortex.

'A description of the distribution of motor responses' (which Penfield and Welch considered to lack a well developed topographical arrangement in man, although they found an organized topographical representation in the supplementary motor area of the monkey) 'is not sufficient to convey a picture of these movements. The character of movement is perhaps more important.' This character was, in their observations, complex and included 'assumption of postures', 'manoeuvres' (such as stepping) and 'rapid incoordinate movements'. In the assumption of postures 'the musculature of both sides of the body is employed appropriately so as to bring about the change of position.' In addition,

It is our impression that many of the postural synergies which result from stimulation of the supplementary motor area would, with more prolonged stimulation, have gone on to become more elaborate and to have approached the full synergic employment of all extremities and the trunk.

A manoeuvre was defined as a 'definite series of movements in complicated pattern' which could be repeated during the stimulation: stepping, waving of the hand, and successive flexion and extension of the fingers and wrist were examples. Bilateral responses were again evident, for example, when stimulation of a single point produced flexion of the right knee and extension of the left leg—a complex, bilateral response which was repeated on successive occasions when the same point was stimulated.

In summarizing their findings for this midline part of the cerebral cortex which they recognized as roughly coincident with the midline extension of Campbell's intermediate precentral area, Penfield and Welch emphasized that

the postures assumed and the rhythmic movements produced are made possible by employment of ipsilateral limbs and body parts, as well as the contralateral parts. The supplementary motor area has control over the musculature of both sides of the body.

They reported that excision of the supplementary motor area produced no permanent deficit in maintenance of posture or capacity for movement.

1.10 LIMITS OF ELECTRICAL STIMULATION STUDIES

A number of the general matters to which Penfield and his colleagues gave detailed attention could not have been resolved with the electrical stimulation methods that were then available. Hence the debates about the extent of the motor cortex and the exclusive involvement of precentral regions in motor function could not be finalized. Penfield's general conclusion was that the 'circuits' that pass through the precentral and postcentral cortex areas were independent of one another.

This is proven by the fact that removal of the postcentral gyrus does not produce paralysis, nor does removal of the precentral gyrus produce loss of cortical sensibility. On the other hand, after removal of the precentral gyrus alone, crude movement may eventually return, and stimulation of the corresponding segment of the postcentral gyrus does produce such movements even in the absence of its Rolandic bedfellow.

Attempts to delineate more accurately, and in finer detail, the maps of motor representation on the cerebral cortex of experimental animals using intracortical microstimulation (ICMS) have been subjected to detailed evaluation in Phillips and Porter (1977, Chapter 5). Serious limitations apply to the use of repetitive ICMS for this purpose, and little more has been contributed to our understanding of the geographical organization of function within the cerebral cortex by its use. This is not to deny that cortical stimulation, including ICMS, is a valuable tool in the identification of structures in the cortex which can be activated by these means, and in indicating connections and processes within spinal systems which must be involved in the production of movements. The results obtained by the use of this electrical stimulation tool, in analysing organizational aspects of cortical outputs in this way, will be dealt with in later sections of this book.

Porter (1987) states that

Electrical stimulation and the observation of muscle contractions is a neurophysiological form of cartography which maps the locations from which certain movements and muscles can be activated under the conditions of that experiment and also allows cortical addresses, sometimes multiple, to be specified for particular motor actions. In this sense, functions for the addresses and for the territories in which the addresses are located may be defined. But the 'wrist flexion' territory, for example, also contains addresses of other movements, as re-evaluated recently in a thoughtful review of the representation of movements and muscles within the motor cortex (Humphrey 1986). Moreover, many of the cartographers, finding no convenient way to map simultaneously those addresses which were excitatory and those which could have been as powerfully inhibitory, gave the latter no locations. More recent work, using intracortical microstimulation in conscious animals trained to maintain constant levels of muscle contraction in particular groups of muscles from which electromyograms (EMGs) were simultaneously recorded, makes it clear that the effects obtained from brief, weak microstimulation of any one point in area 4 can be excitatory to some muscles and inhibitory to others. In addition, rebound excitation often follows a period of inhibition of the EMG and could have been interpreted, in palpation of muscle contractions, as a direct excitatory effect from the stimulated cortical locus (Schmidt & McIntosh, 1984). The effects produced can be complex and they depend on the phase of the task that the animal is performing when the stimulus is delivered (Cheney & Fetz, 1985).

Moreover, as is now obvious from studies in human subjects, the instructions given to a person and the attention directed to movement outcome can greatly modify the responses obtained from stimulation of the brain, presumably by modifying the excitability of the output elements in the cortex.

1.11 CORRELATIONS BETWEEN HISTOLOGY AND MOVEMENT
RESPONSES

The parallel progress of studies which employed electrical stimulation of
the brain, and those which sought ever more minute parcellation of the
cyto- and myelo-architectural features of the cortex, conditioned a general
expectation in the first half of this century that identifiable histological
features would be associated with recognizable functional characteristics.
Clearly electrical stimulation of the brain's surface with repetitive pulses or
sinusoidal currents, even in conscious patients who were able to communi-
cate with the surgeon/experimenter was altogether too crude a tool to allow
natural functions to be revealed. Hence it was necessary for Penfield and
Rasmussen (1952, p. 20) to state that the cortical areas defined and num-
bered by Brodmann, 'except for areas such as 4, 3 and 17', should not
necessarily

be considered as functional units. Partly because there is less pretence to complete
mapping, and partly because those areas that are outlined correspond to some extent
with the functional frontiers that are developing in the cortex of man, we find the
cytoarchitectonic areas of the Vogt's (1919) useful.

The Vogt's had conducted careful, detailed cytoarchitectural examination
of the brains of monkeys which had previously been subjected to 'mapping'
experiments using electrical stimulation under light anaesthesia. Then, in
work similar to that of Campbell (1905), they performed cytoarchitectural
analysis of the human cortex to define zones analogous to those which had
been described in the monkey. Their cytoarchitectural map of the human
brain revealed regions that corresponded very closely with those defined by
Foerster (1936) as a result of his studies using electrical stimulation of the
brain in surgical patients. This correspondence emphasized the essential
similarity of the findings of Foerster and Penfield and strengthened the
general conclusions about the cortical map of motor responsiveness in the
human brain and about its internal organization.

1.12 PREMOTOR CORTEX

Some controversy surrounded the issue of motor responses evoked by electrical stimulation of the 'premotor' region — area 6 of Brodmann (6a alpha
of the Vogt's) which corresponds in general to the intermediate precentral
cortex of Campbell (1905) on the convexity of the hemisphere. Foerster
attempted directly to examine the functions of separate cytoarchitectonic
zones of the human cortex, which zones he delineated in general by their
inclusion within particular cerebral gyri. He used both electrical stimulation
within each zone and local excision of these in a large number of patients.

His experience was summarized in the ninth Hughlings Jackson lecture (Foerster 1936). He described flexor synergies, limited to the contralateral musculature, as the characteristic movements produced by stimulation of premotor cortex. In addition, he reported that 'the motor effects of stimulation of the superior parietal lobe, area 5, are very similar to those obtained from area 6a beta.' The main difference was that 'ipsilateral spasms' followed soon after the contralateral ones.

The studies in patients undergoing neurosurgical operations shed no light on theories concerning the organization of suppressor strips such as area 4s, proposed by Hines (1944) on the basis of electrical stimulation studies in animals. Nor, in view of the vagaries, instability, and complications which accompany electrical stimulation and which have been mentioned in the descriptions of Brown and Sherrington (1912), should it be expected that this method would provide reliable evidence concerning their existence or the explanation for their effects. Excitatory and inhibitory circuits are now known to be intermingled and interconnected within even minute zones of the cerebral cortex and their apparent segregation in separate strips must have resulted from experimental artefact.

1.13 OUTPUTS ACTIVATED BY ELECTRICAL STIMULI

As has been pointed out by Phillips and Porter (1977), while electrical stimulation cannot be a tool for evoking natural function in a projection area of the cerebral cortex, it can be utilized to exhibit 'the outputs that are available for selection by the intracortical activities that it cannot itself evoke'. An output which provides the major common connection with the motor apparatus resident within the spinal cord is the pyramidal tract. Figure 1.12 indicates the status of this projection pathway and its relative location as well as its relationship to cortical organization and to cerebellar and basal ganglia involvement in cortical connectivity. The diagram does not attempt to indicate the intricacies of the intracortical connectivities which could assist in the 'selection' of outputs referred to above. Anatomical observations relevant to intracortical organization will be considered in Chapter 2.

The diagram in Fig. 1.12 does indicate that the cerebral cortex is intimately associated with those other brain structures whose operations are related to movement performance. Profuse corticopontine projections issue from all regions of the cerebral cortex, and not least from the motor cortex itself. Local intracortical mechanisms in each cortical region will determine the actions that are directed along these corticopontine pathways to interact with cerebellar networks and hence to influence the resultant signals that return from the cerebellum, via the thalamus, to become part of the intracortical machinery for generation of corticospinal outputs from the motor

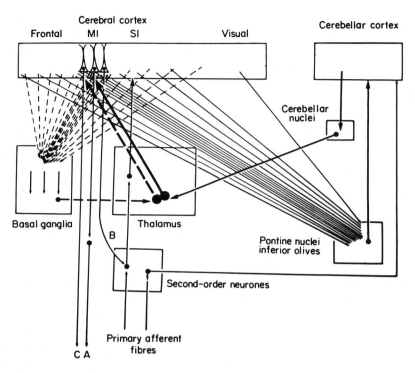

FIG 1.12   The status of the pyramidal tract is revealed by its connections. This diagram is reproduced with permission from Fig. 1.2 of Phillips and Porter (1977). It indicates some of the connectivity of the pyramidal tract which is relevant to the function of corticospinal systems in the control of voluntary movement. M1 and S1: primary motor and sensory cortex; A: cortico-reticulo-spinal projections; B: projections controlling sensory input to the CNS (dorsal horn, trigeminal nucleus, dorsal column nuclei etc.); C: corticospinal projections.

cortex. Similar re-entrant circuits direct cortical outflows through corti-costriate pathways to the processing machinery of the basal ganglia from which the motor cortex again receives part of the input to its intracortical operations. The spinal machinery for movement is available to be accessed by these large and important supraspinal structures, principally by way of the corticospinal projections from the motor cortex.

1.14 STRUCTURE AND FUNCTION IN THE SPINAL CORD

Whether conducted to the spinal cord directly through corticospinal fibres (C in Fig. 1.12) or whether they reach the spinal cord indirectly after synaptic interruption in the brainstem (A in Fig. 1.12), the influence of the corticospinal outflow must be expressed by affecting the inbuilt spinal machinery for movement. It is in the spinal cord that unequivocal relationships between structure and function can be defined and where the functional significance of connectivity has been most categorically established both in experimental animals and in man. Hence the motoneurones function to *cause* contraction of motor units in the specific muscle which their axons innervate (Sherrington's 'final common path'). Individual afferent fibres in the dorsal roots function to convey into the central nervous system signals which are *caused* by specific activation of peripheral receptors with which the afferent is connected. Because of their relative accessibility to physiological investigation, detailed information exists about these receptors in muscle, joints, tendons, fascia, and skin, and about the particular imposed stimuli which are transduced by them to generate the afferent signals which are then carried along segregated pathways into the spinal cord.

At least for the most directly connected of these afferent fibres, the sign and meaning of the connections which are made with other neuronal elements, segmentally and at other levels, have been understood by examining the reflexes that are produced by their activation (Lloyd 1943). Direct analysis of the mechanisms underlying the functional consequences of this connectivity, studied by intracellular registration of transmembrane responses, has allowed the details of synaptic transmission at these connections to be documented (Eccles *et al.* 1957). A number of general principles which then apply to the functional results of connectivity in the spinal cord have been developed. These indicate the physiological propositions that will need to be explored at other sites of synaptic interaction — within the cerebral cortex and between the outputs of the cerebral cortex and the structures to which these project. Because of their remoteness from the motoneurones whose actions can be specified unequivocally, the certainty with which motor functions can be ascribed to connections at these other sites will depend upon the detailed understanding of the interactions which occur between particular connected elements, and on the consequences of these interactions in associated structures in the brain, which will be influenced inevitably by the changes in neural activity at any site.

1.15 PRINCIPLES OF SPINAL CORD ORGANIZATION

Baldissera *et al.* (1981) have summarized some of the elements of the complex spinal circuitry, relatively directly connected with motoneurones, which must be engaged by any signals which produce discharge of the motoneurones and hence muscle contraction. Some aspects of the operation of this 'wiring diagram' during the production of a voluntary movement can be examined in conscious animals or human subjects: others must be inferred. Most of the detailed information about connectivity between the elements of the 'wiring diagram' has been discovered by examination of the spinal cord of the cat. Enough results have been obtained, however, from other animals, including the monkey, and from direct and indirect studies in man, to make it clear that a series of principles, based on examination of the cat's spinal cord, can serve as the basis for investigation of their applicability to the understanding of voluntary movement in man.

The simplified schematic diagram of Fig. 1.13 is meant to provide a framework for later discussion of particular influences of descending fibre systems on the spinal cord machinery for movement. It identifies only some of the elements within the segmental arrangement of connected structures; the ones that can most readily be assigned to a category using conventional electrophysiological methods, and which have been shown to act as inhibitory interneurones, albeit acting on different populations of motoneurones. A whole variety of other interneurones conceivably exist, some of them potentially excitatory in action, in receipt of selected afferent signals and making organized connections with particular output elements in the spinal cord. Moreover, propriospinal neurones serve to interconnect

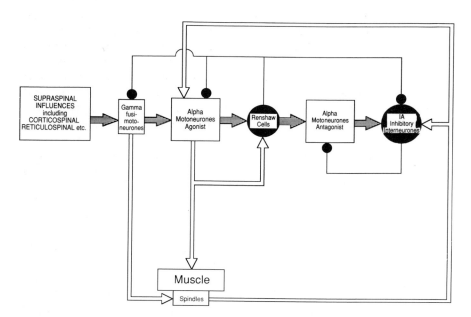

FIG 1.13   A simplified diagram of the basic segmental organization which can influence motoneurone function at a spinal level. Descending projections to the spinal cord, and especially corticospinal influences from the motor cortex, are included as horizontal arrows impinging on the various species of spinal neurones.

neurones across several segments of the spinal cord. A category of proprio-spinal involvement in motor function will be discussed fully in a later chapter.

1.16 RECURRENT INHIBITION

The principle of recurrent inhibition (Renshaw 1941) followed from the demonstration that antidromic impulses in motor axons reduce the excit-ability of motoneurones projecting to the same or synergistic muscles. Interneurones, situated in the medial part of the ventral horn of the spinal cord, receive synaptic connections from the recurrent collaterals of motor axons. These excitatory synapses cause the interneurone (Renshaw cell) to discharge impulses which project an inhibitory influence upon moto-neurones. Recurrent inhibition depends upon access, by collaterals of motor axons, to interneurones, which access is also available both to supraspinal influences and to segmental afferents. The Renshaw cell is no exception to the general rule of convergence on to interneurones. The con-vergence may, however, be discriminate, so that particular projections are able to select organized assemblies of interneurones. In addition to their excitation from recurrent axon collaterals, Renshaw interneurones receive excitatory and inhibitory synaptic inputs from many other sources, including synapses from descending fibre systems, among them the cor-ticospinal pathways. Because of this convergence, part of it arising in supraspinal structures, the inhibitory action of particular Renshaw cells and the effects exerted on selected motoneurones may be flexible and capable of control by higher centres. The same may be said for other populations of spinal interneurones, such as the common Ia inhibitory interneurone.

Although the schema of Fig. 1.13 is intended to provide a general frame-work, it is important to recognize that specializations exist within each category of neurone identified here. Motoneurone properties differ, and a given muscle may be innervated by groups of motoneurones belonging to one or more of several classes with axons conducting impulses at differ-ent velocities (Burke 1981). Although a given Renshaw cell may receive convergent excitation from the axon collaterals of many motoneurones (Eccles 1964; Ryall 1970), the inhibitory action of the Renshaw cell may be restricted to a group of agonist motoneurones and possibly only to those in a particular functional class. Not illustrated in the diagram is the fact that dorsal root afferents are able to engage and excite Renshaw cells, perhaps via polysynaptic paths, and that inhibition may also be observed in these cells following dorsal root stimulation (Curtis and Ryall 1966).

Renshaw cells may also be influenced by supraspinal systems (horizontal shaded arrows in Fig. 1.13). Inhibitory and excitatory effects have been produced by stimulation of the cerebral cortex (Maclean and Leffman

1967), the internal capsule (Koehler *et al.* 1978) and the reticular formation (Hasse and van der Meulen 1961), as well as other brain structures. The precise linkages which provide for these influences require further analysis and their functional significance for movement performance requires evaluation. That these descending connections may be operating to modulate Renshaw cell excitability during voluntary movement has been suggested by the studies in man by Hultborn and Pierrot-Deseilligny (1979).

Recurrent inhibition of fusimotor neurones has been revealed (Brown *et al.* 1968; Ellaway 1971). Recurrent inhibition of the Ia inhibitory interneurone (affecting antagonist motoneurones) has also been demonstrated to involve Renshaw cells excited over axon collaterals of agonist motoneurones (Hultborn *et al.* 1971). These are clearly important elements of the 'wiring diagram' which must be considered in any examination of the functional significance, and the relevance for movement performance, of anatomical connectivity within the spinal cord (Hultborn *et al.* 1979).

1.17 THE MONOSYNAPTIC REFLEX: RECIPROCAL INNERVATION

The reflex pathways from muscle spindle afferents have been the spinal structures most thoroughly studied since the definition by Lloyd (1943) of monosynaptic excitation of motoneurones by rapidly conducting (group I) muscle afferents. This excitation is directed both to homonymous and to synergistic motoneurones. In conjunction with it may be revealed a concurrent inhibition of 'antagonist' motoneurones, utilizing a disynaptic pathway through what is now demonstrated to be a 'common' inhibitory interneuronal system accessible to a number of convergent projections (Hultborn and Udo 1972; Illert and Tanaka 1978). These connections, illustrated in the greatly simplified schema of Fig. 1.13, provide one anatomical substrate for *reciprocal innervation.* Although an influence of group II afferents on fusimotor neurones (gamma motoneurones) and polysynaptic projections to these from Ia fibres have been described (Grillner 1969), no monosynaptic excitation of gamma motoneurones has been found to derive from group Ia afferents (Eccles *et al.* 1960). Therefore no connection from muscle spindles to gamma motoneurones is illustrated in the simplified schema of Fig. 1.13.

It is clear that supraspinal systems are able to engage this segmentally organized machinery. Lundberg and Voorhoeve (1962) demonstrated corticospinal facilitation of reciprocal Ia inhibition of motoneurones. In the monkey, Jankowska *et al.* (1976) demonstrated a monosynaptic action of corticospinal fibres on the Ia inhibitory interneurone. This may be the principal route, or perhaps the only route, by which corticospinal actions inhibit spinal motoneurones. Vestibulospinal connections also facilitate Ia inhibitory interneurones (Grillner and Hongo, 1972) in the cat.

1.18 GOLGI TENDON ORGANS: REFLEX INHIBITION: OTHER AFFERENTS

Our greatly oversimplified schema does not include indications of other systems which undoubtedly have significance for regulation of muscle contractions and control of movements. The reflex inhibition of a muscle's own motoneurones which is produced by activation of group Ib afferents arising in Golgi tendon organs is mediated by interneurones which are also accessible to higher centres of the brain (Lundberg 1975). The corticospinal tract has been shown to facilitate transmission in inhibitory and excitatory pathways activated by Ib afferents with a latency that indicates a mono-synaptic projection from the cortex to the interneurones involved in these processes (Illert *et al.* 1976b).

Local influences of cutaneous receptors must also be taken into account when seeking an understanding of the spinal machinery for movement production or of the effects exerted on that machinery by a movement which is initiated by supraspinal nervous signals. Moreover, the spinal cells of origin of many of the ascending pathways which convey inputs from peripheral receptors to brainstem nuclei, to the thalamus and to the cere-bellum may be influenced by supraspinal descending pathways.

1.19 STUDIES IN MAN

A series of investigations in conscious human subjects has set out to examine the function, during voluntary movement, of separate interneuronal groups of defined elements in the spinal cord, such as those indicated in Fig. 1.13 (Stephens *et al.* 1976; Fournier *et al.* 1986; Malmgren and Pierrot-Deseilligny 1987; Pierrot-Deseilligny 1989). By examining, in repeated presentations, the effects of an imposed stimulus on the discharges of a motor unit which is being activated voluntarily, such effects being assessed by constructing a post-stimulus time histogram of the motor unit spikes in relation to the timing of each stimulus, changes in firing probability of the motor unit which are time locked to the stimulus will be revealed. The temporal profile of these changes in probability can be correlated with the timing and sign (excitatory or inhibitory) of the synaptic actions exerted on the moto-neurones by the imposed stimulus (Fetz and Gustafsson 1983). Applying these methods in man allows an estimate of the functional significance of the synaptic machinery to be assessed in relation to voluntary motor func-tion. Such experiments, when taken together with the anatomical evidence obtained in the cat and the monkey and with the details of the discharges recorded from identified neuronal elements in the conscious monkey, have great implications for the topic of this book and will be dealt with more extensively in later chapters.

1.20 CORTICAL ACTIONS ON SPINAL MECHANISMS

Our purpose in the preceding section has been to set the scene for a more extensive discussion of recent work that explores particularly the influences of descending projections from the cerebral cortex on spinal elements in the context of the schematic summary of Fig. 1.13. We shall examine how these corticospinal projections are organized at a supraspinal level and how particular outflows may be selected via cortico-cortical interactions. Their demonstrated effects on spinal cord elements will then be examined as a prelude to a description of the experimental observations, made in monkey and in man, which contribute evidence concerning voluntary management, by these interacting systems, of muscle contraction. We do not intend to reiterate all the discussion of experimental work analysed in Phillips and Porter (1977). Rather, we shall attempt to concentrate on the evidence accumulated since the publication of that book, except, where it is necessary for the logical development of our account, to refer back to issues which were explored in depth earlier.

1.21 STROKE, AND THE EFFECTS OF LESIONS IN MAN

We have already referred to the fact that it was Broca's description of a left frontal lesion in the brain of his aphasic patient that established the fact of localization of motor function in the cerebral cortex of man. We have also referred to Campbell's histological descriptions of the brains of patients with motor aphasia and with agraphia. He considered that his intermediate precentral field which contained Broca's area must be involved in the higher level control of the motor signals which must issue from the precentral motor cortex in an organized way to produce articulate speech. He also proposed that this intermediate precentral region must be involved in the ordering of other movements, such as in spontaneous writing and copying from dictation because these behaviours required the elaboration of skilled movements and hence the organization of appropriate outputs from the motor cortex. Penfield and Rasmussen (1952) summarized their results on removal or destruction of cortical regions in a cerebral hemisphere with the diagram that is reproduced as Fig. 1.14. Similar summaries could have been produced from Foerster's observations or from other clinicopathological examinations of neurological patients.

As a result of a generalized or localized disorder in cortical function or an interruption to some of the outflow pathways from the cerebral cortex, most commonly caused by a cerebrovascular accident or stroke, disturbances (disintegration) of motor performance may be produced, and some parts of the musculature may be completely paralysed and unable to be employed

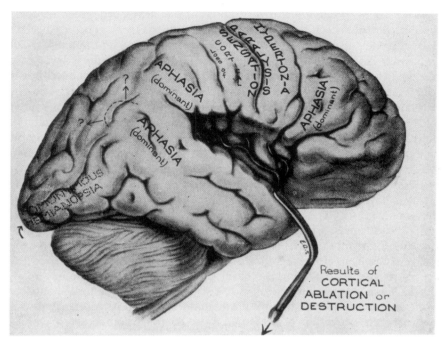

FIG 1.14   A schematic indication of the functional deficits produced by lesions to local areas of the cerebral cortex in man. This summary is reproduced with permission from Fig. 108 of Penfield and Rasmussen (1952).

in voluntary movement. Cerebral embolism or cerebral thrombosis can cause the abrupt onset of hemiplegia. Cerebral haemorrhage may be accompanied by headache at the onset and the more gradual development of neurological deficits. Sahs *et al.* (1979) characterize the afflicted patient, after recovery from the acute disturbance and unconsciousness, to appear with 'a sagging face, a dangling arm, a wobbly gait, and all too frequently a speech impediment which interferes with useful communication'. There is, of course, an extensive neurological literature that deals with the signs and symptoms of stroke, and of related disorders, and that allows the precise set of signs and symptoms that apply to that patient to be used to diagnose the location of the diseased site in the brain or to identify the particular vascular territory within which the disease has occurred.

Aphasia or language disturbances characteristically occur in those with a lesion of the dominant (usually and predominantly the left) hemisphere. It may be possible to reveal receptive or expressive components of this language disorder and particular regions of cerebral cortex have been associated with the processing of separable aspects of language function.

Hence a series of classifications of aphasias has developed which describe the disorder of speech as anomic, semantic, global, and so on, and relate these disorders to a specific step in language processing and possibly to an associated region of cerebral cortex (Kertesz 1979). While it is usually accepted (Fig. 1.14) that there are two major speech areas in the left hemisphere, one in frontal cortex (Broca) and one in temporal/parietal cortex (Wernicke), damage to the first being associated with a poverty of speech and loss of fluency while damage to the second produces difficulty in understanding of speech, lesions outside these boundaries may also result in disabilities in using or producing language (Luria 1970; Hécaen and Albert 1978). In the same manner as dissociation of the organized flow of processing for language production in the brain may be interfered with by regional cortical lesions, say in the parietal lobe, so the organization of movement performance using the limbs may be disrupted similarly giving rise to clumsiness and apraxia resulting from regional cortical lesions. Even when the motor outflow from the cerebral cortex itself seems to have escaped damage, movement performance may be grossly disordered, as occurs in diseases affecting the basal ganglia and the cerebellum.

The classic signs and symptoms of a stroke affecting the motor outflow from the cerebral cortex involve a unilateral weakness in voluntary movements. More recovery is possible and more demonstrable return of voluntary strength occurs for the musculature acting about proximal joints of the limb than for those operating at distal joints. Moreover, some muscle groups, for example those involved in elbow extension, may remain much weaker than their antagonists throughout recovery. Tendon jerk reflexes, which may be depressed in the acute phase of the stroke, become exaggerated on the hemiplegic side, and the tone of the affected muscles as tested by extension of a joint may be increased to produce spasticity. Yet reflexes which depend on polysynaptic connections and the excitability of interneurones in the spinal cord (e.g. the abdominal reflexes produced by cutaneous stimulation) are absent. The extensor plantar response (Babinski sign) is used as an indicator of interruption to corticospinal connections. In babies, when corticospinal connectivity is still being established, the plantar response is normally an extensor one. It becomes a flexor response, during normal development in children, as those components of motor behaviour, which are demonstrated to be dependent on corticospinal influences, develop.

It should be possible to provide an explanation for the various manifestations of central nervous system damage or disease which is based on our knowledge of the connectivities of affected regions and of the functions subserved by those connections. Denny–Brown's efforts to elucidate the mechanisms of such phenomena as the reflex changes, differential recovery, and spastic paresis resulting from stroke are described in his Sherrington Lectures (1966). Since then it has become possible, using microneurography and new methods of examining the human brain, to apply a series of direct and indirect measurements to the study of these phenomena in human subjects and to make longitudinal observations in patients which will allow the experimental questions to be constrained and the functions of particular parts of the brain in aspects of movement elaboration to be addressed.

1.22 SUMMARY

In this chapter we have reviewed, very briefly, the historical basis on which the concept of the localized nature of the representation of movement on the cerebral cortex was established. We have shown that, in primates, the maps of motor function are organized to provide a fixed sequence in this localization, with movements of the hindlimb most medially situated on the contralateral precentral gyrus, followed by movements of the forelimb and then the face. The localization of movement representation coincides very closely to the region in which the lamina V pyramidal cells of origin of the corticospinal tract are most densely aggregated. Not all movements achieve equal representation: the areas, and presumably the number of output connections, associated with movements of the contralateral great toe, thumb and index finger, angle of the mouth and tongue are enormously greater than those devoted to movements about the more proximal joints of the limb.

Electrical stimulation of the cerebral cortex of conscious human subjects reveals that complex synergistic movement responses, which can be bilateral, are obtained from areas outside the precentral motor cortex. Hence the intermediate precentral cortex of Campbell, which includes premotor zones and the supplementary motor area seems to be associated with the ordering of patterned outputs from the cerebral cortex. Damage to these regions of cerebral cortex, as to some areas of parietotemporal cortex, may be associated with disintegration of the smoothly controlled execution of movement performance. Damage to the precentral cortex or its outflow through the corticospinal tract produces motor disturbances characterised by unilateral weakness of voluntary movement and greatest disability in relation to the power of voluntary movements about the distal joints of the limb.

While there are serious limitations to the interpretations of the results of electrical stimulation experiments and of the information which can be deduced about normal function from the disabilities produced by disease, a framework is provided by these observations which allows us to proceed to further study of the anatomy and physiology of the output system operating through the corticospinal tract and of the influences of its impact on the spinal cord machinery for the production of movement.

2

Anatomical substrates for movement performance: cerebral cortex and the corticospinal tract

---

Although the function of a particular cortical area is determined not so much by its intrinsic structure as by its *extrinsic* connections, its inputs and outputs (Mountcastle 1978), it is important to review the intrinsic structure of the motor cortex with which these inputs, and the determinants of its functions, must interact. Intrinsic networks are available for selection by different inputs and are utilized in the organization of cortical outputs to the multiple sites which receive these projections. We shall concentrate on the features of the motor cortex which distinguish it from other cortical areas. We shall describe in detail the sources of the inputs which operate on its intrinsic networks and we shall give special attention to the organization of its corticofugal outputs. In hierarchical models of mammalian motor systems, the motor cortex, and in particular its corticospinal output, are seen as executive structures. Nevertheless, it is now abundantly clear that the motor cortex is not independent and self sufficient in these executive functions: it is itself under the influence of a large variety of different inputs, including some originating in the periphery.

All regions of the cerebral cortex appear to have the same general structure (Rockel *et al.* 1980). What then are the special characteristics of the primary motor cortex? The density of neuronal packing is lowest in the motor cortex; in monkeys there are about 110 neuronal cell bodies in a rectangular block, 30 μm square at the surface, cut through all six cortical laminae (Sholl 1956; Rockel *et al.* 1980). Although similar counts have been made in other cortical areas, the motor cortex is substantially thicker than the cortex of the association and primary receiving areas, and, while its cell packing is therefore considerably lower, there is a larger volume available for neuropil and synaptic interactions. Rockel *et al.* (1980) indicate that, in both man and macaque, motor cortex is about 1.6 times thicker than primary visual cortex and about 1.3 times thicker than association cortex. According to Phillips (1981), 'its widely-spaced neurones are separated by large masses of neuropil, which could provide for the very rich and flexible synaptic connections between the neurones'. An important function of the motor cortex, and of any motor system which will be adaptable to different tasks, is to allow a flexible linkage between input and output. Linkages must exist which provide, for example, the machinery for a particular muscle or group of muscles to be activated by a wide variety of different inputs. This is quite unlike the relatively 'hardwired' processing of afferent signals that must be carried out by the primary receiving areas of the cerebral cortex.

2.1.1 Pyramidal neurones

Ramón y Cajal (1909, 1911) originally identified the two basic cellular elements of the neocortex: pyramidal and non-pyramidal cells. Pyramidal neurones provide the anatomical substrates for the important output functions of area 4. There is a greater range of pyramidal cell sizes in area 4 than in any other region of the cortex; if the area of sections through pyramidal cell bodies is measured, there is a tenfold range in monkey motor cortex compared to only fourfold in the postcentral gyrus (Jones and Wise 1977) and this diversity reaches its greatest degree in the human motor cortex, where the distinctive Betz cells can have soma diameters of up to 120μm (Meyer 1987). In the macaque monkey, corticospinal somata range from 10μm to 58μm (Murray and Coulter 1981) and the broad spectrum of fibre sizes within the corticospinal tract presumably reflects this variety (see Section 2.8).

The characteristic feature of the motor cortex is that pyramidal cells, most of which project to other cortical or subcortical regions, are found to be distributed through all cortical laminae from II to VI. The majority of pyramidal neurones is located in laminae III and V. Comparison of the cerebral cortex in animals such as the mouse, rat, cat, macaque, and man reveals a dramatic overall increase in its size and complexity. Accompanying this is an increase in cortical thickness from mouse to man; in the motor cortex this is generated most significantly by the increase in the breadth of the expanded laminae III and V. Lamina V exhibits lower cell packing than any other cortical layer with the exception of lamina I (Sloper *et al.* 1979). Most estimates indicate that there are around 20–25 cells per 100μm^3 within lamina V (Humphrey and Corrie, 1978). Very few of these will be large pyramidal cells; Powell has estimated that a cylinder of baboon's motor cortex 1 mm^2 in area at the pial surface would contain approximately 90 large and 18 000 small pyramidal cells (Landgren *et al.* 1962b). Only about 10–20 per cent of the lamina V neurones will be pyramidal tract or corticospinal neurones sending their axons into the spinal cord.

The apical and basilar dendrites of the pyramidal cells are covered with spines and these spines receive the majority of synaptic inputs, of both the asymmetric and symmetric variety (presumed excitatory and inhibitory, respectively). Counts of as many as 63 synaptic contacts per 10μm of apical dendrite have been made (Feldman 1984), and Cragg (1975) has estimated that there may be as many as 60 000 synapses upon a single pyramidal cell.

The morphology of pyramidal cells has been reviewed by Peters and Jones (1984) and by Feldman (1984). Using the Golgi method to stain cellular elements of the cerebral cortex, Sholl (1953) and Kemper *et al.* (1973) detailed the branching patterns, spine density, and length of dendrites of pyramidal neurones in different laminae of the motor cortex of the cat and monkey. The method of intracellular injection of HRP into neurones whose identity and connections can be studied electrophysiologically allowed the complete reconstruction of dendritic and axonal processes of individual cells, for which the output target and synaptic input had been determined. Moreover, myelinated axons, which are not revealed in the Golgi studies, can be followed. Pyramidal tract neurones (PTN) in area 4 of the cat's cerebral cortex have been studied in this way by Deschênes *et al.* (1979b) and Landry *et al.* (1980). Several morphological features were observed which distinguished PTNs in the cat's motor cortex from other pyramidal neurones and from lamina V neurones in other regions of the cerebral cortex (Gilbert and Wiesel, 1979). Thus the axon collaterals of lamina V PTNs in the cat's motor cortex (Fig. 2.1) were distributed only in the deeper cortical laminae V and VI (Landry *et al.* 1980; Ghosh *et al.* 1988). Deschênes *et al.* (1979b) reported that the spines on the apical dendrites of 'fast' PTNs (with rapidly conducting axons) were much more sparsely distributed than those on 'slow' PTNs, and this has been recently confirmed (Yamamoto *et al.* 1990). Aspiny pyramidal cells have not been found in other cortical regions. A differential distribution of spines is yet to be studied at the electron-microscopic (EM) level. A relative lack of spines on fast PTNs might underlie some of the distinctive biophysical and physiological differences between fast and slow PTNs; all of the latter display spiny dendrites (Takahashi 1965; Yamamoto *et al.* 1990). Relatively few presumed

---

FIG 2.1   Camera lucida reconstructions of the somata, dendrites, and axon (A), in the left-hand panels, and of the soma, axon, and intracortical axon collaterals in the right-hand panels, of two pyramidal tract neurones (PTN) with slowly conducting axons. Both these cells were impaled with an HRP-filled microelectrode. Both were situated in the anterior sigmoid gyrus of the cat's cerebral cortex. The antidromic responses of these neurones to electrical stimulation of the cerebral peduncles (PP) are illustrated as superimposed recordings in each instance. The orientation of the sections from which the reconstructions were drawn is parasagittal, anterior to the left. Most of the intracortical axon collaterals of these slowly conducting PTNs were distributed within lamina V. Note the long 'tap root' dendrite of the slow PTN illustrated in (a). (From Ghosh *et al.* (1988), p. 299. Copyright © 1988. Reprinted by permission of Wiley-Liss, a division of John Wiley and Sons Inc.)

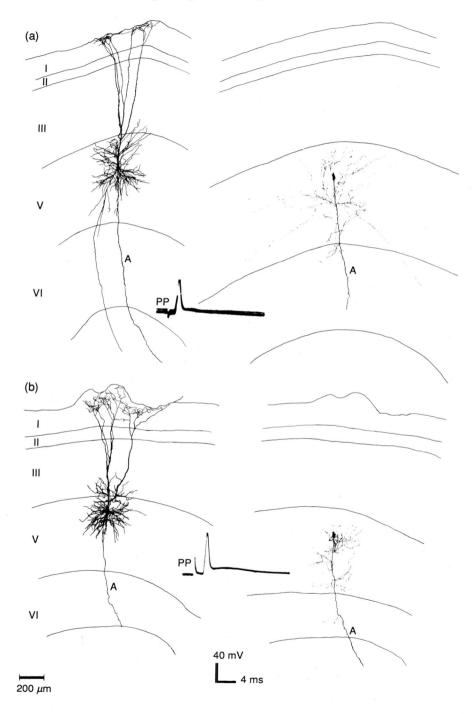

(a)

I
II

III

V

A

VI

PP

A

(b)

I

II

III

V

PP

A

VI

A

200 μm

40 mV

4 ms

excitatory synaptic contacts are found on the cell somata of pyramidal cells when portions of these are examined in EM sections.

In the motor cortex, pyramidal cells are distinctly clustered (Sloper 1973; Jones and Wise 1977; Murray and Coulter 1981). Each cluster gives rise to a group of closely associated ascending apical dendrites which follow the fundamental radial architecture of the cortex to the most superficial layers (Feldman 1984). These dendritic bundles are probably a rich site of communication between pyramidal cells. It remains to be demonstrated whether or not the members of the cluster belong to the same or different functional groups, especially with regard to their output targets (see Chapter 8).

Ghosh *et al.* (1988) examined the morphology of single neurones filled with HRP and situated in each of laminae II, III, V, and VI of area 4 gamma of the cat's motor cortex. In contrast to the restricted distribution of the axon collaterals of lamina V neurones, lamina III pyramidal neurones had extensive short and long axon collaterals which provided synaptic boutons within all laminae of the cortex. These morphological differences between cortical pyramidal neurones in different laminae were also seen in identified cells located in the monkey's precentral motor cortex and similarly stained by intracellular injection of HRP (Ghosh and Porter 1988a). Here again, the intracortical axon collaterals of lamina V pyramidal neurones, including fast and slow PTNs, were limited in their distribution to lamina V and VI, while the lamina III neurones exhibited great variation in their intracortical axon collateral arbors. The largest lamina III intracortical collaterals spread through all cortical laminae and covered about 3 mm of cortex mediolaterally (see also DeFelipe *et al.* 1986). The smallest lamina III intracortical collateral arbor was restricted to lamina III.

In the monkey, antidromic volleys from the pyramidal tract evoked monosynaptic excitatory postsynaptic potentials in fast PTNs, predominantly inhibitory responses in slow PTNs and either excitatory or inhibitory responses in other pyramidal neurones in lamina V. Antidromic volleys from the peduncles produced mainly excitatory effects on all classes of neurones presumably over recurrent axon collaterals (see Fig. 2.2). Some of the inhibitory responses could be explained by a disynaptic effect produced on the receiving cell by impulses in the recurrent axon collaterals of fast PTNs. These inhibitory connections may serve to prevent synchronization of the corticofugal output. The lamina III pyramidal neurones that were identified morphologically in this work were inhibited by the recurrent collaterals of PTNs.

In the cat, two adjacent PTNs, one with a fast-conducting axon $(27.5 \, \text{m·s}^{-1})$ and one with a slowly conducting axon $(19.2 \, \text{m·s}^{-1})$ were studied intracellularly and both subsequently visualized by filling with HRP when they were found to be separated by about $100 \mu \text{m}$. There was considerable intermingling of the dendrites and axon collateral arbors of the two cells. Close crossings were observed at several points between axon collat-

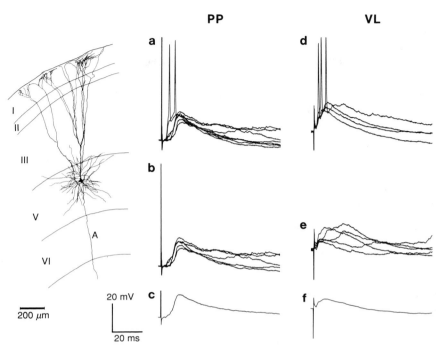

FIG 2.2   Synaptic influences revealed by intracellular recordings in a lamina V
pyramidal neurone in the anterior sigmoid gyrus of the cat. This neurone could not
be activated antidromically by stimulation of the cerebral peduncles. However,
stimulation of the peduncles (PP) evoked EPSPs (some suprathreshold (a)). Average
of five sweeps in (c). The EPSPs produced by stimulation of the ventrolateral
thalamus (VL) were more complicated. At high stimulus intensity (d) these also
could evoke firing of the cell. Average 14 subthreshold sweeps in (f). The neurone
possessed a complex dendritic tree, revealed in this reconstruction, and its axon (A)
gave off three intracortical collaterals (not illustrated in this figure) which were
limited in their projection to arborizations within laminae V and VI. (From Ghosh
et al. (1988), p. 304. Copyright © 1988. Reprinted by permission of Wiley-Liss, a
division of John Wiley and Sons Inc.)

erals of one neurone and basal dendrites of the other and with oil immersion
microscopy, a terminal bouton arising from a collateral of the slow PTN
was found closely opposed to the shaft of the basal dendrite of the fast PTN
(Fig. 2.3).

In addition to the obvious differences in the extent of distribution of the
intracortical axon collaterals of lamina V and lamina III neurones, lamina
V neurones, in general, seemed to have more apical shafts, and to spread
their apical and basal dendrites over wider territories than the lamina III
neurones. A method for developing an index of morphological 'complexity'
in the images of neural elements arises from concepts developed in the

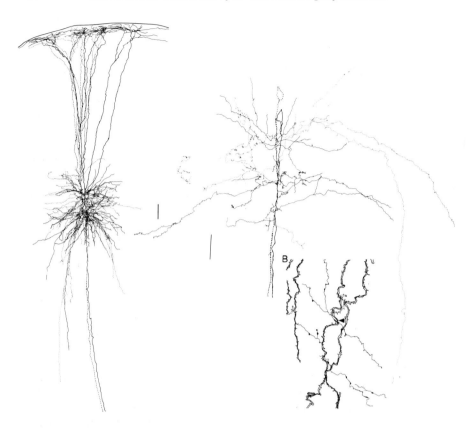

Fɪɢ 2.3   At the left are illustrated the camera lucida reconstructions of the somata, dendrites, and axons of two adjacent pyramidal tract neurones (PTNs) from the cat's motor cortex. The slow PTN is drawn with continuous lines and the outline of the fast PTN, with its soma 100 μm more superficially situated, is drawn with interrupted lines. The intracortical axon collaterals of the two cells, which are not included in the left-hand drawings, are illustrated as they issue from the pair of somata in the upper right reconstruction. Vertical bars for both these illustrations extend for 100 μm. The extent of the overlap of the profuse dendritic and axonal branches of these two cells, although exaggerated by the two-dimensional recon-structions and the compression of these arborizations into a single plane, allows for a multitude of close crossings between them. The inset (B) reveals a reconstruction, using an oil immersion objective for microscopy, of a probable synaptic contact (arrow head) between a terminal bouton of a fine branch of an axon collateral of the slow PTN and the shaft of a basal dendritic branch of the fast PTN. Horizontal calibration is 10 μm for this inset. (Adapted from Ghosh *et al.* (1988), pp. 306–7.)

fractal geometry of Mandelbrot (1982) and has been employed by Smith *et al.* (1989) to study the complexity of neuronal structures. A computer algorithm coupled with image processing capability was developed to trace the boundaries of reconstructed neurones revealed by HRP filling and to derive a fractal dimension which would provide an index of complexity of the morphology of the neurone. When this was applied to cultured glial cells, grown on a planar surface, increasing complexity which accompanied growth and differentiation of the glial elements was clearly revealed and the fractal dimension increased progressively (Smith *et al.* 1991). By summing up the geometric detail of an object revealed by examining that object against many scales and with different magnifications, a single number, D, the fractal dimension, was obtained which was related to the addition of detail revealed with increasing magnification. The slope, S, of a graph obtained by plotting the logarithm of the length of the border against the logarithmic length of the measuring element enables the fractal dimension, D, to be obtained:

$$D = 1 - S$$

The fractal dimension, D, will have a value between 1 and 2 when referring to the complexity of two-dimensional images. An increase in fractal dimension indicates an increase in complexity of the image and since changes in slope determine the fractal dimension, a change from 1.1 to 1.2 represents a doubling in structural complexity.

The two dimensional reconstructions of the cortical pyramidal neurones examined by Ghosh *et al.* (1988) and Ghosh and Porter (1988a) were treated as images for fractal analysis. All the fractal dimensions of cortical neurones were similar and there were no statistically significant differences between different groups in different laminae or between pyramidal neurones in the cat and the monkey (Porter *et al.* 1991). Moreover, no statistically significant correlations were revealed between D and the total extent of the dendritic spread or other measured features of the cells. In general, however, the morphology of lamina III neurones in the monkey appeared to be more complex (mean D of 1.53 ± 0.02 SD) than that of lamina V pyramidal cells, including the fast and slow PTNs (mean D of 1.46 ± 0.06). The complexity of the intracortical axonal arbors was less than that of their dendritic branching (mean D of 1.43 ± 0.09 for lamina III neurones and mean D of 1.34 ± 0.07 for lamina V neurones). This index, obtained from the fractal geometrical analysis, is at least consistent with the subjective impressions gained by examining these filled and stained profiles by microscopy (Fig. 2.4).

It is of some interest that, in this small sample of pyramidal neurones from the motor cortex of cat and monkey, differences between the two species were observed. Whereas, in the monkey, lamina III neurones were found to be more complex than lamina V neurones, the reverse was the case

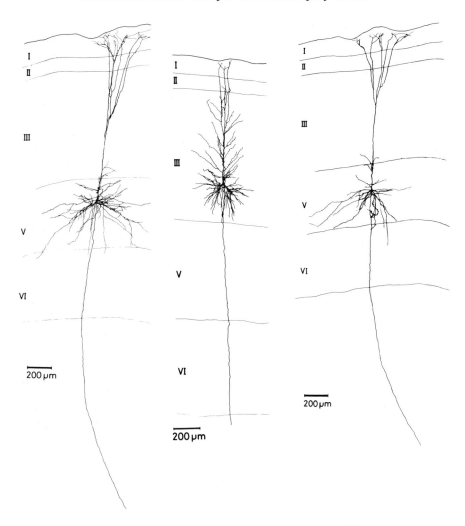

FIG 2.4   Camera lucida reconstructions of representative lamina III and lamina V
pyramidal neurones, to illustrate dendritic territories occupied, and the complexity
of dendritic arborizations, revealed by intracellular injection of HRP into cells
located in the precentral motor cortex of the monkey. Although the intracortical
axon collateral branches were also revealed by this technique, they have not been
included in this diagram, which contrasts the appearances of a fast PTN (left-
hand illustration), a slow PTN (right-hand illustration) and a lamina III (presumed
cortico cortical) neurone, in the middle. A full description of all these cells is to
be found in Ghosh and Porter (1988a).

in the cat. Moreover, the lamina V neurones, including PTNs, were more complex in the cat than in the monkey. The higher level of complexity in a cat lamina V PTN may signify a larger number of computational operations to be accommodated on its many complex, spine covered, dendritic branches. In the thicker, more extensive motor cortex of the monkey, with many more PTNs, less densely packed, some of the computational operations may be subserved by separate cells rather than by different dendritic branches of the same cells. Different functions may be performed by separate neurones, in the monkey's motor cortex, each with lesser requirements for morphological complexity.

2.1.2 Non-pyramidal neurones

Although Sloper *et al.* (1979), in their EM study, found similar proportions of non-pyramidal (28 per cent) and pyramidal neurones (72 per cent) in both motor and sensory cortex, it is not possible to distinguish a separate lamina IV in the motor cortex. The small spiny stellate cells, which in most cortical areas form lamina IV and which are the principal targets of thalamic input, are rarely identified in the motor cortex. Much more common are the large aspinous stellate, or basket cells (Sloper *et al.* 1979; Meyer 1987). These are found chiefly in layers III, IV, and V, and their dendritic trees are also organized radially. The axonal targets of basket cells, like other non-pyramidal neurones, are almost exclusively intrinsic to the cortex. Basket cells make inhibitory GABAergic synaptic contacts with pyramidal neurones (Jones 1983) and are prime candidates for the inhibitory effects exerted by the intracortical collaterals of corticofugal neurones. Their axon systems, which are myelinated, are predominantly horizontal in orientation. Smaller, neurogliaform cells have a much more localized connectivity which is thus integrated within the general radial organization of the cortex. GABA antagonists have now been shown to produce effects on the output map of the motor cortex in rats (Jacobs and Donoghue 1991, Chapter 8).

2.1.3 Intrinsic connectivity

Radial organization is the principal structural feature of all regions of the neocortex. The majority of synaptic inputs to both pyramidal and non-pyramidal neurones is probably derived from local, intrinsic sources (Gatter and Powell 1978), and much of it is expected to be inhibitory (Jones 1983). In the motor cortex, several physiological studies using spike-triggered averaging or cross-correlation analysis have confirmed that synaptic connections are much more frequently found between neighbouring neurones than between remote pairs (Renaud and Kelly 1974; Allum *et al.* 1982; Kwan *et al.* 1987; see review by Fetz *et al.* 1990). The amplitude of the cross-correlation, taken to be an indication of synaptic strength, decreased with

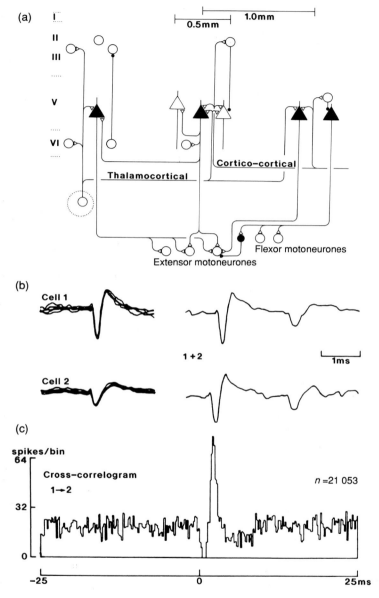

FIG 2.5 (a) Summary diagram of synaptic connections between motor cortex cells revealed by cross-correlation features. Cells are characterized by location in cortical laminae and by their projections: non-pyramidal cell neurone (circle), pyramidal neurone (open triangle), and CM cell (filled triangle). Inhibitory linkages are shown by a solid synapse and excitatory by an open synapse. Note that CM cells exciting flexor motoneurones are shown to inhibit extensor motoneurones via an inhibitory

increasing distance between the pair of sampled neurones (see Fig. 2.5). Direct morphological evidence for these connections between neighbouring pyramidal neurones has been found by Ghosh *et al.* (1988) (see Fig. 2.3). The significance of close crossings of dendritic branches of adjacent cells requires further investigation. The demonstration of presumed excitatory synaptic contact between axon collaterals of a slow PTN and basal dendrites of a fast PTN is consistent with physiological evidence for excitatory coupling between these classes of cells.

Smith (cited in Fetz *et al.* 1990) recorded from neighbouring motor cortex cells in monkeys performing alternating wrist movements. He found that 84 of 215 pairs of neurones showed significant cross-correlation features, 90 per cent of which were consistent with both neurones receiving a common input; serial effects, indicating that one neurone either inhibited (5 per cent of pairs) or excited (5 per cent) the other, were rare. An example of synaptic interaction between a PTN and an unidentified neurone is shown in Fig. 2.5. Fast PTNs in the cat motor cortex are now known to receive recurrent EPSPs from collaterals of both fast and slow PTNs (Ghosh and Porter 1988a). Spike-triggered averaging (STA) of intracellular records is generally recognized to be a more sensitive technique for revealing intrinsic cortical connections than is cross-correlation of extracellular spike activity; Kang *et al.* (1988, 1991) have used STA to determine the amplitude of the unitary EPSPs underlying these effects. They found a mean EPSP size of 111 μV. The rise time of recurrent EPSPs in fast PTNs generated by discharge of fast PTNs was shorter than for those produced by activation of slow PTNs, suggesting, on average, a more remote dendritic location for the synaptic terminals from the slower PTNs. Intracortical conduction velocities in the fine collaterals can be extremely slow (0.1 m·s^{-1}) (Fetz *et al.* 1990), so that effects generated transsynaptically by intracortical stimulation can result in substantial delays at the level of the corticospinal output (see Section 8.2).

Matsumura Sawaguchi and Kubota (cited in Fetz *et al.* 1990) have succeeded in making intracellular recordings from PTNs in awake, behaving monkeys. They found evidence of both excitation and inhibition originating from a number of reference cells recorded in one track and used to compile STAs of intracellular recordings from a single cortical cell in lamina V (see

---

spinal interneurone. (From Fetz *et al.* 1990. Reproduced with permission.) (b, c) Cross-correlation of activity from two motor cortex neurones recorded from an awake monkey by one microelectrode. Cell 1 was identified as a pyramidal tract neurone (PTN). Superimposed records shown in (b) on left. Cell 1 often fired before cell 2, as illustrated in the single sweeps on the right. The cross-correlogram is shown in (c). Spikes from cell 2 were sampled with respect to 21 053 reference spikes from cell 1, which discharged at time zero. Cell 2 activity was clearly raised 1–2 ms after spike 1 had fired. (From Lemon (1990). Reproduced with permission.)

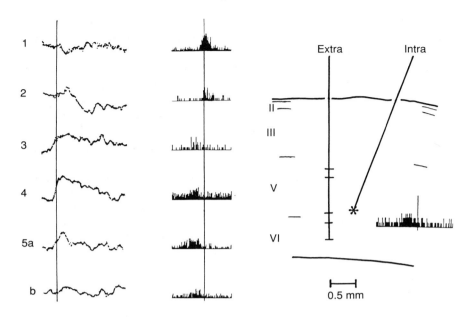

FIG 2.6 Synaptic interactions between motor cortex cells in the awake monkey revealed by STA. Diagram at right indicates location of five different neurones recorded extracellularly in a vertical track near an intracellularly recorded cell (*). Records 1–5 at left are STAs of the membrane potential of this cell produced by trigger spikes from each of the extracellularly recorded neurones. Discharge of trigger cell shown by vertical line. STAs reveal presence of postsynaptic inhibition from superficial layer V cells (1 and 2) and a common excitatory input from deeper cells (3, 4, and 5a). Histograms (centre) illustrate firing patterns of cells during a conditioned wrist movement (at centre vertical line). Note that cells 1 and 2 fired *after* the intracellularly recorded cell (activity histogram at far right). From the work of Matsumura, Sawaguchi and Kubota. (From Fetz *et al.* (1990). Reproduced with permission.)

Fig. 2.6). Common excitatory inputs were most common in cells with similar task related patterns.

The strength of local interactions confirms the basic radial architecture of the motor cortex. While the functional implications of this organization have been long established in the primary receiving areas, their significance within the motor cortex is not clear. This is chiefly because we do not know what operations might be carried out in the radial arrangements of the motor cortex. Asanuma and his colleagues suggested that the radial arrangements might function as the basic input–output modules for the control of single muscles (Asanuma and Sakata 1967; Asanuma and Rosén 1972; Rosén and Asanuma 1972). More recent studies, however, suggest that the organization of both input and output is considerably more complex, and that a given radial zone might be more likely to be concerned with multiple muscle control (see Section 8.4).

A further characteristic feature of motor cortex is the profuse horizontal connectivity provided by axons of intrinsic neurones which run mainly at the junction of lamina II/III border, and deep within lamina III. These intrinsic projections are orientated mainly in the parasaggital plane, and spread for up to 3 mm away from the column (Gatter and Powell 1978; DeFelipe *et al.* 1986; Ghosh *et al.* 1988; Huntley and Jones 1991); they would presumably allow for a considerable amount of synaptic interplay between different radial arrangements, and form part of the flexible synaptic organization so distinctive of the motor cortex. Further horizontal communication is provided for by the axon collaterals of corticofugal pyramidal cells (see below). Vertically orientated fibres within the radial organization were considered by Gatter and Powell (1978) to be chiefly afferent or efferent, rather than intrinsic fibres.

2.1.4 Afferent connections

As investigators clarified the position of the motor cortex in a number of key central nervous system loops involving the cerebellum and the basal ganglia, as well as other areas of the cortex, so has the importance of these afferent inputs become fully appreciated. The evidence now coming from the study of single axonal arborization patterns within area 4 suggests that these inputs are organized in a highly specific fashion with dense clusters or patches of termination in target areas, and with few if any terminals in intervening regions (see, for example, Shinoda and Kakei 1989).

Thalamocortical afferents

The absence of a clear lamina IV does not mean that neurones of the motor cortex do not receive thalamic inputs. Thalamocortical terminals were found by Strick and Sterling (1974) and by Sloper and Powell (1979) in all layers of motor cortex, being densest in lamina III and at the III/IV border, with a second dense band in the deeper part of lamina V. Most thalamo-cortical afferents appear to terminate directly on the dendritic spines of pyramidal neurones, where they make asymmetric (type 1) contacts, which are presumed to be excitatory. This has been confirmed by electrophysio-logical studies which have shown monosynaptic EPSPs generated in pyramidal tract neurones by thalamic stimulation (Amassian and Weiner 1966; Deschênes *et al.* 1979a; Ghosh *et al.* 1988; Yamamoto *et al.* 1990). An example is shown in Fig. 2.2. In the cat, thalamocortical axons have been shown to arborize widely within the motor cortex, with a tangential spread of up to 3 to 4 mm, and with synaptic boutons in laminae III and VI (Deschênes and Hammond 1980); similar patterns of arborization were reported by Asanuma *et al.* (1974), and by Shinoda and Kakei (1989) using intra-axonal injection of tracers to study single identified afferents.

Cortico-cortical afferents

These projections, which arise chiefly from pyramidal cells in laminae II and III, terminate in all cortical layers, and often make widespread connections in lamina IV of granular cortex and more specific 'patchy' or columnar patterns of termination in the upper layers (Jones *et al.* 1975). Corticocortical inputs terminate on both pyramidal and non-pyramidal neurones, on dendritic spines of the former and on dendritic shafts of the latter (Sloper and Powell 1979). Electrophysiological evidence for these connections in monkey motor cortex has been obtained by Ghosh and Porter (1988b).

An attempt has been made to quantify the relative contributions of the supplementary motor areas (SMA), premotor cortex and the somatosensory cortex (areas 3, 1, 2) by counting the neurones retrogradely filled with HRP after small injections of HRP into a limited region of the hand area of the precentral motor cortex in the monkey (Ghosh *et al.* 1987). This study confirmed that most of the connectivity is local, from within the arm region of area 4. Thereafter, the cortico-cortical inputs are dominated by those from SMA, premotor cortex, and areas 1, 2, and 5 (see Jones *et al.* 1975 and Chapter 7).

Callosal afferents

These inputs arise from pyramidal cells in the deeper part of lamina III in the homotopic part of area 4 of the opposite hemisphere and terminate in layers I through III, almost entirely on dendritic spines (Lund and Lund 1970; Sloper and Powell 1979). The lower border of the dense degeneration of commissural connections corresponds to the upper border of the dense band of thalamocortical afferents. It will be important to analyse the precise neuronal elements on which these terminals make contact because, of course, the ascending dendrites of even the deepest layer cells traverse these laminae. Callosal interconnections avoid the motor representations of the most distal extremities (Jones and Powell 1969; Gould *et al.* 1986).

2.2 MICROPHYSIOLOGY OF PYRAMIDAL NEURONES

The use of intracellular recording electrodes to study the microphysiology of the cells of origin of the corticospinal tract in anaesthetized cats was pioneered by Charles Phillips (1956a, b; 1959). Phillips (see Fig. 2.7) showed that these cells had 'resting' membrane potentials of the order of $-70\,\text{mV}$, and that the action potentials generated in them by antidromic activation or by synaptic or electrical depolarization were of very brief

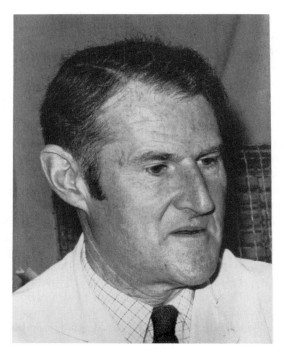

Fɪɢ 2.7   Charles G. Phillips was educated at Magdalen College, Oxford and St Bartholomew's Hospital, London. He was a Captain in the RAMC during World War II and served with the distinguished neurologists and neurosurgeons who dealt with head injuries and other war wounds. He was successively a Fellow of Trinity College, Oxford and of Hertford College, Oxford when, after a distinguished career as a physiologist in the University Laboratory of Physiology, Oxford, he was elected to Dr Lee's Professorship of Anatomy at the University of Oxford. He served the British Medical Research Council and The Physiological Society and was Editor of Brain from 1975 to 1981. This photograph was taken in 1971 during one of his visits to Monash University in Australia. His meticulous, detailed experiments on corticospinal neurones and particularly his pioneering intracellular recordings from Betz cells in the anaesthetized cat's motor cortex, have provided the background knowledge on which much present thinking about voluntary movement is based.

duration and 'overshot'. Not only when the cells had been impaled, but also when recordings were made from corticospinal axons in the spinal cord, without any possibility of damage or mechanically produced depolarization of cortical elements by microelectrode puncture, it was clear that these neurones could respond to an excitatory drive by firing at very high frequencies (Phillips and Porter 1977, pp. 57–62).

Using intracellular recording techniques in anaesthetized cats, Creutzfeldt *et al.* (1964), Takahashi (1965), and Koike *et al.* (1968a, b; 1970; 1972) attempted the examination of the basic membrane properties of the cortical neurones that could have contributed to these individual responses. Takahashi (1965) showed differences in the duration of the action potentials and in the form of the spike afterpotentials in fast PTNs compared with the same measures in slow PTNs. Such results suggested a biophysical basis for the separation of PTNs into these two categories (Bishop *et al.* 1953). On the one hand, large cells with a large surface area seemed to have a low total membrane resistance, and to exhibit a brief spike duration and a brief afterhyperpolarization. These cells contributed corticospinal axons with fast conduction velocities. The smaller cells, with a smaller surface area, had a high total membrane resistance, a longer spike duration and afterhyperpolarization. Their corticospinal axons were slowly conducting.

In recent years it has become possible to study the membrane properties of the large pyramidal neurones in lamina V of the cat's motor cortex *in vitro* by using brain slice preparations taken from lateral cruciate cortex of pentobarbitone anaesthetized animals (Stafstrom *et al.* 1984a, b). These cells cannot be classified according to the destination of their axons (which are interrupted by the preparation of the slice). However, their laminar location and their microscopical structure can be defined by the injection into them of HRP or biocytin (Spain *et al.* 1991b). Thus the geometry of the cells and the properties of their membranes can be compared with those identified neurones studied in intact cerebral cortex (see also Woody *et al.* 1989). More importantly, the *in vitro* preparation allows the maintenance of stable intracellular recordings for long periods during which the controlled use of current and voltage clamping methods (Finkel and Redman 1985) and the manipulation of superfusing solutions with differing ionic compositions and a variety of pharmacological agents can be employed to study the dynamic behaviour of ion channels in each cell (Schwindt *et al.* 1988a, b; 1989).

It has been shown by the team of scientists led by Wayne Crill that pyramidal neurones in lamina V possess a variety of potassium channels in their cell membranes (Foehring *et al.* 1989; Schwindt *et al.* 1988a, 1989). Manipulation of the composition of the superfusing solutions has allowed the functional significance of these channels to be explored. Separate potassium currents which are activated either by increases in intracellular calcium or by intracellular sodium have been shown to have relatively slow kinetics and also to be modulated by known neurotransmitters (Schwindt *et al.* 1988a, 1989; Foehring *et al.* 1989). In addition, the use of these techniques has allowed the definition of two transient voltage-gated potassium currents (Spain *et al.* 1991a). The activation and inactivation characteristics of these potassium currents were different, as were their voltage dependence. While the two currents were insensitive to blockade of calcium influx, they differed in sensitivity to tetraethylammonium (TEA), 4-aminopyridine (4-AP) and cobalt. A larger role for the slower of these two transient potassium currents in the functional repolarization of the pyramidal neurones was illustrated by a greater prolongation of the action potential in the presence of 4-AP. Rapid repolarization is related to the frequency of discharge of which the cell is capable, and interference with repolarization can induce epileptic bursts of discharge.

Because both transient currents were activated by cell membrane depolarizations well below the threshold for action potential initiation, it was suggested that both currents could influence the time course of post-synaptic responses (EPSPs) or the rise of membrane potential towards spike threshold (Fetz *et al.* 1990). Hence these transient voltage-dependent currents could have a significant influence on pyramidal neurone excit-ability by affecting the total synaptic depolarization drive to action potential generation. The influences of such intrinsic properties of mammalian neurones on their functional capacities is discussed by Llinás (1988). It is likely that such inherent characteristics underlie the measured properties of pyramidal neurones which have been documented using modern electrophysiological recordings from *in vitro* preparations of the cat's motor cortex (Table 2.1).

Spain *et al.* (1991b) examined the influence of a preceding, conditioning period of membrane hyperpolarization upon the repetitive firing evoked by a test current pulse in layer V pyramidal neurones in a cat's cortical slices prepared from the motor cortex. The conditioning hyperpolarization, ranging from −60 up to −100 mV, influenced the firing rate of the test neurones in response to a depolarizing current. The initial firing rate to the same imposed depolarization became faster as the pre-pulses were made more negative in 13 of the 87 cells tested. This was regarded as post hyperpolarization excitation. These cells also had the shortest duration action potentials, and the lowest input resistance. In 55 others, the initial firing rate to the imposed current became slower as the conditioning pulses were made more negative (post-hyperpolarization inhibition). In 12 other neurones, mixed responses, exhibiting both excitatory and inhibitory phases, were obtained.

TABLE 2.1 Representative properties of motor cortex pyramidal cells (from Spain *et al.* 1991a).

Property	Mean ± SD	n
Resting potential (mV)	−70 ± 4	86
Spike height (mV)	96 ± 9	72
Spike duration (ms)*	0.65 ± 0.2	71
Input resistance (MΩ)**	11 ± 4	39

*Measured at action potential threshold; **measured at 200 ms during injection of a −1 nA current pulse

Neurones were filled with HRP or biocytin; although only seventeen of the cells could be reconstructed histologically, they were all located within lamina V and all were pyramidal neurones. The cells which had shown post-hyperpolarization excitation or a mixed response had fewer spines on their main apical dendrites and larger somata than the cells which demonstrated post-hyperpolarization inhibition. They also possessed prominent oblique tap-root dendrites. On the basis of other morphological (Deschênes *et al.* 1979b) and electrophysiological evidence obtained from experiments on the motor cortex of anaesthetized cats, it was suggested that these excitation responses to a period of membrane hyperpolarization were characteristic of cells with rapidly conducting axons. However, one morphological characteristic, the possession of a prominent oblique tap-root dendrite, is not confined to fast PTN, as the cell illustrated in Fig. 2.1 demonstrates.

Conditioning hyperpolarization affected only the transient, initial phase of the firing of the cells in response to a depolarizing current. Moreover, the effects were only obvious when the depolarizing current was adjusted to evoke low tonic firing rates. Ionic currents were measured under voltage clamp conditions following conditioning hyperpolarizing pulses. It was possible to attribute post-hyperpolarization excitation to activation of the hyperpolarization activated cation current described by Spain *et al.* (1987), because the time and voltage dependence of both were similar. Both post-hyperpolarization inhibition and the two transient voltage-dependent potassium currents referred to above were found to have similar voltage dependence. However, the time course of the inhibition of neuronal discharge following a hyperpolarizing influence corresponded only to the slow inactivation kinetics of the slow transient potassium current. This effect was also reduced by 4-AP.

While these findings in brain slice preparations cannot be related directly to measurements made in PTNs with slowly and rapidly conducting axons, they strengthen the case for the existence of a variety of cell types in the motor cortex whose functional responses to synaptic drives will depend on the intrinsic properties of their cell membranes as well as on the magnitude of the excitatory and inhibitory synaptic influences converging on to them. In particular, these recent observations suggest that inhibitory influences, hyperpolarizing cortical neurones, will set the background from which different pyramidal cells will respond with different temporal patterning of their output discharge, to excitatory drives that reach them over common routes from the thalamus or from other cortical regions. In addition, of course, this range of responsiveness must influence all the behaviours of these cells and must complicate interpretations of cortical outputs which will be generated by such things as intracortical microstimulation (ICMS) which will produce synchronous complex synaptic actions on a large number of cortical elements (see Section 8.2).

2.3 TRANSMITTERS IN THE CORTICOSPINAL SYSTEM

Despite the importance of the corticospinal system, we still know comparatively little about the neurotransmitters in it. Central to modern ideas of motor cortex function is the temporal coding of activity within the corticospinal tract for the efficient control of movement performance. The corticospinal system would thus be expected to employ one of the 'fast' type of rapidly inactivated neurotransmitters. All the earliest responses to corticospinal volleys, whether in recurrent collaterals within the cortex or in target spinal interneurones and motoneurones are excitatory (Phillips and Porter 1977, p. 144).

The most likely candidate excitatory transmitters are aspartate and glutamate. GABA, an inhibitory transmitter, is found only in non-pyramidal cells. In guinea pigs, Potashner (1988) showed that ablation of the sensorimotor cortex caused a specific depression of D-[^{3}H]-aspartate uptake and release in the contralateral spinal cord. It is also known that corticostriatal, corticothalamic, and corticobulbar fibres have a high-affinity uptake system for D-aspartate and will transport it retrogradely back to the cortical cell bodies (Rustioni and Cuénod 1982; Jones 1984). Most of the glutamate and aspartate immunoreactive cell bodies are pyramidal cells in laminae III, V, and VI. Giuffrida and Rustioni (1989) recently succeeded in showing that at least 65–75 per cent of identified corticospinal neurones exhibited this immunoreactivity. We still know little about the characteristics of the postsynaptic receptors that are activated by these putative neurotransmitters.

Extension of the use of *in vitro* slice preparations (see Section 2.2) will surely allow the examination of transmitter and receptor microphysiology to be extended within the motor cortex in a variety of mammals. It is technically feasible to record simultaneously from two connected neurones under stable conditions, to examine the unitary synaptic events caused in one by discharges in the other, and to employ pharmacological tools to further evaluate the contributions of NMDA (*N*-methyl-D-aspartate) and non-NMDA excitatory amino acid receptors to these events and processes (Thomson 1986; Thomson *et al.* 1989a). There is also evidence that glycine may enhance NMDA-receptor mediated synaptic potentials in neocortical slices (Thomson *et al.* 1989b). More detailed information about the microphysiology of synaptic events within the interconnected networks of the cortex itself may allow refined study of the mechanisms underlying such changes as temporal facilitation, which seems to occur at cortico-motoneuronal synapses (Phillips and Porter 1977, pp. 65–79) and may also be a property of the synapses formed by intracortical collaterals of such corticospinal fibres. In addition, if long-term potentiation (LTP) or other temporal modifications of synaptic effectiveness which could alter the functional state of the motor cortex occur here, their mechanisms could be examined in detail as they have been in hippocampal slices (Sayer *et al.* 1989; Friedlander *et al.* 1989). Asanuma and his colleagues have advanced evidence for prolonged changes in synaptic efficacy akin to LTP produced by repetitive activation of cells in the motor cortex and have related this to motor learning and memory (Iriki *et al.* 1990; Asanuma and Keller 1991; see Section 8.8).

2.4 LAMINAR ORGANIZATION OF SUBCORTICAL PROJECTIONS FROM THE PRIMARY MOTOR CORTEX

Although the corticofugal projections from the primary motor cortex possess special features, such as the cortico-motoneuronal component of the cortico-spinal system and the corticorubral projection, in other respects the sub-cortical targets of motor cortex output are similar to those from other cortical areas (Kuypers 1981; Jones 1984). It is now well established that these subcortical projections are all derived from pyramidal cells in lamina V. There are two exceptions to this rule: the majority of corticothalamic fibres arise from lamina VI, and some corticostriate fibres arise from lamina III (Goldman-Rakic and Selemon 1986).

As shown in Fig. 2.8, lamina V is organized such that the more superficial cells project to the striatum, while progressively deeper lying neurones project to the midbrain, brainstem, and spinal cord (see Fig. 1.12 for a summary of these projections, and Table 2.2). Thus projections to the claustrum and striatum arise from small pyramids in the upper parts of lamina V. Some corticothalamic fibres arise from lamina V and project bilaterally to the intralaminar nuclei (Catsman-Berrevoets and Kuypers 1978), but the majority come from lamina VI and project to the VL and VPL nuclei (Künzle 1976). Corticostriate fibres from areas 4 and 6 project to the putamen (Goldman-Rakic and Selemon 1986).

Projections to the mesencephalon (red nucleus), together with those to the brainstem (corticopontine, corticobulbar, and corticonuclear fibres) arise from small to medium-sized pyramidal cells in the middle or deeper parts of lamina V. There is evidence that some of the projections to the magnocellular red nucleus are derived from deeper lying pyramids (Catsman-Berrevoets *et al.* 1979). Finally, corticospinal projections are derived from medium to large-sized neurones in the deeper parts of layer V.

2.5 THE CORTICAL AREAS OF ORIGIN OF DIFFERENT SUBCORTICAL PROJECTIONS

As well as exhibiting differences in their *laminar* origin, it is now clear that projections to different subcortical targets arise from different, sometimes

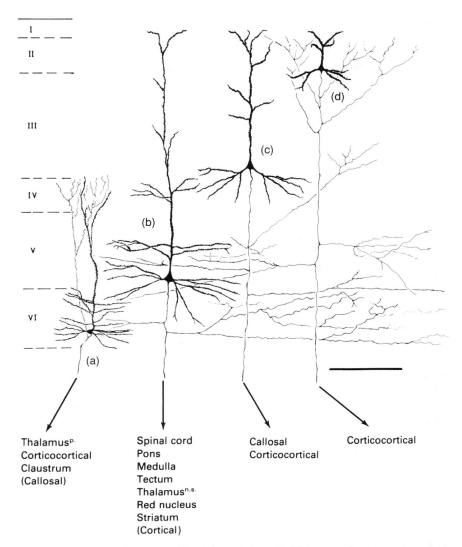

I

II

III

IV

(b)

V

VI

(a)

(c)

(d)

Thalamus^{p.}
Corticocortical
Claustrum
(Callosal)

Spinal cord
Pons
Medulla
Tectum
Thalamus^{n.s.}
Red nucleus
Striatum
(Cortical)

Callosal
Corticocortical

Corticocortical

FIG 2.8 Schematic diagram of laminar origins of efferent projections of cortical cells, based mainly on data from the monkey. Parentheses indicate a projection may not arise from the layer indicated in all species or in all areas. Thalamus$^{P., n.s.}$: principal relay and non-specific nuclei, respectively. (From Jones (1984), p.535. Reproduced with permission.)

overlapping, regions of the sensorimotor cortex. The origin of projections to different cell groups in the monkey is illustrated in Fig. 2.9, taken from Kuypers (1981). It shows that the fibres descending to the VL nucleus of the thalamus, and to the parvocellular and magnocellular red nucleus

TABLE 2.2 Laminar origin of corticofugal neurones in primate motor cortex (adapted from Jones and Wise 1977).

Lamina	Corticofugal neurones
I	
II	
III	Cortico-cortical
	Corticocallosal
	Corticostriate
V-a (upper)	Corticostriate
	Corticorubral
	Corticoreticular
	Corticopontine
	Corticobulbar
	Corticonuclear
V-b (lower)	Corticospinal
VI	Corticothalamic

are almost entirely derived from the precentral gyrus (area 4 and lateral area 6; see Fig. 2.13). There are far more numerous projections to the rostral, parvocellular red nucleus than to the caudal, magnocellular division, from which the rubrospinal tract originates (Fig. 2.9(b, e)). Humphrey *et al.* (1984) estimated the parvocellular projection to comprise 90 per cent of the total corticorubral system. While the magnocellular neurones appear to be dominated by cerebellar inputs from the interpositus nucleus, parvocellular neurones receive a much stronger cortical input. The dendritic locations of synaptic inputs from these two sources may influence their effectiveness (Allen and Tsukahara 1974). The projection to the magnocellular division is derived from more caudal parts of the precentral gyrus, while that to the parvocellular division has a more widespread and rostral origin (Catsman-Berrevoets *et al.* 1979; Kuypers 1981; Humphrey *et al.* 1984). Corticopontine fibres from area 4 terminate in distinct rostrocaudally orientated slabs or lamellae, with a somatotopic organization (Brodal 1978).

A comparison of corticobulbar projections in different species reveals a pattern of termination which parallels that seen in the corticospinal projection (see Section 2.9). Thus in mammals such as the goat, cat, and rat, the corticobulbar projection is directed chiefly to the sensory nuclei, such as the principal and spinal trigeminal complex, with no projections to the cranial motor nuclei. In these animals, most corticospinal projections terminate in the dorsal horn and intermediate zone of the spinal cord. However, in primates, there are direct projections to the cranial motor

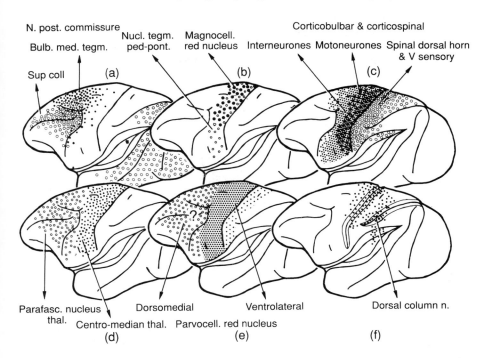

N. post. commissure
Nucl. tegm.   Magnocell.   Corticobulbar & corticospinal
Bulb. med. tegm.   ped-pont.   red nucleus   Interneurones Motoneurones Spinal dorsal horn
& V sensory

Sup coll   (a)   (b)   (c)

Parafasc. nucleus   Dorsomedial   Ventrolateral   Dorsal column n.
thal.   Centro-median thal.   Parvocell. red nucleus
(d)   (e)   (f)

FIG 2.9 Origin of cortical projections to different cell groups in the brainstem and spinal cord of the monkey. Note that cortical projections to superior colliculus, nucleus of posterior commissure, bulbar medial tegmental field (shown in (a), parafascicular thalamic nucleus (d), and dorsomedial part of parvocellular red nucleus (e) are derived mainly from frontal areas rostral to the precentral gyrus. Note that projections to magnocellular red nucleus (b), nucleus tegmenti pedunculopontis (b), centromedian thalamic nucleus (d), and ventrolateral part of parvocellular red nucleus (e) are primarily derived from the precentral gyrus. Note also that cortical projections to bulbar lateral tegmental field and spinal intermediate zone (small dots in (c)) are derived from precentral gyrus and rostrally adjoining areas, whereas those terminating in the bulbar and spinal motoneuronal cell groups are mainly derived from caudal part of precentral gyrus (asterisks in (c). Note further that cortical projections to spinal V complex and spinal dorsal horn (c), and to the dorsal column nuclei (f) are derived mainly from postcentral and parietal areas and secondary sensory cortex but that projections to dorsal column nuclei are also derived from caudal part of precentral gyrus. (From Kuypers (1981), p. 635. Reproduced with permission.)

nuclei, and particularly crossed projections to the oral part of the facial nucleus, and bilateral projections to the trigeminal motor nuclei and hypoglossal nuclei (Kuypers 1958a,c, 1981; Iwatsubo *et al.* 1990). Interestingly, these direct projections arise from the caudal part of the precentral gyrus, as do the cortico-motoneuronal projections to the spinal cord (see below).

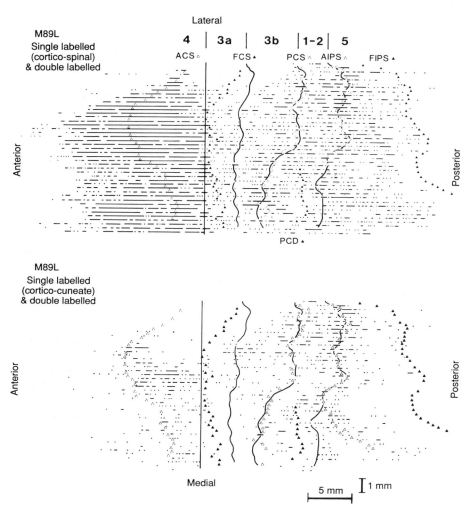

FIG 2.10 Unfolded reconstruction of the distribution of labelled corticospinal (above) and corticocuneate populations (below) in the left pre-and postcentral gyri of a macaque monkey which had previously received injections of retrograde fluorescent tracers into the corticospinal tract (on the right side at C2–C3 spinal level) and into the right cuneate nucleus. Each dot corresponds to one labelled cortical neurone. Where labelled neurones are close together individual dots join to form a horizontal bar. Open and closed triangles correspond to gross anatomical references identified by the abbreviations ACS, FCS, and PCS (anterior bank, fundus, and posterior bank of the central sulcus, respectively), AIPS and FIPS (anterior bank and fundus of the intraparietal sulcus, respectively). PCD: postcentral dimple. For instance, the row of closed triangles subjacent to FCS indicates the position of the central sulcus on each horizontal line corresponding to one

There are no direct projections from motor cortex to the extraocular motor nuclei.

Corticoreticular projections arise from wide areas of the cortex (Keizer and Kuypers 1984; see Fig. 2.9(a, b)), including the rostral parts of the precentral gyrus (area 6, Catsman-Berrevoets and Kuypers 1976). These fibres are distributed ipsilaterally to the pontine and bilaterally to the medullary reticular formation. Their targets include the raphe nuclei and the reticular nuclei which give rise to the reticulospinal tracts (Brodal *et al.* 1960; Peterson *et al.* 1974; Alstermark *et al.* 1983a, b).

There is a somatotopic projection from the motor cortex to the dorsal column nuclei. The projection fibres are derived from small pyramidal cells, and, in the cat, they conduct at different velocities depending on whether they are destined for the gracile or cuneate nucleus, a property which may be related to the relative times of central arrival of sensory input from the forelimbs and hindlimbs (Cole and Gordon 1976). The fibres leave the pyramidal tract below the decussation and then take a recurrent course into the cuneate and gracile nuclei (Kuypers 1958b; Valverde 1966). Here they tend to avoid the cell cluster zones which give rise to the medial lemniscus; and it has been suggested therefore that they exert their effects on sensory transmission by influences on interneurones (Kuypers and Tuerk 1964, Cheema *et al.* 1983; 1984a). In both the cat and the monkey, the cortico-cuneate projection originates from the caudal part of the precentral gyrus (areas 4 and 3a), from the postcentral gyrus (areas 3b, 1 and 2) and from area 5 (Weisberg and Rustioni 1979; Bentivoglio and Rustioni 1986, see Figs. 2.9(f), 2.10). The projection from postcentral zones is particularly strong in primates, in which there has been a progressive reduction in the corticospinal projection to the spinal dorsal horn. There are very few corticonuclear projections to the *external* cuneate nucleus, which transmits proprioceptive information to the cerebellum (Kuypers 1958b; Weisberg and Rustioni 1979).

2.6 CORTICOFUGAL COLLATERALS FROM THE MOTOR CORTEX

From the above account, it will be clear that there is some overlap in the areas of origin of some corticofugal projections (see Fig. 2.9). In addition,

---

unfolded cortical section. The vertical, straight, and continuous line (between ACS and FCS) corresponds to the position of the boundary between area 4 and area 3a. The three continuous, curved lines posterior to the straight line corresponds to the boundaries between the indicated cytoarchitectonic areas. Note the high density of corticospinal neurones in area 4 compared to the postcentral areas; in contrast, a large proportion of corticocuneate cells were found postcentrally. (From Bentivoglio and Rustioni (1986), p. 269. Copyright © 1986. Reprinted by permission of Wiley-Liss, a division of John Wiley and Sons Inc.)

despite the general laminar organization of the cells of origin of different outputs, there is a degree of radial overlap within lamina V (Jones and Wise 1977). The overlap in cortical origins raises the possibility that single corticofugal neurones project to multiple subcortical sites. The first description of the collaterals that would provide for such multiple projections was made by Ramón y Cajal; their existence was confirmed by electrophysiological studies using antidromic invasion from the two collateral branches (Tsukahara *et al.* 1968; Endo *et al.* 1973). In 1977, Phillips and Porter commented that 'much combined microscopical and electroanatomical work will be needed before we have a complete catalogue of the pyramidal tract collaterals'. Much of this work was done by Kuypers (Fig. 2.11) and such

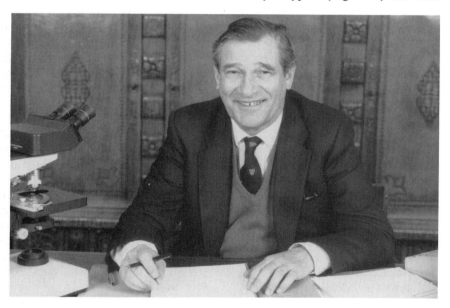

FIG 2.11   Henricus (Hans) Kuypers (1925–89). Kuypers studied medicine at Leiden University in the Netherlands. After first specializing in neurology, he trained as a neuroanatomist under W. J. H. Nauta. He worked for many years in the USA, and then returned to Rotterdam, the Netherlands. In 1984 he was elected to the Chair of Anatomy in Cambridge. He was a pioneer of multidisciplinary neuroscience, and a founder member of several European neuroscience associations. He introduced a number of exciting new neuroanatomical tracing techniques, including double-labelling with fluorescent tracers, and the use of transneuronal viral probes for examining inputs to motoneurones. But he was chiefly interested in utilizing the information provided by these new methods to better understand the organization of the descending motor pathways and the steering of hand and arm movements by the brain. He carried out careful lesion studies to test his hypotheses, and was particularly successful in establishing a functional role for the direct corticomotoneuronal connections.

studies made up an important part of his profound contribution to our understanding of the organization and function of the descending pathways. Kuypers showed that collateralization of corticospinal fibres to other subcortical centres represents a significant feature of the cortical output in all species studied. This collateralization presumably subserves the copying of cortical output signals to several different structures, so that the same information about corticospinal output is available to each of them. The pattern of branching to connect with subcortical targets appears to be specific, and is unlikely to have arisen due to errors during development (Killackey *et al.* 1989). There is evidence that collateral branching is more pronounced amongst PTNs with large, rapidly conducting axons (Humphrey and Corrie 1978).

Another aspect of this question concerns the proportion of the total corticofugal projection to a given structure which is derived from branched pyramidal tract axons: this would appear to be the majority in the case of the corticonuclear projection in the monkey, whereas parts of the red nucleus and reticular formation, for example, have a largely independent, 'private line' projection from the cortex.

The most important breakthrough in the study of collateralization was the introduction by Kuypers and his colleagues of the fluorescent retrograde double labelling technique (van der Kooy *et al.* 1978). Two or more different fluorescent tracers are injected into putative target structures of a given corticofugal system, and, after retrograde transport back to the parent cell bodies, the tracers are visualized, either by fluorescence under different wavelengths of light, or revealed at the same wavelength but in different compartments of the same neurone (e.g. the tracers Fast Blue in the cytoplasm and Nuclear Yellow in the nucleus, respectively) (Kuypers and Huisman 1984). The existence of divergent collaterals has also been established by other retrograde labelling techniques (Hayes and Rustioni 1979) and by careful electroanatomical studies. One of the most complete studies is that by Humphrey and Corrie (1978) who analysed in detail the subcortical branching of PTNs recorded in a defined subregion of the macaque motor cortex, which when stimulated gave rise to wrist flexion or extension. A schematic diagram of the complex branching of corticospinal collaterals is shown in Fig. 2.12, from the review by Wiesendanger (1981a).

2.6.1 Corticorubral collaterals

Catsman-Berrevoets *et al.* (1979) found some double labelled cells in the caudal part of the motor cortex after injections in the spinal cord and magnocellular red nucleus. Although they showed that the number of cortical cells projecting to the parvocellular red nucleus was far greater, very few of these projection cells were double-labelled corticospinal cells. Hence the parvocellular red nucleus can receive 'private' inputs from the motor

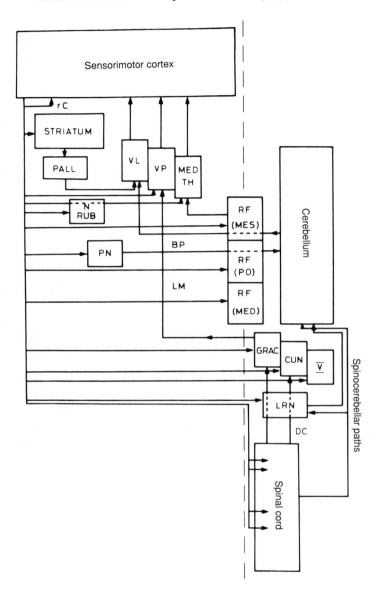

FIG 2.12   Schematic representation of the collateralization of the pyramidal tract. The first set of collaterals are given off as recurrent collaterals (rC) within the cortex. Subcortical targets of pyramidal tract collaterals include the striatum, the specific (VL, VP) and non-specific (MED) thalamic nuclei, the red nucleus (N. RUB), the pontine nuclei (PN), the mesencephalic (MES), pontine (PO), and the medullary (MED) reticular formation (RF), the dorsal column and trigeminal nuclei (GRAC, CUN, V), and the lateral reticular nucleus (LRN). Further collateralization

cortex. Several electrophysiological studies have reported a large proportion of rapidly conducting (modal peak 30–40 m·s^{-1}) corticorubral fibres, most of which appear to be collaterals of pyramidal tract fibres. Thus Humphrey and Rietz (1976) found that 54/63 (86 per cent) of corticorubral cells could be antidromically activated from the pyramid, and Humphrey and Corrie (1978), in the converse experiment, showed that 20 per cent of fast corticospinal neurones could be activated antidromically from the red nucleus. However, since slowly conducting (modal peak 12–14 m·s^{-1}) corticorubral fibres are far more numerous, and since very few of these are collaterals of the pyramidal tract (9 per cent) (Humphrey and Rietz 1976), the corticorubral projection can be considered to be largely independent of that to the spinal cord. The significance of cortical projections provided by fibres of different diameter is not known.

2.6.2 Corticopontine collaterals

The existence of these collaterals is technically difficult to establish because of the proximity of the pontine nuclei to the bundles of corticospinal fibres passing through them. Electrical stimulation of, or injection of transportable agents into, the pontine nuclei without involving stem corticospinal axons is hazardous. Early electrophysiological investigations clearly suggested branching (see Wiesendanger 1981a). In the cat, Ugolini and Kuypers (1986) were able to label the collaterals after injections of Fast Blue into the corticospinal tract, and they concluded that, because the density of labelling obtained in these experiments was similar to that obtained in other experiments after *anterograde* labelling of the corticopontine projections from the motor cortex, a 'major portion of the pericruciate corticopontine connections is established by corticospinal and pyramidal collaterals'.

2.6.3 Corticoreticular collaterals

Keizer and Kuypers (1984) made an extensive examination of the corticospinal and corticobulbar projections to the medial medullary reticular formation (MMRF) in the cat. The cortical origins of these two populations overlapped to a large extent and between 5 and 30 per cent of the retrogradely labelled neurones were double-labelled depending on the site of the injection in the MMRF, with a larger percentage of collaterals reaching the

---

occurs within the spinal cord. The targets of pyramidal tract collaterals are in turn the source of re-entrant loops, among which are the lemniscal system (LM), the cerebellar projections to the VL thalamus, and the pallidal (PALL) projections from the basal ganglia. (From Wiesendanger (1981a), p. 446. Reproduced with permission.)

most medial part of the MMRF. The double-labelled neurones were mainly located in those regions of the cortex involved in movements of the trunk, neck, and shoulder. Motoneurones innervating muscles involved in these axial and proximal movements receive monosynaptic inputs from reticulospinal fibres arising in the MMRF (Peterson *et al.* 1974) and this suggests that there is a dual control of this group of motoneurones through corticospinal and reticulospinal pathways (see below). A similar conclusion was reached following examination of the pattern of corticoreticular organization in the monkey by Keizer and Kuypers (1989).

2.6.4 Corticonuclear collaterals

These collaterals are probably important for control of afferent transmission through the cuneate and gracile nuclei, and have been implicated in the 'cancellation', by efference copy signals, of sensory inputs generated by voluntary commands (Ghez and Pisa 1972; Coulter 1974; Prochazka 1989; Chapman *et al.* 1988; Jiang *et al.* 1990). There would appear to be a clear species difference in the organization of descending influences directed to the dorsal column nuclei. In the cat, both anatomical (Rustioni and Hayes 1981) and electrophysiological (Gordon and Miller 1969) studies have suggested that the proportion of corticospinal fibres contributing to the corticonuclear input is very small (14–16 per cent) (Rustioni and Hayes 1981). However, clear evidence for corticospinal arborization within the cuneate nucleus was found after intraxonal injections by Cheema *et al.* (1984a). In the monkey, Bentivoglio and Rustioni (1986) and Humphrey and Corrie (1978) found that the majority (up to 60 per cent and 72 per cent, respectively) of the corticonuclear projection is derived from corticospinal collaterals. Humphrey and Corrie (1978) estimated that about 8 per cent of all corticospinal axons had corticonuclear collaterals. According to Bentivoglio and Rustioni (1986), a higher proportion of postcentral corticocuneate cells were branched than were the axons of cells located in the precentral motor cortex (see Fig. 2.10). This probably reflects the pattern of areal origin of corticospinal projections to different regions of the spinal grey (see Section 2.6). Species differences may also be recognized in this pattern of organization, since the corticospinal projection from the motor cortex in primates, and especially in man, appears to avoid the dorsal horn.

A branched type of organization may be involved in the control of afferent input needed for precise tactile resolution of spatiotemporal cues generated in a moving limb. During 'active touch', the control of afferent, and particularly cutaneous, feedback, conceivably would be better regulated, temporally, if it were derived from the same output system which would be activated in generating the exploratory movements. It is probably also important to note that the primate motor cortex appears to receive a far greater input from cutaneous mechanoreceptors than is the case in the cat, where the input to cortex is dominated by proprioceptive signals (see Chapter 6). Hence, in the primate, cutaneous cues may have more direct access to specific output cells involved in the performance of the exploratory movement, and sensory–motor interaction may be accommodated more significantly at a cortical level.

Other cortico-subcortical connections have been described, for example projections to the lateral reticular nucleus and the inferior olive. The components of such connectivity served by collaterals of corticospinal fibres is, however, less well documented.

2.7 THE CORTICAL ORIGIN OF THE CORTICOSPINAL TRACT

In every mammal studied, the primary motor cortex contributes more fibres to the corticospinal tract than any other region. But there are also substantial projections from other frontal and parietal areas (Nudo and Masterton 1990a; see Figs. 2.9(c), 2.13). Taken together with the clear differences in the patterns of termination of fibres derived from these several cortical areas, these overall observations suggest a multiplicity, rather than a single, function for the corticospinal tract.

In man, Holmes and May (1909) using the retrograde degeneration technique, had originally concluded that the entire corticospinal tract was derived from the motor cortex. This was based on studies of the cortex of patients with spinal damage. Jane *et al.* (1967) counted the number of fibres in the pyramidal tract of a 51 year old patient in whom the precentral gyrus had been removed surgically 20 years earlier. The ipsilateral pyramid had a fibre count that was 40 per cent of the intact, contralateral pyramid, suggesting that about 60 per cent of the tract must be derived from the precentral region (areas 4 and 6) (see Wiesendanger 1969).

For experimental studies in animals, the classical approach was to make surgical lesions in specific areas of the cortex, and then to await complete degeneration of all the damaged axons issuing from that region. It would then become possible to compare fibre counts of the pyramidal tract on the intact and lesioned side (van Crevel and Verhaart 1963; Russel and DeMyer 1961). More recently, the distribution of retrogradely labelled neurones after injections of HRP or fluorescent tracers in the spinal cord or pyramidal tract has been plotted. Table 2.3 shows the proportions of corticospinal tract cells that have been found in different cytoarchitectonic areas in a number of these different investigations. Table 2.4 shows the detailed analysis of the corticospinal origin from the frontal lobe recently carried out by Dum and Strick (1991).

There is a considerable variation across studies. In the tracer studies, some of the variability may result from differences in the effectiveness of

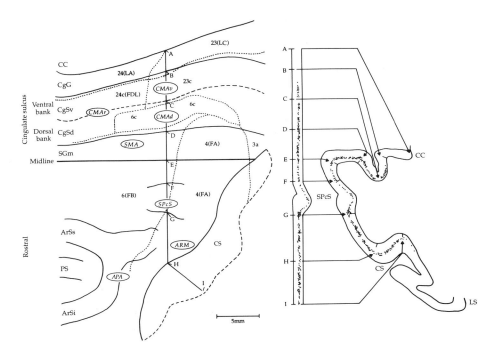

FIG 2.13   Schematic diagram of motor areas in the macaque frontal lobe. Individual coronal sections of cortex (far right) were straightened (middle) to form a flattened reconstruction (left) of the frontal lobe. Dots indicate retrogradely labelled corticospinal neurones. The vertical line on the reconstruction indicates the level of the section displayed at the right. Capital letters (A–I) on the middle panel and on the vertical line in the reconstruction indicate the major points of unfolding (e.g. at sulcal boundaries). Cytoarchitectonic regions are identified both by numbers (according to Brodmann) and by letters in parentheses (according to von Bonin and Bailey). Dotted lines indicate borders between these cytoarchitectonic regions. A dashed line indicates the fundus of each unfolded sulcus. The centres of the different areas in the frontal lobe that contain retrogradely labelled corticospinal cells after tracer injections in the spinal cord are indicated by the circled lettering: APA, arcuate premotor area; ARM, arm representation of the primary motor cortex; SPcS, superior precentral sulcus; SMA, supplementary motor area; CMAd, caudal cingulate motor area, dorsal bank; CMAv caudal cingulate motor area, ventral bank; CMAr, rostral cingulate motor area. Other abbreviations: ArSs and ArSi, superior and inferior arcuate sulci; CC, corpus callosum; CgG, cingulate gyrus; CgSd, cingulate sulcus, dorsal bank; CgSv, cingulate sulcus, ventral bank; CS, central sulcus; LS, lateral sulcus; PS, principal sulcus; SGm, superior frontal gyrus, medial wall. (From Dum and Strick (1991). Reproduced with permission.)

TABLE 2.3 Cortical areas giving rise to the corticospinal tract

Species	Reference	Technique	Frontal lobe (areas 4, 6)			Parietal lobe (areas 3a, 3b, 1, 2, 5, and SII)			
				4	6	3,1,2		5	SII
Man	Jane *et al.* (1967)	Fibre degeneration	60%			40%			
Monkey	Russell and DeMyer (1961)	Fibre degeneration	60%	31%	29%	40%			
	Murray and Coulter (1981)	HRP	40%	35%	5%	60%[1]			
	Toyoshima and Sakai (1982)	HRP	63%	51%	12%	37%	13	12	12
Cat	Groos *et al.* (1978)	HRP	59%[2]			41%	35	4	2
	Keizer and Kuypers (1984)	HRP, fluorescent tracers	80%[3]			20%			

[1]includes 25% of labelled neurones in area 3a; [2]these authors did not report labelling in area 6; [3]includes area 3a

TABLE 2.4 Distribution of corticospinal neurones in the frontal lobe of the monkey (from Dum and Strick 1991).

Region	Area (mm^2)	WGA–HRP in C4–T2 ($n = 42, 912$ neurones) (%)	WGA–HRP in C2–T1 ($n = 71, 128$ neurones) (%)
Primary motor cortex (MI)	84	48.5	49.7
Sup. precentral sulcus (SPcS)	20	7.0	9.9
Arcuate premotor area (APA)	18	4.0	9.6
SMA	44	18.5	12.2
Cingulate motor areas: dorsal (CMAd)	22	10.5	8.0
ventral (CMAv)	14	6.8	6.1
rostral (CMAr)	24	4.0	2.9

Results of retrograde labelling of corticospinal neurones in 2 animals after injections of WGA–HRP in the cervical grey matter. Small numbers of neurones found in area 6DR are not included in this table

the injected label, individual differences between animals in the number of corticospinal axons, and in the extent of the injection sites (see Dum and Strick, 1991). Because different areas of the cortex project preferentially to specific regions and laminae of the cord, injections limited to particular regions of the spinal grey may have labelled disproportionately high numbers of neurones in some cortical areas (for instance, injections in the dorsal horn will tend to label a higher proportion of postcentral than precentral neurones). Even when large injections of tracer are made into the upper cervical spinal cord (so as to fill unilaterally both grey and white matter), the number of corticospinal cells that have been labelled has usually been substantially smaller than might be expected on the basis of published fibre counts for the pyramidal tract in the same species (Toyoshima and Sakai 1982; Keizer and Kuypers 1984). This raises the possibility that an incomplete and perhaps unrepresentative sample of the total corticospinal population had been labelled. The single exception of which we are aware is the study by Toyoshima and Sakai (1982) who labelled over 500 000 cells after application of HRP to the cut medullary pyramid of the monkey. But even in this case there must have been the possibility that some of the HRP spread to label additional corticopontine and corticobulbar fibres.

2.7.1 Origin of the corticospinal tract in the monkey

In the frontal lobe, in addition to the corticospinal projections from the primary motor cortex, substantial contributions from the arcuate premotor area, SMA, and cingulate gyrus have been identified. These different regions are shown in Fig. 2.13, taken from Dum and Strick (1991).

Primary motor cortex (area 4) is the origin of the major projection (30–50 per cent of the total projection, according to the particular study). The density of corticospinal neurones is greatest in area 4, and this is particularly marked in the caudal parts of the precentral gyrus, where the cells are grouped in clusters, rather than distributed evenly throughout the cortex (see Fig. 2.14). The existence of these clusters is typical of motor cortex and has been reported in both electrophysiological and anatomical studies (e.g.

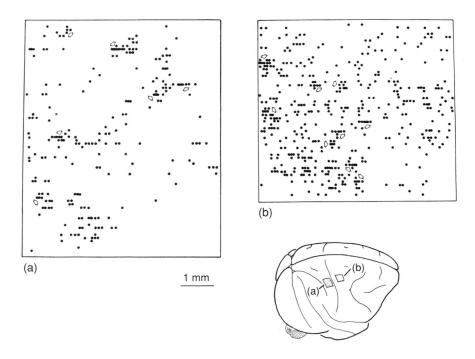

FIG 2.14   Plots showing an enlarged view of the clustering of labelled corticospinal neurones in the SI cortex (a) and the MI cortex (b), following spinal injections of HRP in two different macaque monkeys: (a) (C_5-T_1 spinal segments), (b) (T_1-T_3 spinal segments). Arrows indicate small clusters of cells which are often parts of larger aggregations of labelled neurones. (From Murray & Coulter (1981), p. 346. Copyright © 1981. Reprinted by permission of Wiley-Liss, a division of John Wiley and Sons Inc.)

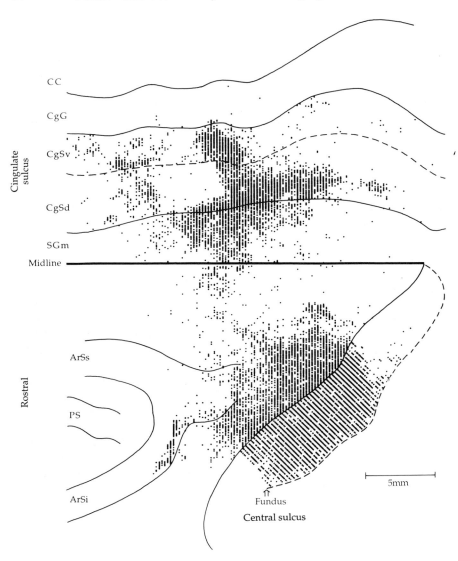

Fig 2.15 Map of corticospinal neurones in the frontal lobe of the macaque monkey. The frontal lobe has been flattened according to the scheme illustrated in Fig. 2.13. WGA-HRP was injected into the contralateral spinal grey matter from C4 to T2. Each retrogradely labelled corticospinal cell is represented by a dot. See Fig. 2.13 for abbreviations. (From Dum and Strick (1991). Reproduced with permission.)

Lemon *et al.* 1976; Humphrey and Corrie 1978; Sessle and Wiesendanger 1982). There is some evidence that the small pyramids located between the clusters are non-corticospinal neurones, that is, in the vicinity of a cluster there are representatives of other pyramidal cell populations projecting to subcortical, but not spinal, targets (Toyoshima and Sakai 1982).

The range of corticospinal cell sizes is greater in area 4 than in any other area, and nearly all the really large (>40 μm soma diameter) corticospinal neurones are located in area 4; lumbar projecting neurones are significantly larger than those terminating in the cervical cord (van Crevel and Verhaart 1963; Jones and Wise 1977; Murray and Coulter 1981).

There is a clear somatotopic organization in the projection from the more caudal parts of area 4; small lesions in the hand area produce intense degeneration in the cervical segments and virtually none in the lumbar enlargement, and vice versa for lesions in the leg area (Kuypers and Brinkman 1970). This has been confirmed with HRP injections into the enlargements (Murray and Coulter 1981). Dum and Strick (1991) made multiple injections of WGA HRP into the spinal grey matter of the entire cervical cord in two monkeys; the injections were made through the dorsal columns to avoid labelling corticospinal axons in the lateral corticospinal tract that were destined for thoracic, lumbar, or sacral levels. The results from one of these animals is shown in Fig. 2.15. These authors identified a strong projection from the region of the superior precentral dimple (SPcS in Fig. 2.13) on the area 4/6 boundary. There are good arguments for recognizing this region as a separate motor area of the frontal lobe (Muakassa and Strick 1979; Godschalk *et al.* 1984).

As shown in Fig. 2.16, the principal target of neurones in area 4 is the dorsolateral part of the intermediate zone and the regions of the lateral motoneuronal cell groups innervating the most distal, hand and foot muscles (Kuypers and Brinkman 1970; Coulter and Jones 1977). This is further illustrated in Fig. 2.17 which shows the findings of Ralston and Ralston (1985) using anterograde labelling of terminals after injection in primary motor and sensory cortex, respectively.

2.7.2 Other premotor areas of the frontal lobe

In the study by Dum and Strick (1991), around 49 per cent of the labelled neurones were located in the primary motor cortex. The distribution of neurones in the other areas is shown in Table 2.4. This also shows the relative surface area of the other areas in the frontal lobe which give rise to the tract. They contribute 12–29 per cent of the fibres in the tract, and, according to Dum and Strick (1991), just over half of the fibres from the frontal lobe arise from these regions. All of them are interconnected with the primary motor cortex. Their different functional contributions are considered in Chapter 7.

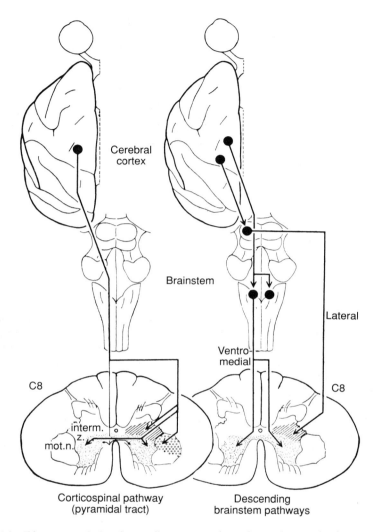

Cerebral
cortex

Brainstem

Lateral

Ventro-
medial

C8   C8

interm.
z.
mot.n.

Corticospinal pathway   Descending
(pyramidal tract)   brainstem pathways

FIG 2.16 Diagrams of the descending connections from the cerebral cortex and
the brainstem to the spinal cord in the macaque monkey. Note that one half of
the brain is connected directly and indirectly (via descending brainstem pathways)
to the dorsolateral (hatched) and ventromedial parts (stippled) of the intermediate zone and to motoneurones (small open circles) of distal extremity muscles
contralaterally, but mainly to the ventromedial parts of the intermediate zone
ipsilaterally. (From Brinkman and Kuypers (1973), p. 624. Reproduced with
permission.)

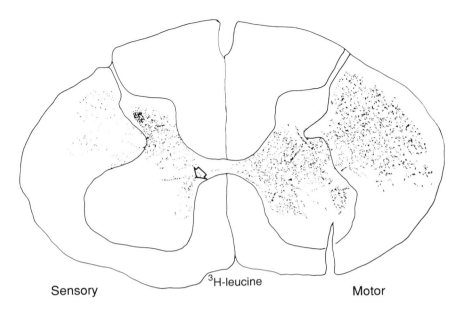

Sensory   ³H-leucine   Motor

FIG 2.17   The projections of the cortex to the spinal cord of the macaque monkey following injection of ³H-leucine into the right sensory and the left motor cortex demonstrated by autoradiography. Note the strong projection to the dorsal horn from the sensory cortex, which is absent for the motor cortex fibres, most of which terminate more ventrally in the intermediate zone and directly among moto-neurones. The sensory cortex projection to the superficial dorsal horn is not revealed by autoradiography. The projections indicated by the arrow in the medial ventral horn on the left are fibres from the motor cortex which cross the midline to terminate in the ipsilateral ventral horn. (From Ralston and Ralston (1985), p. 329. Copyright © 1985. Reprinted by permission of Wiley-Liss, a division of John Wiley and Sons Inc.)

The *arcuate premotor area (APA)* is located in the caudal bank of the arcuate sulcus, in its lower limb and spur (Figs. 2.13, 2.15). The *supplementary motor area (SMA)* has long been recognized as an important part of the motor system, and the area of origin of its corticospinal fibres corresponds well to its definition by other means. Both the APA and the SMA appear to have a somatotopic representation (Sessle and Wiesendanger 1982; Macpherson *et al.* 1982 a,b; Godschalk *et al.* 1984; Hutchins *et al.* 1988). The arm area of the SMA appears to be confined to the superior frontal gyrus. Lumbar projecting neurones have been identified in the dorsal bank of the cingulate sulcus (Murray and Coulter 1981; Dum and Strick 1991).

The *cingulate motor areas*: corticospinal neurones have been identified in three separate regions of the cingulate sulcus: in the dorsal bank of the cingulate sulcus (referred to as CMAd in Fig. 2.13) and lying within cytoarchitectonic area 6; in the ventral bank of this sulcus rostrally (CMAv), that lies within area 23c, and finally within a more rostral region (CMAr), that lies within area 24. These projections, which are also organized somatotopically (Hutchins *et al.* 1988), provide evidence for a limbic contribution to the corticospinal system. There are no corticospinal projections from the frontal eye fields.

Projections from the more rostral parts of the precentral gyrus, including area 6, appear to be distributed more to the ventromedial part of the intermediate zone of the spinal grey matter (Fig. 2.16), and many of these projections are bilateral (Kuypers and Brinkman 1970). This part of the intermediate zone gives rise to long propriospinal connections which contribute to the control of muscles of the trunk and girdles, via bilaterally projecting fibres (see Kuypers 1981). Two further points of interest are that, in the monkey, it is this same region of the intermediate zone which receives descending connections from brainstem pathways influenced by cortico-bulbar fibres originating from the *same*, rostral parts of the precentral gyrus (see Section 2.5 above). Secondly, these more rostral regions of the precentral gyrus, which project bilaterally to the spinal cord, are in receipt of the bulk of the callosal input to area 4.

2.7.3 Corticospinal projections from the parietal lobe

Area 3a contains some of the largest corticospinal neurones outside area 4, and projections from both areas 3a and 4 appear to overlap within the spinal cord. Area 3a is a transitional region between primary motor and sensory cortex (Jones and Porter 1980) and in this respect it is interesting that it appears to project slightly more dorsally within the spinal grey than does area 4 (Coulter and Jones 1977). *Areas 3b, 1 and 2* have a rather sparse projection from small-diameter pyramids (Murray and Coulter 1981). These neurones appear to be primarily concerned with the control of afferent transmission: they terminate chiefly in the dorsal horn (Kuypers and Brinkman 1970; Coulter and Jones 1977), and many of them branch to innervate the dorsal column nuclei (see Section 2.5 above). Finally, there are some projections from areas 5 and 7 and from the second somatosensory area (SII).

Ipsilateral projections are far less numerous than contralateral. In areas 4 and 6, Toyoshima and Sakai (1982) estimated ipsilaterally projecting corticospinal neurones to be 5.9% per cent and 1.8 per cent, respectively, of the corresponding contralateral population. There have been a number of reports of PTNs whose activity is related to ipsilateral body movements and some of them may have ipsilaterally-, or more likely, bilaterally-projecting axons (Lemon *et al.* 1976; Matsunami and Hamada 1978; Tanji *et al.* 1987; see also Chapter 5). It will be necessary for specific experiments to assess the precise physiological actions, directed to particular spinal neurones, which are produced by these ipsilateral corticospinal projections.

2.7.4 Origin of the corticospinal tract in the cat

A similar pattern of organization applies in the cat corticospinal system, with the important exception that medial area 6 (area 6aα, the presumed equivalent of the SMA in primates) contributes very few fibres to the tract (van Crevel and Verhaart 1963; Groos *et al.* 1978; Keizer and Kuypers 1984). This is also the case in the racoon (Sakai 1990). There is a major, somatotopically organized projection from area 4 in the cat, which gives rise to 90 per cent of the large fibres in the pyramidal tract (Van Crevel and Verhaart, 1963). As shown in Fig. 2.18, the fibres originating from lateral and medial regions of the pericruciate cortex project mainly contra-laterally to the cervical and lumbosacral enlargements, respectively. In between these 'specific' zones is a 'common' zone which projects to both enlargements, via both uncrossed and crossed corticospinal tracts

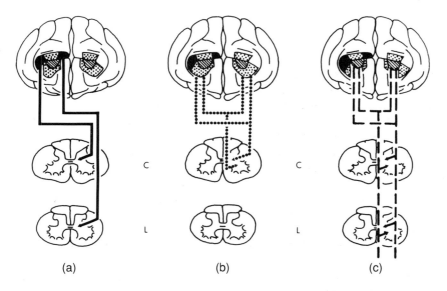

Fig 2.18 Schematic diagram of the various corticospinal projections originating in different parts of area 4 in the cat: (a) specific crossed corticospinal projections to the cervical (C) or lumbosacral (L) enlargement, via the dorsolateral funiculus; (b) specific bilateral projections for one enlargement, via the dorsolateral and ventral funiculi; (c): common bilateral corticospinal projections to both enlargements, via the dorsolateral and ventral funiculi. (From Armand (1982). Reproduced with permission.)

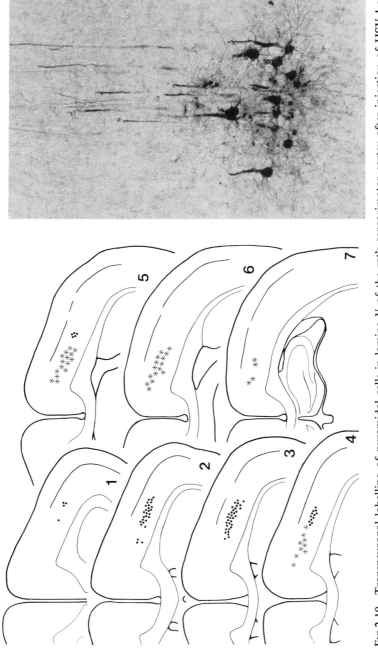

FIG 2.19 Transneuronal labelling of pyramidal cells in lamina V of the rat's sensorimotor cortex after injection of HSV-1 virus into the contralateral median and ulnar nerves 3.5–4 days previously (right). The distribution of labelled neurones, which were revealed by immunohistochemical conjugation with HRP, is shown on the left. The label was concentrated in the forelimb representation after ulnar and median nerve injections (dots in sections 1 to 4) and in the hindlimb representation following injections into the contralateral tibial nerves (asterisks in sections 4 to 7). (Adapted with permission from Ugolini *et al.* (1989) and Kuypers and Ugolini (1990).)

(Hayes and Rustioni 1981; Armand 1982; Armand *et al.* 1985). This is an important observation since it suggests that the degree of axonal branching within the spinal cord may vary according to the location of the cortical origin of the axon (see Section 4.12).

2.7.5 Origin of the corticospinal tract in the rat

Most of the corticospinal neurones are located in the sensorimotor cortex. In the rat there is considerable overlap between somatosensory and motor cortex, although the latter, as defined by low threshold ICMS, is equivalent to the lateral agranular field (AG_l; Wise and Donoghue 1984). This agranular field has a clear somatotopic organization. Corticospinal neurones are found throughout this field, and also extend laterally into the adjacent granular (SI) cortex.

In all of the anatomical studies to date it has been possible to identify regions of the spinal cord to which a given cortical area projects. However, this cannot provide specific information about the control of particular interneurones and motoneurones innervating a designated group of muscles. In 1989, however, corticospinal neurones involved specifically in the control of distal forelimb and hindlimb muscles in the rat were identified by Ugolini *et al.* using a retrograde transneuronal viral labelling technique. Herpes simplex virus, injected into either forelimb median and ulnar nerves, or into the hindlimb tibial nerve, resulted in labelling of clusters of pyramidal cells with a clear medio-lateral somatotopy (Fig. 2.19). This exciting technique promises to be extremely useful for unravelling the fine structure of the corticospinal projection to different spinal targets (Ugolini 1991).

Small numbers of neurones have also been found in the visual, limbic, and prefrontal areas (Miller 1987). These neurones may represent a remnant of the transient corticospinal projection from wide regions of the cortex that has been observed in neonatal rats (Stanfield and O'Leary 1985; see also Section 3.2).

2.8 THE COMPOSITION OF THE CORTICOSPINAL TRACT

With the exception of Francois Françk (1887), the early investigators of the cortical output leading to movement were generally not interested in the mechanisms that linked the motor cortex with the spinal cord and the musculoskeletal apparatus for movement execution. Our aim here is to provide a general anatomical description of these linking outputs in terms that make their functions more easily intelligible. The detailed description of the corticospinal tract is important because its structure and organization serve as a guide to understanding what the output from the cortex means

for the motor apparatus of the limb. In addition, the structure of corticospinal connectivity places a constraint on the number of possible output
arrangements that can be employed by the cortex. It is the proper study
of these outputs that promises better insight into the functions that are
subserved by the arrangements of neuronal networks that exist for selection
in different combinations within the cortex.

As we have already indicated, all the cortical outputs to subcortical structures arise from laminae V and VI, and in all mammals studied, the cerebral
cortex has a greater number of neurones projecting to the spinal cord than
does any other supraspinal structure (Nudo and Masterton 1988). All of
these output fibres travel in the internal capsule and descend in the cerebral
peduncle. Although the corticospinal component of the peduncle is relatively small (approximately 18 per cent by area (Lankamp 1967), but only
5.3 per cent by fibre count (Tomasch 1969)), it is of undoubted significance
because it represents the principal means whereby the supraspinal apparatus,
including the cerebral cortex itself, the cerebellum, and the basal ganglia,
can gain access to the motor apparatus of the spinal cord. We shall concentrate on those anatomical features of the pyramidal and corticospinal
tracts that can be demonstrated to be directly related to the key function
of corticospinal involvement in the management of muscles controlling
voluntary movement. The correlation between corticospinal structure and
function will be dealt with separately in Chapter 3.

2.8.1 Number of fibres

All primates possess a large pyramidal tract containing many corticospinal
fibres (over 1 million in the case of man). Towe (1973) demonstrated that
there is a precise relationship between body weight and the number of corticospinal fibres. Data from all the species he investigated fell on a line,
with the exception of the ungulates and marsupials, which fell below it.
Fibre number is poorly correlated to dexterity (Chapter 3). Table 2.5 lists
the number and average size of corticospinal fibres in a small selection of
representative species. For these species it also gives the level within the
spinal cord to which the tract extends within the spinal grey matter in which
corticospinal terminals are found to penetrate.

Most of the data presented in Table 2.5 were obtained in studies using
the light microscope (LM). More recently a number of electron microscope
(EM) studies have been published, all of which have demonstrated higher
numbers of fibres than were previously counted. The chief differences arise
because of the large numbers of unmyelinated fibres that can be revealed
at the EM level, and which confirm the slowly conducting nature of most
of the fibres in the tract (see below). In the rat, unmyelinated fibres by far
outnumber myelinated fibres (133 000 and 91 000 respectively; Leenen *et al.*
1982; see also Harding and Towe 1985). The total number of fibres by far

TABLE 2.5 Light microscopic details of the pyramidal tract in different mammals.

Species	Body wt. (kg)	Number of fibres	Area of tract (mm²)	Largest fibre (µm)	Mean fibre size (µm)	Spinal penetration	Deepest lamina
Man	70	1 101 000	11.43	22	1.03	Coccygeal	IX
Chimpanzee	44	807 000	7.77	–	0.96	Coccygeal	IX
Macaque	8.3	400 000	2.89	12	0.72	Coccygeal	IX
Cat	3.5	186 000	1.13	5	0.60	Sacral	VIII
Rat	0.4	137 000	0.14	5	0.10	Sacral	VIII
Goat	80	260 000	0.57	5	0.21	C7	VI

Details refer to a single pyramidal tract bundle. 'Average fibre size' derived by dividing tract area by number of fibres. For full details see Heffner and Masterton (1975) exceeds those in the light microscopic study of Brown (1971) (see Table 2.5). Similarly, Thomas *et al.* (1984) counted 414 965 fibres in the cat. These new data call for a re-evaluation of the body weight/fibre number relationship once the results of more EM studies in other species become available.

2.8.2 Size of fibres

In all species the great majority of pyramidal tract fibres are of small diameter, although many of these small fibres may not reach the spinal cord (see Section 2.7). In the cat 93 per cent of pyramidal fibres have axon diameters of <4 μm. In man, 92 per cent are <4 μm, and only 2.6 per cent are larger than 6 μm. Many of the largest fibres are probably derived from the giant Betz cells, of which there are about 30 000 in the human motor cortex (Lassek 1948). Although there is an increase in the size of the largest fibres from the lower mammals up to man (see Table 2.5), there is no correlation of fibre size with either phylogenetic status or digital dexterity (Heffner and Masterton 1975, 1983; see also Chapter 3). The largest fibres reported (25 μm) have been found in the seal (Lassek and Karlsberg 1956).

In the rat, about 60 per cent of the pyramidal fibres appear to be unmyelinated (Leenen *et al.* 1982). In the cat, this proportion is estimated at 12 per cent by Thomas *et al.* (1984). But some doubts as to the nature of these very fine elements were raised by Ralston *et al.* (1987) who have claimed, on the basis of longitudinal rather than transverse sections of the tract, that the profiles classified as unmyelinated fibres are, in fact, astrocytic processes rather than axons. These authors claim that only 1 per cent of monkey tract fibres are unmyelinated. Poor quality of fixation of post-mortem material has so far precluded satisfactory EM studies of unmyelinated fibres in man (Graf von Keyserlingk and Schramm 1984). None of the electrophysiological studies in several animal species has found corticospinal fibres conducting at velocities less than 5 m·s^{-1} (Humphrey and Corrie 1978; Tan *et al.* 1979; Mediratta and Nicoll 1983). This might be because cells with very fine axons have a small soma size and would be difficult to sample electrophysiologically (Towe and Harding 1970; Humphrey and Corrie 1978), although this has not been a problem in recording from cells of origin of other central tracts with much slower conduction velocities (Waxman and Swadlow 1978).

2.8.3 Funicular trajectories

In the monkey, according to Humphrey and Corrie (1978), about 75 per cent of the larger, myelinated fibres descend into the spinal cord, the remainder terminating in the medulla (Kuypers 1958a,b,c). In different species the corticospinal tract descends through dorsal, ventral, and lateral funiculi

(Phillips and Porter 1977, p. 11-13; Armand 1982), although in most carnivores and in all primates the majority of the fibres are found in the dorsolateral funiculus, with a smaller number of fibres in the anterior (ventral) corticospinal tract. According to the results obtained by retrograde transport of HRP in the cat, 92 per cent of the dorsolateral fibres at C7 are crossed, whereas only 63 per cent of the ventral fibres are crossed (Armand and Kuypers 1980). Uncrossed fibres make up around 10-15 per cent of all corticospinal fibres in the cat (Armand and Kuypers 1980), and similar values are quoted for the monkey (Verhaart 1970). Satomi *et al.* (1989) have reported a few corticospinal fibres in the dorsal funiculus of the cat. Barnard and Woolsey (1956) searched for a topographical localization of fibres within the pyramidal tract of the rat and monkey by examining the pattern of degeneration at different levels after localized lesions of the motor cortex. Only above the cerebral peduncle was there any evidence for any such segregation of fibres according to area of cortical origin; below the peduncle the fibres were completely intermingled with each other (see Nathan and Smith 1955). In man, Weil and Lassek (1929), by measuring the area of the lateral tract at different levels, concluded that 50 per cent of the corticospinal fibres terminate in the cervical cord, 20 per cent in the thoracic, and 30 per cent in the lumbosacral cord. In man there are considerable variations in the form and distribution of the lateral tract at different levels of the cord; fibres extend throughout the lateral funiculus and are not confined just to the dorsolateral region (see Fig. 2.22). There are substantial asymmetries in the area of the lateral tract on the two sides, and there appears to be a reciprocal relationship between the area of the lateral and anterior (uncrossed) tracts (Nathan *et al.* 1990). In some cases the anterior tract is small and cannot be identified below the upper thoracic level.

2.9 PENETRATION OF THE TRACT WITHIN THE CORD AND PATTERNS OF SPINAL TERMINATION

In his description of the organization of descending pathways, Kuypers (1973) wrote: 'When considering the connections of the descending pathways . . ., it should be realised that their motor capacities are not so much determined by the location of their cells of origin . . . as by . . . the motor capacities of the interneurons and motoneurons on which these pathways terminate'. As well as commenting on the function of different pathways originating in different supraspinal structures within a species (e.g. vestibulospinal and corticospinal pathways), this important point helps us to understand differences in corticospinal organization in different species. On the basis of differential projections to the dorsal horn, to different regions of the intermediate zone and to different motoneuronal cell

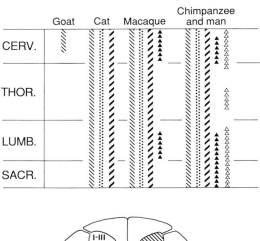

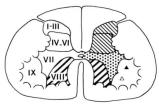

FIG 2.20   Schematic diagram illustrating the termination of corticospinal fibres in four different representative species: goat, cat, macaque monkey and chimpanzee/man. The upper diagram indicates the spinal level (cervical to sacral) reached by projections to different parts of the spinal grey matter, as shown in the section below. The symbols represent terminations: in the dorsal horn (laminae I –III and IV–VI, thin hatching); in lamina VII (dots) and VIII (thick hatching) of the intermediate zone; and cortico-motoneuronal projections to lamina IX (triangles). Note the bilateral projection to lamina VIII, the absence of CM projections in the cat and goat, and the presence, in chimpanzee and man, of CM projections to both dorsolateral motoneurones innervating muscles of the extremity (filled triangles) and to ventromedial motoneurones of the axial and truncal muscles (open triangles). (Adapted from Armand (1982).)

classes, Kuypers (1981) divided mammalian species into four main groups (see Figs. 2.20, 2.21).

Group 1: Mammals with corticospinal fibres extending only to cervical or mid-thoracic segments and terminating in the dorsal horn. In this group of animals, which includes the ungulates (such as the goat), the rabbit, and most of the marsupials, a majority of the corticospinal fibres terminate in the cervical enlargement. Here they are chiefly directed to the dorsal horn (Rexed lamina IV and medial parts of laminae V and VI) and the dorsal parts of the intermediate zone (lateral parts of laminae V and VI), with a

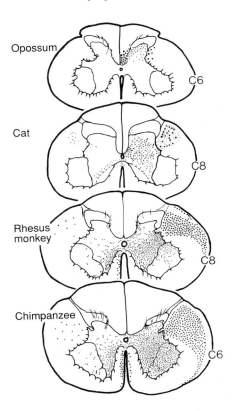

FIG 2.21   Distribution of corticospinal fibres from left hemisphere to low cervical spinal grey matter in opossum, cat, rhesus monkey, and chimpanzee. Drawings based on findings from a number of studies reviewed by Kuypers (1981). The corticospinal projection in the opossum is restricted to the dorsal horn. Note the large extent of the tract within the lateral funiculus in the monkey and chimpanzee, and the very much denser CM projection in the latter species. (From Kuypers (1981), p. 630. Reproduced with permission.)

few fibres in lamina VII. There is a progressive ventral shift of corticospinal termination from polyprotodont (kangaroo) to diprotodont marsupials (phalanger: Tasmanian brush-tailed possum), which may be a reflection of different contributions of the corticospinal connections to the control of limb movement in the latter species (Martin *et al.* 1972; Hore and Porter 1972; Armand 1982). For example, a greater role of corticospinal connections in the precise control of the forelimb for reaching and grasping was inferred from the results of pyramidal tract section in the brush-tailed possum (Hore *et al.* 1973). In the elephant, two-thirds of the pyramidal tract fibres terminate in the region of the facial nucleus (innervating its large trunk), and relatively few fibres reach the spinal cord (see Nathan and Smith 1955).

Group 2: Mammals with corticospinal fibres extending throughout the spinal cord and terminating in the dorsal horn and intermediate zone. This group includes the procavia, and carnivores such as the cat and dog, the rat, and some New World monkeys, such as the marmoset. Fibres terminate mainly contralaterally in the dorsal horn (laminae III–IV), although there is now clear evidence for some projections to the most superficial laminae (I,II; Cheema *et al.* 1984b; Casale *et al.* 1988). There are dense projections to laminae V, VI, and VII, and anterograde WGA–HRP transport indicates some projections to lamina VIII (Cheema *et al.* 1984b). Some fibres, which travel in the anterior corticospinal tract, are distributed bilaterally to the medial part of lamina VIII, from whence they are thought to influence motoneurones innervating trunk and girdle muscles. These fibres are derived from cortical regions separate from those giving origin to fibres terminating in the dorsolateral parts of the intermediate zone, which is thought to influence motoneurones innervating muscles of the extremity (Kuypers 1973, 1981; Armand 1982; Armand *et al.* 1985).

Direct cortico-motoneuronal (CM) connections in these species are absent or sparse (Valverde 1966; Brown 1971; Wise and Donoghue 1984; Kuang and Kalil 1990). Elger *et al.* (1977) claimed that cortical stimulation in the rat produced short-latency EPSPs in forelimb motoneurones. However these could not have been corticospinal in origin because the conduction time (as short as 1–1.5 ms) was far too short even for the fastest corticospinal fibres in the rat (range $11–19 \, \mathrm{m.s}^{-1}$; McComas and Wilson 1968; Mediratta and Nicoll 1983; Stewart *et al.* 1990). It is most likely that the uncontrolled cortical stimuli used by Elger *et al.* (1977) activated subcortical structures. For this reason, we consider that it is inappropriate for this paper to be cited as evidence of cortico-motoneuronal connections in the rat. Other workers (e.g. Bannister and Porter 1967) have been unable to detect monosynaptic EPSPs in motoneurones following pyramidal tract stimulation in the rat.

Group 3. Mammals with corticospinal fibres extending throughout the spinal cord and terminating in the dorsal horn, intermediate zone, and dorsolateral parts of the lateral motoneuronal cell groups. This group includes most of the New and Old World monkeys. In addition to the dorsal horn and intermediate zone, cortical fibres are distributed directly to the dorsolateral parts of the lateral motoneuronal cell groups which innervate the muscles of the extremity. This projection is almost entirely crossed. According to Molenaar and Kuypers (1978), the dorsolateral part of the intermediate zone is the source of short propriospinal fibres which chiefly influence the motoneurones of the extremity, i.e. the same motoneurones which receive the direct CM projections. There are also bilateral projections

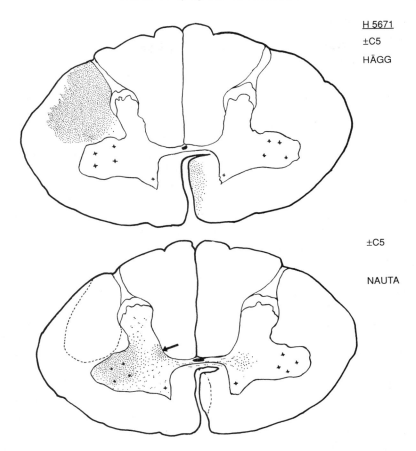

H 5671
±C5
HÄGG

±C5

NAUTA

FIG 2.22 Human post-mortem material. Diagrams of the human spinal cord at C5. In the upper diagram, pyramidal tract fibre degeneration is revealed in Häggqvist-stained material. The crossed fibres occupy the dorsal part of the dorsolateral funiculus, separated by the dorsal spinocerebellar tract from the periphery, while uncrossed fibres are diffusely spread near the midline in the medial part of the anterior funiculus. This degeneration was found in the spinal cord of a 56-year-old woman who died 6 weeks after an extensive cerebrovascular accident.

The lower diagram reveals the Nauta-stained pre-terminal degeneration in the spinal grey matter. This is most dense in the lateral parts of the anterior horn amongst those motoneuronal columns which supply the distal musculature. The arrow indicates the area in which the fibres from the anterior funiculus terminate. In saggital sections many of these fibres are seen to leave the anterior funiculus through the anterior commissure and run for a short distance longitudinally to terminate within the contralateral grey matter. (From Schoen 1964).

to the ventromedial parts of the intermediate zone (lamina VIII). Direct CM projections are relatively sparse in prosimians such as the galago (bushbaby) and lemur, but are well established in the macaque. Although a specialized carnivore, the racoon has been included in this group (Armand 1982). Cortico-motoneuronal projections to the motoneuronal cell groups are sparse and there is scant electrophysiological evidence for such a direct projection (Gugino *et al.* 1990).

Group 4. Mammals with corticospinal fibres extending throughout the spinal cord and terminating in the dorsal horn, intermediate zone, and both dorsolateral and ventromedial parts of the lateral motoneuronal cell groups. In this group corticospinal fibres are distributed profusely both to motoneurones innervating distal extremity muscles and to ventromedial motoneurones innervating more proximal muscles, including those acting on the girdle. This group includes man and the great apes. The pronounced ventral expansion is accompanied by less dense projections to the dorsal horn (see Fig. 2.22).

The principal conclusions from this analysis are that the influence of the cerebral cortex over the spinal cord via the corticospinal tract is largely restricted to the upper parts of the spinal cord in the lower mammals, and that, in these species, its principal action must be exerted on the sensory mechanisms of the dorsal horn. The ventral shift of connections in the higher mammals provides access, first to those regions of the intermediate zone which control the motoneurones innervating distal muscles (probably via propriospinal interneurones with short axons; Kuypers 1978, 1981) and subsequently directly to these motoneurones, via the cortico-motoneuronal (CM) connections. There is also a parallel development, in higher mammals, of bilateral corticospinal projections to the ventromedial intermediate zone, and also directly to the motoneurones innervating proximal limb and girdle muscles.

2.10 SUMMARY

The corticospinal fibres, the majority of which have their origins from a restricted region of the cerebral cortex, are provided by the axonal processes of pyramidal cells within lamina V. While having many features in common, such as prominent apical dendrites and profuse spinous projections from the branches of their dendritic trees, pyramidal neurones exhibit a range of morphological characteristics which have now been detailed with intracellular labelling of functionally identified members of the class. Attempts to quantify the complexity of the geometry of these pyramidal neurones suggest variations between the cat and monkey which may reflect differences in the number of computational functions performed by these cells in the two species.

Pyramidal neurones within the motor cortex are interconnected by intracortical axon collaterals which allow each neurone to influence defined laminae and specific territories within its region. The intracortical axon collaterals of lamina V neurones tend to be limited in their projections to lamina V and closely adjacent regions of lamina VI. Lamina III neurones have a much wider range of collateral distribution and this is more variable from cell to cell. One third of the neurones in the cortex are non-pyramidal cells and these are also involved in the networks of local connectivity. It is through the interactions of extrinsic connections from other brain structures engaging these intracortical networks that the outputs of the motor area are selected and specified.

Corticofugal projections may innervate only a localized territory or they may provide branches to other brain structures along their trajectory towards that territory. The degree to which the projections are limited to one target region (corticorubral to the parvocellular red nucleus or corticospinal) or distributed to several regions by collateralization (corticospinal fibres with collaterals to the pons or the medial medullary reticular formation) has been examined particularly effectively using double labelling techniques. There are clear species differences in the extent of collateralization of corticospinal projections. Moreover, specific targets appear to be linked by particular subpopulations of the corticospinal projection. Hence those corticospinal fibres derived from the sensory cortex and destined to innervate dorsal horn regions within the cervical spinal cord have been shown to provide corticonuclear collaterals to the cuneate nucleus.

In primates a majority of corticospinal fibres derives from pyramidal neurones in the precentral gyrus, and some of these fibres make direct cortico-motoneuronal contacts with spinal motoneurones. It is possible to make a broad classification of mammals into groups with a variety of trajectories of corticospinal projections and a range of patterns of spinal termination of these projections. In lower mammals, corticospinal fibres extend only to cervical or mid-thoracic regions of the cord and terminate in the dorsal horn, while in higher groups, the fibres extend through the whole length of the spinal cord and make extensive cortico-motoneuronal connections in the ventral regions of the cord.

On the basis of anatomical organization and connectivities, corticospinal fibres must be capable of contributing to an extensive range of functions. Different weightings given to the wide variety of multiple connectivities which are demonstrated for some of these corticospinal projections would imply a capacity for a variable range of influences on many aspects of sensation and movement. Some corticospinal fibres, and particularly the cortico-motoneuronal connections in the higher apes, may have the capacity to exert highly specific, localized actions on a limited population of functionally related neurones at a single target site.

3

Correlations between corticospinal connections and function

3.1 INTRODUCTION

Motor behaviour has been studied extensively both under natural conditions and also in experimental test situations in the laboratory. Descriptions of motor performance in a variety of animals, and the accurate measurements of such elements of performance as dexterity, have been aided by the analysis of high-speed cinematographic records of motor behaviour. We are now in a position to seek correlations between some measures of motor performance and a number of observed anatomical and physiological elements of brain development in those same animal species. In the corticospinal system, there are differences in the cortical areas of origin, in the number and sizes of fibres, their course within the spinal cord, and their patterns of distribution and termination within the spinal grey matter. In recent years the relationship of these features of corticospinal tract organization to motor capacity has been subjected to detailed tests (Towe 1973; Heffner and Masterton 1975, 1983; Nudo and Masterton 1990a, b). These investigations have provided a rigorous analysis of the involvement of the corticospinal tract in the control of fine finger movements, which had been proposed by several early investigators (e.g. Lassek and Rasmussen 1940). Within a single species, further evidence relating the corticospinal tract to control of movement performance has been gained by establishing parallels between the rate of postnatal development of the corticospinal system and the timing of maturation of motor behaviour in that species. Finally, correlations between structure and function have been sought by making experimental lesions of the corticospinal system both in the adult animal and in the infant at a specified stage of its development. A large number of tests has then been carried out to determine the deficits in motor performance which could be detected after the lesions were made. These different approaches to discovering the functional contribution to movement performance of the corticospinal system will now be considered in turn.

3.2 FEATURES OF CORTICOSPINAL ORGANIZATION RELATED
TO FUNCTION

Heffner and Masterton (1975, 1983) investigated the corticospinal features
which were best correlated with an index of digital dexterity for 69 different
mammals. The index of dexterity accorded to different mammals is based
on the scheme presented in Table 3.1. They concluded that fibre number,
mean fibre size, and the size of the largest fibres were all poorly correlated
with dexterity in the different species they studied. In fact, many of these
features seem to be related simply to the body weight of the species concerned (Towe 1973). But even after factors related to body weight had been
removed, the correlations with these features of corticospinal organization
were still poor.

Heffner and Masterton found that the two factors that were strongly
correlated with dexterity were the level to which the tract penetrated and
the presence of cortico-motoneuronal projections reaching into the deepest
spinal lamina (the motoneuronal cell groups of lamina IX). Those animals
in which the tract terminates in more dorsal spinal laminae have fused digits
or do not use the digits independently. It is, of course, difficult to arrive
at an index of dexterity that adequately describes the motor capacities of
all species, and recent X-ray studies of paw movement in the cat challenge
the idea that it is incapable of independent digit movement (Caliebe *et al.*
1991). It may thus be too sweeping a generalization to suggest that cortico-

TABLE 3.1   Index of dexterity in different mammals (from Heffner and Masterton
(1983); based on Bishop (1964) and Napier (1961).

Function	Dexterity index	Digit type
Specialization for locomotion	1	Fused or restrained digits
	2	Separate digits that do not converge when flexed
Primitive hand	3	Convergent but not prehensile (not capable of holding an object in one hand)
Specialization for manipulation	4	Prehensile digits, non-opposable thumb
	5	Prehensile digits, pseudo-opposable thumb
	6	Opposable thumb, capable of power and limited precision grips
	7	Opposable thumb, capable of precision grip in opposition to each finger

TABLE 3.2   Correlation of corticospinal tract parameters with digital dexterity in mammals (from Heffner and Masterton 1975).

Parameter	Correlation coefficients	
	Digital dexterity	Digital dexterity, body weight factors removed
Number of fibres	0.26	0.40
Largest fibre size	0.26	0.31
Average fibre size	0.42	0.53
Area of medullary tract	0.34	0.71*
Penetration down cord	0.71*	0.72*
Deepest lamina reached	0.66*	0.71*

* = $p < 0.01$

motoneuronal projections are the *sine qua non* of independent digit movements.

However, it is clear that the index of digital dexterity is highest in animals with abundant cortico-motoneuronal projections (mammals of groups 3 & 4; see Section 2.9). These same species have large corticospinal fibres with axon diameters greater than $12 \,\mu m$, and electrophysiological studies have shown conclusively that these fast axons establish cortico-motoneuronal connections (Phillips and Porter 1977, pp. 139–147). However, it is by no means certain that it is only the largest fibres that make cortico-motoneuronal connections. The relatively poor correlation between maximum fibre diameter and dexterity (Table 3.2) could be taken to suggest that some of the slower fibres may also contribute to the cortico-motoneuronal system and to the capacity for independent finger movements and digital dexterity. Evidence that this is indeed the case is now available (see Section 4.11). Nevertheless, it is clear that fibres making cortico-motoneuronal connections make up only a proportion of the whole corticospinal tract, and, disappointingly, this proportion is as yet undetermined. It may be quite small in some species, and it is interesting that Nudo and Masterton (1990b) found that the total amount of cortical tissue which gave rise to the corticospinal tract in different species was not well correlated with dexterity; dexterity was in fact better related to the total amount of neocortex present than to any other quantitative measure.

3.3 THE EVOLUTION OF THE CORTICOSPINAL TRACT IN PRIMATES: CORRELATION WITH DIGITAL DEXTERITY

To what extent is corticospinal development accompanied by the evolution of motor skill, and particularly digital dexterity, in the primate group? The hands of most primates bear a remarkable resemblance to each other (Fig. 3.1), but there are large differences in dexterity (Bishop 1964; Schultz 1968; Phillips 1971).

The tree-shrews (Tupaioidea) with a dexterity index of 3 (see Table 3.1) and marmoset (Leontocebus; index: 4) exhibit whole-arm control and a relatively crude gasping action in prehension. In social grooming, the marmoset may use its hand to part fur, but specks of dirt are removed by the lips and teeth (Bishop 1964). Both animals lack cortico-motoneuronal projections. Among the prosimians, the lemur (index: 5) is skilled at

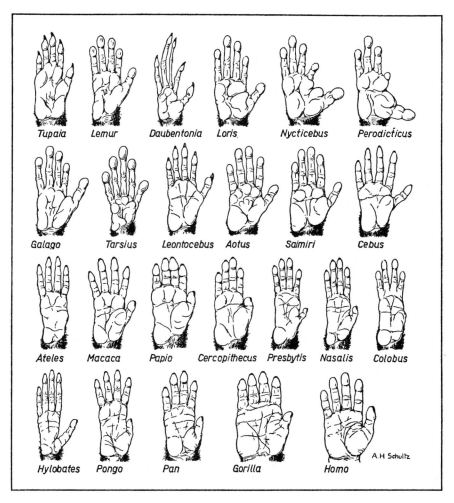

FIG 3.1 Palmar views of the right hands of some adult primates, all reduced to the same hand length. (From Schultz (1968).)

prehension, but does not manipulate objects in the hand. Some New World monkeys, such as the squirrel monkey (Saimiri), are capable only of whole-hand control (Fragazy 1983), while others such the capuchin (Cebus) grip small objects between the sides of the digits, and Costello and Fragazy (1988) state that these monkeys can make thumb–index opposable precision grips. Although they do not possess a truly opposable thumb, Cebus are expert tool-users (Antinucci and Visalberghi 1986) and have well-developed cortico-motoneuronal projections (Bortoff and Strick 1990). Spider (Ateles) and woolly (Lagothrix) monkeys have a large number of cortico-motoneuronal projections to motoneurones innervating their prehensile, glabrous-tipped tails (Petras 1968).

In the Old World monkey, such as the macaque (index: 6), there are clearly observable differences between power and precision grips (Napier 1961). The latter is characterized by a highly fractionated pattern of muscle activity, particularly during *movement* of the digits into the precision-gripping posture (Long and Brown 1964; Muir 1985; Chao *et al.* 1989). The grip itself is associated with a pattern of muscular co-contraction involving many different muscles (Smith 1981), but with different levels of activity organized into a specific pattern (Darling and Cole 1990). Examples of different grips are shown in Fig. 3.2, based on a classification of human manipulative movements proposed by Elliott and Connolly (1984).

In the chimpanzee (index: 7), although the locomotor adaption of the hand for knuckle-walking '. . . may have restricted the range of anatomical positions that the thumb and index finger can adopt in relation to one another, the *functional* (i.e. cerebral) ability to perform precision patterns and grips has not been compromised' (Phillips 1971) (see Fig. 3.1).

In their study of digital dexterity in different primates, Heffner and Masterton (1983) found a significant correlation between dexterity and the cross-sectional area of the pyramidal tract, once body weight factors had been taken into account (see Table 3.2). In other words, the increasing size of the corticospinal tract that accompanies the ascent of the phylogenetic scale is greater than would be expected from the parallel increase in body weight. In man there are considerable asymmetries between the cross-sectional area of the tracts on the right and left sides, with the right tract being larger in three-quarters of the cases studied, although this does not appear to be related to handedness (see Nathan *et al.* 1990).

Cortico-motoneuronal projections are far more numerous in the great apes and in man than in the macaque monkey (Kuypers 1981; see Fig. 2.20) and there are also important differences amongst the New World monkeys which appear to correlate well with dexterity (Heffner and Masterton 1983; Bortoff and Strick 1990). These results confirm the suggestion, originally put forward by Bernhard *et al.* (1953) and by Kuypers (1962) of the importance of the cortico-motoneuronal connections for independent finger movements. Such a conclusion has gathered a wide degree of support from

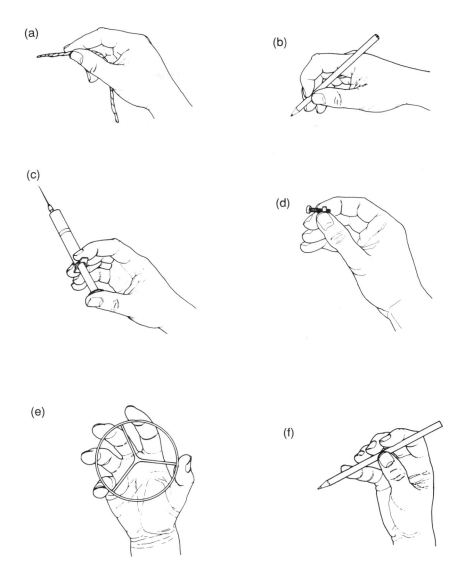

FIG 3.2 Classification of manipulative hand movements. (a)-(c) show simple synergies in which movements of all digits are convergent: (a) pinch, thumb, and index extended; (b) dynamic tripod, simultaneous flexion, and extension movements of thumb, index and digit 3 manipulate pen; (c) squeeze, simultaneous flexion of thumb, index, and digit 3 will drive plunger into barrel. (d)-(f) show reciprocal synergies in which movements of the thumb are independent of those of the fingers: (d) 'twiddle', thumb in full abduction; (e) 'rock', ventral view of hand gripping a petri dish, with thumb in partial abduction; (f) 'rock', pencil held transversely, in radio ulnar-axis. Thumb is stationary and digit 3 movements are much reduced compared with those of the ring and little fingers. (From Elliott and Connolly (1984). Reproduced with permission.)

the study of the electrophysiology (Chapter 4), development (Section 3.4) and behavioural capacities (Section 3.5) of the cortico-motoneuronal system.

Wood Jones (1920) has written: '. . . it would be difficult to name any movement that is possible in the human hand which is not equally possible in the hand of the Old World monkeys, but anyone may name a host of purposive actions habitual to Man, which are not included in a usual repertoire of a monkey.' and 'The difference between the hand of a man and the hand of a monkey lies not so much in the movements which the arrangement of muscle, bones, and joints makes it possible for either animal to perform, but in the purposive volitional movements which . . . the animal habitually exercises'. This highlights the essential contribution of the cortex itself, and of other supraspinal centres, in determining the commands that are finally directed to the motor apparatus by the corticospinal and cortico-motoneuronal systems. It is the connections which these descending systems make with the motor apparatus that define and constrain the structure of the output system upon which these centres can play.

3.4 DEVELOPMENTAL ASPECTS OF THE CORTICOSPINAL SYSTEM

3.4.1 Origin of the corticospinal tract

Abnormal development of descending motor systems is associated with a number of movement disorders, and yet our knowledge of how these pathways develop is still very limited. For developmental studies, an animal model is essential, but also problematic since the rate of development in different species is very different, and the maturity of different species at birth may vary considerably (Passingham *et al.* 1983; Passingham 1985a). Nevertheless the clear anatomical identity of the pyramidal and the corticospinal tracts have made them attractive models for the study of development, mostly in the cat and in rodents. Wise *et al.* (1977) made a study of the prenatal development of motor cortex projection using anterograde tracing methods in the cat. They found that the corticospinal projection could be identified as early as 50–55 days after gestation, before there was any clear sign of laminar organization in the cortex and before other efferent projections, for instance to the tectum or pons, could be recognized. Small pyramidal cells were first recognized in lamina V at 57 days, with large pyramids appearing shortly afterwards. Wise *et al.* (1977) considered that this early appearance was followed by a 'waiting period' before the cells finally invaded their zones of termination. This waiting period coincides with the entry of thalamocortical afferents to the developing cortex. Such developments may explain the changes in the synaptic responsiveness of these cells in early postnatal life (Oka *et al.* 1985; Tolbert 1989).

Oka *et al.* (1985) also showed that kitten pyramidal tract neurones are still undergoing changes postnatally and do not show a mature form of responsiveness until around 4 weeks after birth. Changes over long periods in rat pyramidal tract neurones were also reported by Wise *et al.* (1979).

The density and proportion of synaptic contacts in the developing macaque motor cortex were studied at the EM level by Zecevic *et al.* (1989). The first synapse was detected at embryonic (E) day E53; at the middle of the gestation period (E89) synapses were present through all cortical layers but at a low density ($5/100 \, \mu m^3$ of neuropil). During the last two months of gestation there was a dramatic eight-fold increase in synaptic density to reach $40/100 \, \mu m^3$ at birth (E165); it reached a maximum of $60/100 \, \mu m^3$ two months postnatally. There then followed a substantial and rapid elimination of synapses, principally of the asymmetric type, until the age of 3 years, after which the density remained at the adult level of around $30/100 \, \mu m^3$. Interestingly, it is during this important postnatal period that there is a reshaping of thalamocortical inputs to the motor cortex, which according to Darian-Smith *et al.* (1991) have a more widespread pattern of arborization in the newborn than in the 6-month-old macaque. There are also changes in cortico-cortical and callosal projections.

In the rat, the origin of the corticospinal tract appears to be much more extensive in the developing than in the adult animal (Bates and Killackey 1984; Schreyer and Jones 1983). Stanfield and O'Leary (1985) showed that injection of the fluorescent retrograde tracer Fast Blue into the pyramidal decussation in newborn rats resulted in a continuous band of labelled lamina V neurones spanning the entire cortex, including the occipital lobe. This type of labelling was not seen in the adult, nor was it seen after injections made on postnatal day 20 or later. Similar results have been obtained in the mouse, hamster, and rabbit (see O'Leary and Stanfield 1986). Corticospinal fibres grow into the pyramidal tract in a staggered fashion, with axons from frontal regions arriving first and those from occipital regions coming last. Most of the 'aberrant' collaterals do not penetrate into the spinal grey matter to make many functional synaptic connections, and may even be electrically silent (Joosten *et al.* 1987; Tolbert 1989). The restriction of the corticospinal neurones to the adult pattern has been attributed both to the elimination of transitory axon collaterals and to cell death (O'Leary and Stanfield 1986; Schreyer and Jones 1988). The withdrawal of collaterals probably accounts for the dramatic loss of fibres from the pyramidal tract during development. In a quantitative EM study in the hamster, Reh and Kalil (1982) showed that the adult tract has only half the fibres found in the newborn.

There is at present no evidence available on the areal distribution of corticospinal cells in the newborn cat or monkey. Biber *et al.* (1978) found an identical pattern of labelling in both young and adult monkeys, although their youngest animal was, at 5 months, probably past any remodelling period. The same is probably also true for the 20-day-old kitten studied by Bruce and Tatton (1981), who found a similar pattern of labelling to that in the adult cat.

3.4.2 Growth of the corticospinal tract

There are marked species differences in the growth of the tract. Thus in the cat, Wise *et al.* (1977) showed that corticospinal fibres have reached the medullary decussation 20 days before birth while, in the rat and hamster, fibres only reach this level at birth and three days after birth, respectively (Jones *et al.* 1982; Reh and Kahil 1981). In the cat, corticospinal fibres have reached all levels of the spinal cord at birth (Leonard and Goldberger 1987b; Theriault and Tatton 1989), and in the monkey they have reached at least to the level of the lower cervical segments (Kuypers 1962). In the rat, this stage is not complete until 15 days after birth (Schreyer and Jones 1983; Joosten *et al.* 1987). There would appear to be a second 'waiting period' before corticospinal axons invade the spinal grey matter, and connections with appropriate targets may be induced by release of a chemotropic factor (Joosten *et al.* 1991). The earliest terminations to appear are in the dorsal horn. In the monkey, the direct cortico-motoneuronal projections do not appear to develop until 6–8 months of age (Kuypers 1962; see Fig. 3.3). This result needs confirmation by the applica-

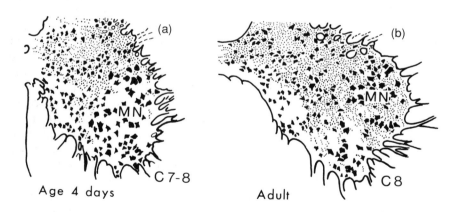

Fig 3.3 Terminal distribution of corticospinal fibres in the lower cervical segments in: (a) 4-day-old infant, and (b) adult rhesus monkey. Terminals were revealed by the Nauta–Gygax stain for anterograde degeneration resulting from large cortical lesions on the contralateral side. Note absence of corticospinal terminals amongst the motoneuronal cell groups in the infant monkey. (Redrawn after Kuypers (1962). Reproduced by permission of Oxford University Press from Lawrence and Hopkins (1976).)

tion of modern tracing techniques to the thorough evaluation of developing corticospinal projections in the primate.

3.4.3 Exuberant branching of corticofugal projections

In common with most developing neurones, immature corticofugal neurones show an exuberant pattern of branching. Thus, in the kitten, axon densities labelled from the pericruciate cortex were widespread through the spinal grey matter, from Rexed lamina I to IX, compared to a much more restricted distribution in the adult (see Section 2.8 above; Theriault and Tatton 1989). Corticospinal branches also crossed the midline at all levels. Other studies have shown that in the newborn kitten, in addition to the ipsilateral projection from the motor cortex to the red nucleus, there is a significant contralateral projection (Leonard and Goldberger, 1987b; Murakami and Higashi 1988). Leonard and Goldberger (1987b) also reported numerous projections to the contralateral VL nucleus of the thalamus.

Many studies have been directed towards the substantial remodelling of the corticospinal projection that occurs after neonatal injury in the rat, hamster, and kitten. These studies have indicated that, for instance, after unilateral section of the pyramidal tract (Castro 1978; Tolbert and Der 1987) or hemispherectomy (Castro 1975; Leong 1976; Huttenlocher and Raichelson 1989; Armand *et al.* 1991) new aberrant pathways develop. In the rat, where nearly all of the pyramidal tract fibres decussate, motor cortex lesions at birth result in the appearance of an ipsilateral, uncrossed projection to the spinal cord from the remaining hemisphere. Aberrant projections to the red nucleus are also found after neonatal cortical lesions in cats (Murakami and Higashi 1988; Villablanca *et al.* 1988). Because these projections resemble those seen in the immature animal, some have suggested that these aberrant projections are somehow preserved by the effects of the lesion, such as failure of projections from the damaged side to displace them or cause them to retract (Leonard and Goldberger 1987a, b). In general, however, the evidence seems to indicate that most of the new projections arise by sprouting of the intact fibres in response to injury (Murakami and Higashi 1988; Villablanca *et al.* 1988). Armand *et al.* (1991) made sensorimotor lesions at birth; subsequent injection of HRP into the intact sensorimotor cortex, revealed widespread aberrant projections, including contralateral projections to the thalamus, red nucleus, and pontine nuclei and ipsilateral projections to the dorsal column nuclei and spinal cord. Some of these may be new, supernumerary fibres. It is clear that several forms of plasticity are necessary for recovery of motor performance and the development of compensatory strategies (Kably 1989).

The extent of such sprouting in adult animals is severely curtailed, as is recovery from lesions. Bregman and Goldberger (1983) have shown that kittens subjected to spinal cord damage have a considerable capacity for reorganization and rerouting of corticospinal fibres, and that this is probably reflected in the recovery of some motor functions such as tactile placing. In contrast, brainstem pathways which developed earlier than the corticospinal tract showed little or no recovery, and the motor patterns which these subserved (e.g. postural reflexes and locomotion) also failed to recover. Armand *et al.* (1991) found that, if sensorimotor lesions were made before postnatal day 30, cats could recover sufficiently to perform complex tasks requiring fine control of both distal and proximal forelimb. These tasks involved accurate reaching and retrieval of a food reward from a narrow tube. Cats operated on between 30 and 60 days of age could recover only the proximal component. If the lesion was made after 60 days no recovery in the performance of these complex tasks was possible.

The evidence for these exuberant projections in the primate is, at present, scarce. Indeed, with the exception of a small projection to the contralateral red nucleus, Sloper *et al.* (1983) could not find any substantial differences from normal distributions in the subcortical projections from the intact sensorimotor cortex in monkeys that had been subjected to ablation of the opposite sensorimotor area at birth. Passingham *et al.* (1983) have suggested that this may be due to the relatively advanced stage of development reached by the monkey at birth. This may also explain why it is that infant monkeys subjected to bilateral pyramidotomy at birth (Lawrence and Hopkins 1976) fail to develop a normal pattern of relatively independent finger movements (see below).

In patients who have undergone hemispherectomy, motor recovery in the contralateral limb is generally better in those whose tissue was removed early in life, than in patients subjected to hemispherectomy after normal maturation of the brain (Benecke *et al.* 1991). Magnetic stimulation of the surviving hemisphere evoked responses in the arm muscles on the ipsilateral side, which were of similar short latency as those recorded from the contralateral limb. There was a clear proximodistal gradient in the amplitude of these ipsilateral responses, being weakest in hand and foot muscles. These ipsilateral responses probably represent a remodelling of the corticospinal output after brain damage in early life; responses of this kind were not observed in patients who sustained brain damage after maturity had been attained.

3.4.4 Myelination of the corticospinal tract

The myelination of the corticospinal fibres occurs postnatally in all species studied: in the rat (Matthews and Duncan 1971), hamster (Reh and Kalil 1982), cat (Huttenlocher 1967, 1970), and man (Yakovlev and Lecours 1967; see Müller *et al.* 1991). According to Jones *et al.* (1982), all

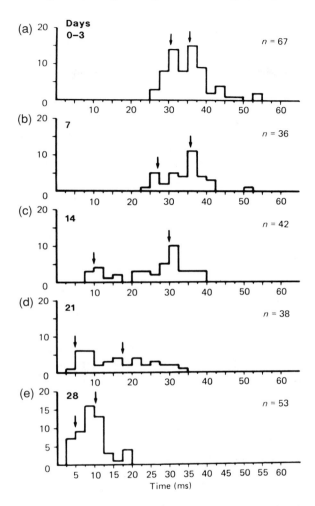

FIG 3.4 Postnatal increases in the conduction velocity of cat pyramidal tract neurones (PTNs). Latency histograms of antidromic responses in PTNs recorded in the motor cortex of kittens at different ages. Antidromic responses elicited by stimulation in the ipsilateral pyramidal tract. (a) Histograms obtained from 67 neurones of zero to 3-day-old kittens. Arrows correspond to the peak latencies of the two positive waves of the pyramidally evoked cortical surface response. (b)–(e) Histograms obtained from 7, 14, 21, and 28-day-old kittens respectively. n = number of neurones recorded in the kittens of different ages. (From Oka *et al*. (1985). Reproduced with permission.)

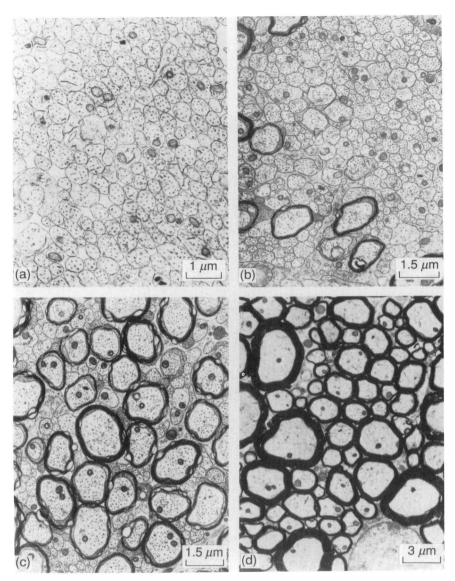

FIG 3.5 Postnatal myelination of the pyramidal tract in the hamster, illustrated by electron micrographs of the tract at four postnatal ages: (a) in the 7-day tract note the copious extracellular space; (b) by 14 days a few myelinated fibres are present and the extracellular space has been filled by insinuating glial processes; (c) at 21 days the tract contains approximately one-half the number of myelinated axons as the adult; (d) the adult pyramidal tract. The different magnifications used show the increase in the size of the axons with age. (From Reh and Kalil (1982). Copyright © 1982. Reprinted by permission of Wiley-Liss, a division of John Wiley and Sons Inc.)

corticospinal axon growth is complete before myelination begins, and in most species, this process is extended over long periods of time. It may take several years in man.

In the cat, myelination is still incomplete at 1 month of age and proceeds slowly to completion at 4–5 months after birth. This process could account for the results of Oka *et al.* (1985), who used the latency of antidromic responses evoked by stimulation of the pyramidal tract to demonstrate a steady change in the conduction velocity of corticospinal axons during the first month of life (Fig. 3.4). At birth, the fastest axons were calculated to conduct at $0.7 \, \text{m.s}^{-1}$, compared to $15 \, \text{m.s}^{-1}$ one month later. It is evident from Fig. 3.4 that the entire population of corticospinal fibres shows a continuous decrease in antidromic latency, although the fastest axons show a particularly marked reduction around two weeks of age, possibly indicating a wave of myelination in which the largest axons are myelinated first (cf. Matthews and Duncan 1971; Reh and Kalil 1982; see Fig. 3.5). Several studies have shown that there is no critical corticospinal axon diameter which predicts whether or not it will become myelinated. In the rat, the corticospinal tract becomes myelinated after the other major motor and sensory pathways are fully myelinated (Matthews and Duncan 1971).

The myelination process not only increases the conduction velocity of the fibres, but may change them in other ways. An immature, unmyelinated axon cannot support the repetitive firing characteristic of the adult neurone (Huttenlocher 1970; McDonald and Sears 1970). Moreover, the opportunity for mutual interaction between axons along the length of their processes must be decreased by the insulating barriers of myelin sheaths.

3.4.5 Electrophysiological and behavioural parallels

Stimulation of the neonatal motor cortex fails to elicit any motor responses comparable to those seen in the adult. When responses do appear, they generally have long latencies and high thresholds. In the kitten, Bruce and Tatton (1980a, b) reported that EMG responses in a variety of facial and upper and lower limb muscles could not be activated by ICMS in the motor cortex until around 37–45 days postnatally (around 110 days gestational age). Even ICMS trains of long duration and high strength (up to $100 \, \mu\text{A}$) were ineffective. At 37–45 days, clear-cut short-latency responses were evident, and were indistinguishable from those in adult cats. Bruce and Tatton (1980b) reported that such responses develop synchronously in all muscles investigated. Interestingly, these authors reported that responses to ICMS appeared before neurones in the motor cortex showed responses to peripheral stimulation, which occurred at around 55–65 days. These input–output changes precede changes in motor behaviour, including the maturation of walking along narrow bridges and forelimb contact placing (Amassian and Ross 1978).

In the monkey, Felix and Wiesendanger (1971) reported that stimulation of the motor cortex in a 7-week-old monkey failed to produce any short latency EMG responses; a 10-month-old animal yielded essentially adult responses. Recently Flament *et al.* (1992c) used magnetic stimulation of the motor cortex to examine, non-invasively, the maturation of short-latency responses in arm and hand muscles of a group of infant Rhesus monkeys (Fig. 3.6). Magnetic stimulation is capable of exciting the entire fast-conducting corticospinal output in the macaque (Edgley *et al.* 1990). In both cross-sectional and longitudinal studies, Flament *et al.* (1992c) found that it was difficult, even with full output of the stimulator, to elicit short-latency responses in monkeys of below 4–5 months of age; thereafter the threshold and latency of the responses decreased steadily, and reached adult values at around 6.5–8 months. Results from two longitudinal studies are shown in Fig. 3.6. In these monkeys, Flament *et al.* (1992c) found that the maturation of these responses parallelled that of relatively independent finger movements. A staggered development of corticospinal projections to forelimb and hindlimb was suggested by Flament *et al.* (1992b) who showed that, in longitudinal studies of infant macaques, cortically-evoked responses in hand muscles could be recorded about one month earlier than those in foot muscles.

In a classic study of the development of motor control, Lawrence and Hopkins (1976) made extensive observations on hand and finger movements in infant Rhesus monkeys. They hand-reared infants from birth; five animals underwent bilateral pyramidotomy 5–28 days after birth, and two served as control animals. The latter were tested on a variety of tasks, including the retrieval of small food morsels from a test board (Fig. 3.7), similar to that used by Lawrence and Kuypers (1968a). The earliest signs of reaching in the control animals was at 3–4 weeks of age. Reaching was inaccurate and grasping of food rewards was part of a rather gross whole arm and hand movement. The retrieval of food was clumsy and, when successful, was achieved by closure of all digits around the reward; release of the food at the mouth was often achieved with difficulty. Smooth reaching occurred in the third month and the first signs of relatively independent finger movements (RIFM) were present in the second to third month. The control animals were judged to have fully mature RIFM at 7–8 months of age. The maturation of RIFM seems to lag the development of tactile discriminative capacity by several weeks (Carlson 1984). Hinde *et al.* (1964) have observed that infant monkeys first begin to groom other monkeys at around six months of age. RIFM are a quintessential requirement for grooming, when often a single hair or a tiny flea must be isolated and gripped (Tower 1940). The developmental time-course of RIFM thus correlates well with the appearance of cortico-motoneuronal projections (Kuypers 1962) and the maturation of short-latency responses to stimulation of the motor cortex described above.

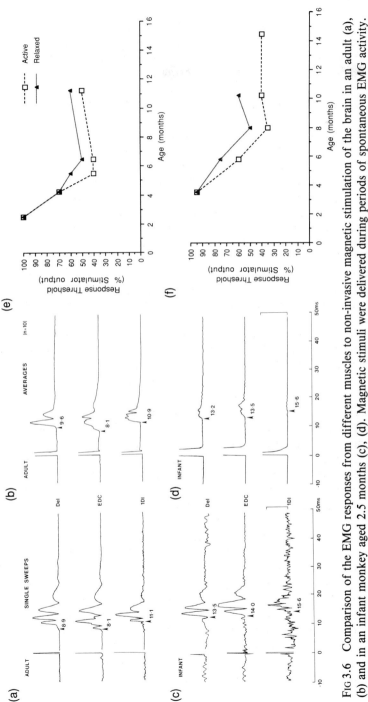

Fig 3.6 Comparison of the EMG responses from different muscles to non-invasive magnetic stimulation of the brain in an adult (a), (b) and in an infant monkey aged 2.5 months (c), (d). Magnetic stimuli were delivered during periods of spontaneous EMG activity. (a), (c): single-sweep responses in adult and infant. (b), (d): average of ten responses. Numbers at arrows are onset latencies (in ms) for responses. In the infant, average responses (d) were small and had long latencies in deltoid (Del) and in extensor digitorum communis (EDC); only one very weak response (shown in (c)) could be recorded from 1st dorsal interosseous (1DI) of this infant, accounting for the very small response in the averaged record. Left vertical calibration for (a) is: Del, 1 mV; EDC, 750μV; 1DI, 500μV For (c): Del, 250μV; EDC, 500μV; 1DI, 30μV. Right vertical calibration for (b) and (d): Del, 750μV; EDC, 750μV, and 1DI, 300μV. (e) and (f), longitudinal study. Thresholds of EMG responses recorded from 1DI following brain stimulation in two infant macaque monkeys. Before 5 months of age the thresholds were high and similar for responses evoked during periods of spontaneous EMG activity (□, active) or during EMG quiescence (▲, relaxed); after this age thresholds fell rapidly and were 10–20 per cent lower when there was spontaneous activity. (From Flament *et al.* (1992c). Reproduced with permission.)

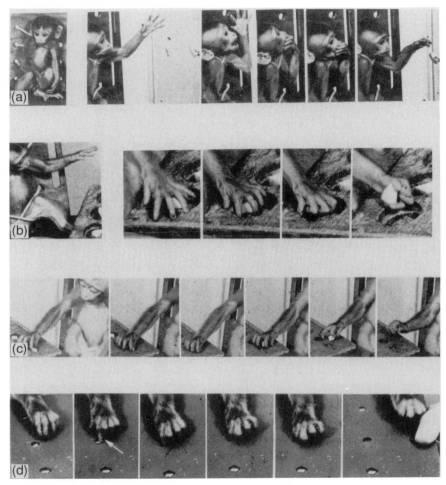

FIG 3.7   Development of motor control in the infant rhesus monkey. (a) Normal animal age 30 days. Reaching for food in forceps. Note inaccuracy of arm movement and grasped snout. After releasing the snout the hand reached accurately for the food. (b) age 35 days. Removal of food from well. Note closure of fingers all together. (c) age 2.5 months. Note ineffective attempts to remove food with index finger alone (first and second frames). (d) age 11 months. Adult level of relatively independent finger movements: note fully extended index finger with other fingers flexed out of the way (second frame). (Reproduced by permission of Oxford University Press from Lawrence and Hopkins (1976).)

Lawrence and Hopkins (1976) found that, in the monkeys pyramidotomized at birth, there was 'no appreciable difference in the development of general motor activity'. They could run, walk, climb, and jump as well as the normal infant animals. Reaching developed in the normal fashion and became smooth and accurate. However, none of the four animals with a complete pyramidotomy ever developed any RIFM; instead food was gripped by flexion of all digits in concert. As might be expected, these animals had great difficulty in extracting small food morsels from the test board and in opening the hand to release the food; these deficits in RIFM persisted into maturity, and could not be overcome by an extensive programme of training.

Although many factors contribute to the mature motor pattern of voluntary hand and finger movements, the above results suggest that the establishment of functional cortico-motoneuronal connections is essential for the full development of RIFM. However, further research will be required to confirm any causal relationship. In man, the maturation of skilled finger movements requires a much longer period of development than in the macaque (Halverson 1943; Forrsberg *et al.* 1991). That this maturation is also dependent on the maturation of corticospinal pathways is suggested by the work of Eyre *et al.* (1991), illustrated in Fig. 3.8. These authors determined the central conduction time (CCT) of responses to magnetic stimulation of the cortex in 308 subjects aged from 32 weeks gestation to 55 years. There was a rapid decline in CCT for the first two years of life, and adult values for CCT in both biceps brachii and the hypothenar muscles were achieved from around 2–4 years of age (see Fig. 3.8 (c) and (d), respectively). Responses were difficult to elicit in relaxed muscles of the youngest subjects, and the threshold for evoking responses in contracting muscles continued to fall up to the 16th year of age (Fig. 3.8(e)). This extended time course was confirmed by Müller *et al.* (1991), and is in keeping with the protracted period during which myelination of the human pyramidal tract continues (Yakovlev and Lecours 1967). Interestingly, maximum fibre size appears to be well correlated with body height at all ages, and the slow process of myelination may subserve the useful function of maintaining a constant central conduction time in the corticospinal pathway during growth (see Eyre *et al.* 1991).

3.5 BEHAVIOURAL CONSEQUENCES OF LESIONS TO THE PYRAMIDAL AND CORTICOSPINAL TRACTS IN DIFFERENT SPECIES

The results of sectioning the pyramidal tract on different aspects of movement performance have been examined both by observation and description of natural performance in experimental animals, or by using specially designed tests. What follows is a review of the effects of experimental

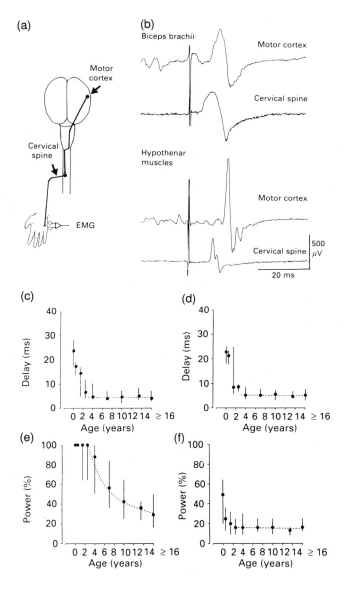

FIG 3.8   Development of responses to non-invasive magnetic brain stimulation in man. In (b), motor evoked potentials were obtained in single trials from biceps brachii and hypothenar muscles in a subject aged 12 years. In each pair of traces the upper record shows the response to stimulation of the motor cortex and the lower record the response to stimulation over the cervical roots (see diagram (a)). In diagrams (c) and (d), central motor conduction delay of the motor evoked potentials in biceps (c) and hypothenar muscles (d) is plotted in relation to age in 308

lesions in monkeys, in which animals pyramidotomy has the most clear cut effects. This work will be used to illuminate the very rare cases of damage confined to the pyramidal tract in man. Finally, reference will be made to some of the observations made in subprimates.

3.5.1 Macaque monkey

Early studies on the effects of pyramidal tract section in monkeys were dominated by the idea that this procedure would serve as a model for the various 'pyramidal' symptoms and signs observed after stroke in man. As a result, a great deal of attention was given to the question of whether spasticity was present (e.g. Denny-Brown and Botterell 1948; Denny-Brown 1950). It is now generally agreed that, in the monkey, neither pyramid-otomy nor lesions confined to area 4 produce the hemiplegic type of spasticity (Lawrence and Kuypers 1968a; Hepp-Reymond 1988), but rather a flaccid paresis, which is most clearly observed in the hand. A detailed account of the various investigations into the effects of pyramidal tract lesions in the monkey has been given by Hepp-Reymond (1988). The following generalized conclusions can be drawn:

1. There is a permanent deterioration in the ability of the pyramidotom-ized monkey to make fine, independent movement of the digits. Tower (1940) commented that the poverty of movement is in proportion to the 'discriminative qualities' of the movement and that 'all fine usage is eliminated'. Most of Tower's animals died within a few days of surgery, and it was Lawrence and Kuypers (1968a) who first established the perma-nent loss of relatively independent finger movements exhibited following long-term survival after bilateral pyramidotomy. In their study, eight out of 39 monkeys were found at post-mortem to have a complete bilateral sec-tion of the pyramids, with minimal involvement of the medial lemniscus or inferior olivary nucleus. Clear deficits were only observed when monkeys were confronted with well-designed test situations. Lawrence and Kuypers found that monkeys had permanently lost the capacity to retrieve small

---

subjects from birth to 55 years. This delay was calculated from the latencies of responses to cortex and cervical spine stimulation. Note marked decrease in the delay at around 18 months of age. Linear regression lines (dashed) shown for the age range 3–16 years. (e) and (f), stimulus intensity (as percentage power output of the stimulator) for evoking responses in the actively contracted biceps brachii following motor cortex (e) and cervical spine (f) stimulation in relation to age. The response threshold for stimulation of the motor roots shows little change after birth, while the threshold for cortically evoked responses is very high for the first two years of life and then shows a rapid followed by a more gradual decline with age. (From Eyre *et al.* (1991). Reproduced with permission.)

food particles from a modified Klüver board. In particular, they could no longer use the index finger, extended at the interphalangeal joints but flexed at the metacarpophalangeal, to winkle the food reward free, and then grip it in pad-to-pad opposition of the food between index finger and thumb. A graphic example of such a deficit is shown in Fig. 3.9 from the work of Brinkman (1974). Both Tower (1940) and Lawrence and Kuypers (1968a) found that pyramidotomized monkeys also had severe problems with releasing the grip on their food, and Schwartzman (1978) noticed that grooming was rarely seen after complete pyramidotomy. It is interesting to speculate whether studies of this scale, in the light of financial and conservationist pressures, will ever be repeated; fortunately some of the results are still available on film and serious efforts should be made to preserve these valuable records and to ensure that they remain available for re-study.

2. There is a permanent loss of contactual hand-orientating responses (Denny-Brown 1966, p. 145). This author commented that the PT is concerned '. . . with those spatial adjustments that accurately adapt the movement to the spatial attributes of the stimulus' (p. 159). The loss of tactile placing should not necessarily be seen as separate from the deficits referred to above. During tactile exploration, for instance, sensory input and relatively independent finger movements are inextricably linked, and it is this sensory-motor linkage which is so much a feature of motor cortex organization (see Chapters 6 and 8). The linkage appears to be disrupted after pyramidal damage (Laursen 1971; Schwartzman 1978). In the monkey, lesions of the dorsal columns at high spinal levels can impair digital control (Vierck 1975, 1978; Brinkman *et al.* 1978; Asanuma and Arissian 1984) and produce deficits not unlike those following pyramidotomy (Davidoff 1989).

3. No *long-term* effects on axial/postural system have been reported (see Hepp-Reymond 1988). Lawrence and Kuypers found that, after the immediate postoperative period, pyramidotomized monkeys could sit, stand, walk, run, and climb normally. Although there was some paresis of the arm and leg immediately after the lesion, this recovered rapidly, so that within a few weeks of the lesion, arm movements, and particularly reaching movements, were fast and reasonably accurate. Lawrence and Kuypers (1968b) went on to show that recovery of these movements after pyramidotomy did not occur if pathways descending from the midbrain and brainstem were interrupted.

4. The severity of the deficit after the lesion varies according to *species*. The paresis of the arm and loss of relatively independent finger movements is much greater in the chimpanzee than in the macaque monkey (Tower 1940). There is also evidence for a greater impairment of more proximal

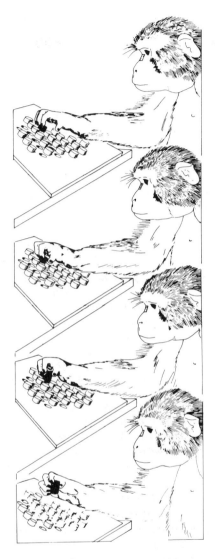

FIG 3.9 Drawings from a film showing a split-brain monkey with a bilateral pyramidotomy taking food from the test board with the right hand under guidance of the contralateral eye. The contralateral hand is brought accurately to the target and dislodges the pellet (black) by means of flexion–extension movements of wrist and fingers. Relatively independent finger movements are not used. (From Brinkman (1974). Reproduced with permission.)

muscles in apes than in monkeys (Leyton and Sherrington 1917; Kuypers, personal communication).

5. As Hepp-Reymond (1988) has pointed out, the degree of recovery from pyramidal tract lesions is related to several factors, including the size of the lesion, the duration and nature of the postoperative period, and the age of the animal at the time of lesion. In the light of recent work on the plasticity of the motor system after damage, it is clear that the behavioural changes after pyramidotomy do not simply result from cutting an important connection between cortex and the spinal motor apparatus: even in the adult animal such a lesion can trigger a large number of morphological and functional changes, many of which occur very rapidly and some of which may contribute to the *recovery* process (Bregman and Goldberger 1982).

An example of the importance of corticospinal plasticity is that, in the monkey, bilateral pyramidotomy produces more dramatic deficits than does a unilateral lesion. Phillips and Porter (1977) wrote that 'Bilateral PT section is certainly more instructive than unilateral, first because it completely denudes each side of the cord of pyramidal synapses; secondly, because the animals cannot rely on a normal hand and are more strongly motivated to overcome their disability' (p. 361). Today we might attach a greater significance to the mechanisms contributing to neural plasticity that may be provided for by the surviving undamaged fibres in the case of unilateral section. The added deficit seen after bilateral lesions is difficult to explain on the grounds of normal connectivity since it is known that the majority of the ipsilaterally descending fibres appear to affect postural and axial muscles, rather than muscles of the hand (Kuypers and Brinkman 1970).

There is also good behavioural evidence, derived from split-brain experiments, that skilled finger movements are particularly dependent upon strictly contralateral projections (Brinkman and Kuypers 1973). However, some PTNs do show activity that is clearly related to ipsilateral hand movements (see Section 5.9), and presumably some of these neurones can continue to contribute to finger movements after unilateral pyramidal tract section. Some investigators report that the cell somata of transected corticospinal neurones survive for as long as 20 weeks post-lesion (McBride *et al.* 1989), although collaterals to other subcortical targets may be involved in sustaining these cell bodies. Finally, there are several observations suggesting that corticospinal tract fibres exhibit collateral sprouting in the months following a unilateral lesion, and that these fibres can recross the spinal cord and influence motoneurones on the contralateral side (Aoki *et al.* 1986; Satomi *et al.* 1988; see Section 3.4 above), although clear changes in the pattern of corticospinal termination after such a lesion were not found by Kucera and Wiesendanger (1985). It is interesting that monkeys with unilateral pyramidotomy display mirror movements of the two hands (Schwartzman 1978), a phenomenon which, in at least some neurological patients, has been shown to be due to branching of cor- ticospinal axons to supply homologous muscles on the two sides (Farmer *et al.* 1990b). This mechanism suggests a very high degree of specificity in the establishment of cortico-motoneuronal connections by a single cor- ticospinal neurone.

Recovery from the lesion is related to the degree of sparing of pyramidal tract fibres (Lawrence and Kuypers 1968a; Hepp-Reymond *et al.* 1974; Schwartzman 1978). Almost complete destruction of all pyramidal fibres was necessary to produce complete abolition of relatively independent finger movements. There was always recovery of these movements with subtotal lesions, although some degree of clumsiness remained. This was confirmed by the study of recovery from unilateral pyramidotomy (Chapman and Wiesendanger 1982). One monkey, in which only 13 per cent of the pyramidal tract fibres were still intact, was able to perform a preci- sion grip, albeit in a somewhat degenerate form. Mitz and Humphrey (1986) reported substantial differences between the motor representation in the precentral gyrus of two monkeys with chronic unilateral section of the pyramid. In one monkey, where section was complete, ICMS was largely ineffective in evoking movement, but in the second animal, with around 15 per cent sparing, ICMS was much more effective.

Lawrence and Kuypers (1968a) maintained that complete bilateral lesions produced a permanent loss of RIFM. But apart from the length of the postoperative period, an important factor is the amount of training or retraining that is given. A number of investigations have attempted to quan- tify the deficit produced by pyramidotomy and most of these have involved retraining monkeys on a task, rather than the simple retrieval of food studied by earlier experimenters. The most detailed experiments are those of Hepp-Reymond and Wiesendanger (1972), Hepp-Reymond *et al.* (1974), and Schwartzman (1978). These authors clearly demonstrated that monkeys can be retrained to perform a precision grip. A paradigm was used in which monkeys were rewarded for producing, in response to a light signal, a minimum force level of 0.5 N exerted upon a small transducer gripped bet- ween the thumb and index finger. After several months of training, reaction time (which had initially increased markedly after the pyramidal tract lesion) came back to within preoperative levels. But there was a permanent increase in the duration of the EMG burst, bringing the performance to the force threshold: movement time rather than reaction time was affected (see Fig. 3.10). The observation that pyramidotomized monkeys can be specifically retrained to produce a precision grip is of considerable signifi- cance for the 'neurorehabilitation' of patients with motor system damage (Bach-y-Rita 1981).

Lawrence and Hopkins (1976) originally criticized the use of the precision grip task as an example of relatively independent finger movements because

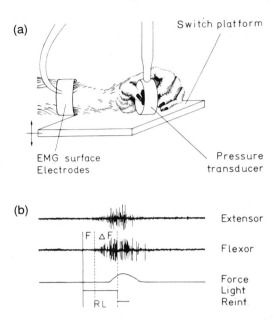

FIG 3.10   Production of force in precision grip by the macaque monkey: (a) Experimental set-up; (b) typical recording with the EMG of finger flexors and extensors, the grip force, the start signal (light), and the reward reinforcing the response (reinf.). After bilateral pyramidotomy monkeys could be retrained to perform this task, although they continued to show a slower rate of change of force and this was associated with a longer EMG summation time (time interval ΔF from EMG onset to force threshold). (From Hepp-Reymond *et al.* (1974). Reproduced with permission.)

'Gripping an object between the thumb and index finger or thumb and other fingers . . . does not take sufficiently into account the activity in the other fingers', i.e. there is no essential requirement for *independent* use of the ulnar digits and the index finger (see Fig. 3.2). This is particularly the case for the side-to-pad grip. It is important to stress that while Lawrence and Kuypers were looking at independent finger *movement*, the more quantitative studies have tended to examine grip posture and grip force. This relates to the important issue of whether it is the fractionated finger movement or the control of grip force that is quintessentially a cortico-motoneuronal feature. In this respect it is perhaps interesting that, in the experimental test situation, it was the dynamic part of the task (the duration of the EMG burst prior to the development of grip force) that was most seriously affected, rather than the ability to maintain a steady grip (Hepp-Reymond *et al.* 1974). Woolsey *et al.* (1972) remarked that monkeys could succeed in picking up small cubes of fruit or candy 'by flexing all fingers together'. Schwartzman (1978) also noted that, although monkeys could depress selectively a series of levers for different fingers and could make a pincer grasp, they had an 'inability to move the fourth and fifth fingers discretely, although most of the time the hand performed normally'.

3.5.2 Man

According to Phillips and Porter (1977, p. 365), 'Pathological processes which are confined to the medullary pyramids are extremely rare'. These authors have given an account of the cases reported in the neurological literature, and further references may be found in reviews by Wiesendanger (1969, 1981a). The fundamental conclusions from the study of such patients is that damage to the pyramidal tract does not cause any marked spasticity, and that it does produce some deficit of individual finger movements. However, one of the best documented cases is that of Bucy *et al.* (1964), in which the pyramidal fibres were sectioned unilaterally at the level of the cerebral peduncle in the case of a patient suffering from hemiballismus, involving the face, arm, and leg on the left side. The central portion of the peduncle, in which the corticospinal fibres are known to travel (Barnard and Woolsey 1956) was divided. The operation resulted in an immediate cessation of the involuntary movements. A flaccid hemiplegia after surgery was rapidly replaced by a 'continuous improvement in strength and coordination' which reached a plateau after seven months. At that time, the patient was able to produce 'fine, individual movements of the fingers fairly well' which 'were only slightly less well executed than on the right side'. There was only mild spasticity present and the Babinski sign was weak. Post-mortem examination of the tissue by DeMyer revealed that only 17 per cent of the fibres in the right medullary pyramid survived the section, and many of these were probably of parietal origin. Bucy *et al.* (1964) pointed out the very substantial differences in the performance of this patient and those with cortical or capsular lesions. They attributed the recovery of their patient partly to the remaining fibres, and partly to ipsilateral connections, but chiefly to the existence of other, indirect or 'extrapyramidal' descending pathways from the cortex. Although, in this case, surgery was carried out only $2\frac{1}{2}$ months after the abnormal movements began, it must be remembered that surgical removal of damaged or functionally disturbed tissue cannot be compared with lesions of intact, healthy tissue in experimental animals. Thus the effects on voluntary movement of hemispherectomy in patients with severe epilepsy are far less striking than, for instance, the sudden inactivation of the hemisphere of normal subjects or the same patients by carotid sodium amytal injections (Wada and Rasmussen 1960; Benecke *et al.* 1991). There is growing evidence for reorganization of ipsilateral pathways from the undamaged hemisphere after stroke (Chollet *et al.* 1991; Fisher 1992).

Pure and complete motor hemiplegia has been reported to occur after vascular lesions producing a unilateral infarct restricted to the pyramidal tract (Ropper *et al.* 1979). This patient still had a weakness of the left arm, slowness of hand movement and a Babinski sign on the side contralateral to the lesioned pyramid. However, recovery was eventually complete, judging by the fact that this patient learnt to play the cello seven years after the lesion! Substantial recovery was also reported in a patient with a lesion affecting the corticospinal fibres as they passed through the basis pontis, although 'precise movements requiring skilled interaction of the digits' were not regained (Aguilar 1969).

Skilled hand movements are suddenly lost as the result of focal ischaemic attacks, including lacunar stroke affecting the internal capsule (Fries *et al.* 1990). In such cases it has been possible to delineate the damage caused to the pyramidal tract by magnetic resonance imaging (MRI) (Danek *et al.* 1990). Such patients often show very rapid recovery; Fries *et al.* (1990) described a patient with complete hemiplegia after a lacunar stroke. After three months, independent finger movements were again possible and after two years there was 'an almost complete restitution of function'. Transcranial electrical stimulation of the damaged hemisphere, two months after the stroke, still evoked responses in the contralateral thenar muscles. These authors have argued that the MRI evidence indicated that restitution of motor function and recovery of motor responses must have involved pathways other than the pyramidal tract. Whether or not this is true depends to a large extent on the interpretation of the MRI scans and whether or not they can indicate reliably the presence of permanently interrupted versus inflamed or oedematous tissue. Another complicating feature may be that, in man, the uncrossed anterior corticospinal tract is often very well developed; it would appear that the principal targets of these fibres are the motoneurones supplying the more proximal limb and girdle muscles (cf. Kuypers 1981). The functional effectiveness of this ipsilateral tract is supported by the observation that patients with stroke often exhibit weakness in these muscles on the side *ipsilateral* to the lesion (Colebatch and Gandevia 1989).

There are thus three factors which should urge caution in our interpretation of the human evidence: the complicated nature of the lesion in most cases, the possibility that substantial changes in motor function may already have occurred before surgical intervention in some cases, and finally that recovery from the initial deficits observed may better reflect the process of compensation within the motor system than the permanent removal of the essential function of the damaged tract (Benecke *et al.* 1991).

3.5.3 Subprimates

Pyramidal tract section in the cat was originally shown by Liddell and Phillips (1944) to produce substantial deterioration in beam-walking in cats. They also noted a characteristic loss of the tactile-placing reaction (cf. Nieoullon and Gahéry 1978), similar to that seen after lesions of the motor cortex (Bard 1938). Cats taught to press on a lever could still do so after a contralateral PT lesion, although the response was slower (Laursen and Wiesendanger 1967). However, the most revealing evidence of the effects of pyramidotomy has come from studies in which specific reaching and food retrieval activities have been examined. Gorska and Sybirska (1980) introduced tasks involving retrieval of small pieces of fish from either a vertical or a horizontal tube. Cats with 'high' pyramidal lesions, at the level of the trapezoid body, were severely impaired in performance of these food-taking movements. Performance returned to normal only in some animals and then only 12–20 months after surgery.

The detailed examination of the reaching and food-taking movement has been the subject of a classic series of investigations by Lundberg, Alstermark and their collaborators, which demonstrated that the reaching and retrieval components were under the control of different neuronal mechanisms. The target-reaching component, which is extremely fast and lasts for around 200 ms (Pettersson 1990), has been shown to be principally under the control of a propriospinal system originating in the C3 and C4 segments. These C3–C4 propriospinal neurones receive a widely convergent input from several descending motor pathways, including reticulo-, tecto-, bulbo-, and corticospinal fibres and they relay these influences to the moto-neurones of forelimb muscles active in target reaching (Illert *et al.* 1977, 1978; see Chapter 4, section 4.5). In contrast, the principal descending systems required for precise organization and execution of the food-taking movement are the corticospinal and rubrospinal inputs which converge upon interneurones within the lower cervical segments and which transmit their signals to the motoneurones of the distal forelimb and digit muscles.

The organization of fibres in the upper cervical cord of the cat allowed Lundberg and his collaborators to make lesions which selectively interrupted the axons of the propriospinal neurones without involving corticospinal or rubrospinal fibres (ventral C5 lesion, see Fig. 3.11) or vice versa (dorsal C5 lesion) (Alstermark *et al.* 1981). Lesions were checked both electrophysiologically and by histological examination. The ventral C5 lesion did not affect food-taking but did cause striking deficits in the accuracy and speed of target-reaching. Initially, cats with this lesion had difficulty with reaching accurately for the horizontal tube containing the fish. 'However, even if the cats could lift and insert the paw into the tube there was . . . a striking ataxic defect in the movement' and 'The paw was

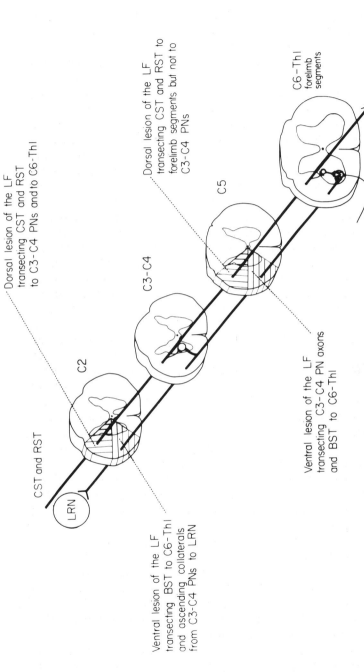

FiG 3.11   Pathways contributing to target reaching and food-taking movements in the cat. Schematic drawing of the cervical spinal cord showing the different lesions and the trajectories of the relevant fibre tracts. CST, corticospinal tract; RST, rubrospinal tract; BST, bulbospinal tracts; PN, propriospinal neurone; LRN, lateral reticular nucleus. A dorsal lesion in the lateral funiculus (LF) interrupted both RST and CST; at the C2 level this lesion abolished inputs from these tracts to both the C3–C4 propriospinal system and to the segmental apparatus at C6–Th1. When the lesion was made at C5, only the latter inputs were interrupted, and the food taking movement was severely affected. Ventral lesions of the LF at C5 cut, among others, propriospinal pathways to the lower cervical segments. The predominant deficit after these lesions was in the target reaching movement. (From Alstermark *et al.* (1981). Reproduced with permission.)

usually placed outside the tube or at the edge of the tube'. This problem persisted for several months after surgery, although long-term recovery was observed after all types of spinal lesion.

The dorsal C5 lesion, cutting cortico- and rubrospinal fibres, produced an immediate deficit in the food-taking movement: the toes were not properly flexed around the food and the wrist supination required to bring the food to the mouth was impaired. Target-reaching was normal in these cats. Food-taking was completely abolished for 2–3 weeks, after which there was a gradual recovery over a period of months. Recovery was complete when the lesion was incomplete. A lesion at C2 which interrupted the corticospinal and rubrospinal input to both the C3–C4 propriospinal system and the lower cervical segments caused severe impairment of both target-reaching and food-taking, with recovery over 3 to 13 weeks.

Subsequent studies have shown that selective lesions of the corticospinal fibres at C4–C5 produced only a transient effect on the food-taking movement (Alstermark *et al.* 1987). These authors assumed that the rubrospinal fibres spared by these lesions could 'take over' the food-taking function completely. Nevertheless, this transient deficit was in striking contrast to the much greater effects caused by interruption of the same fibres at the 'high' pyramidal level (Gorska and Sybirska 1980). The considerable collateralization of the pyramidal system as it descends through the brainstem (Kuypers 1958b; see Section 2.6) might well suggest that section of the pyramids at different levels would produce different effects because of sparing of collaterals at different levels. Alstermark *et al.* (1990a) showed that 'low' pyramidal section, just rostral to the decussation, was also more severe than section of corticospinal fibres at the C5 level; they attributed this specifically to the interruption of fibres to the lateral reticular nucleus, and, perhaps more significantly, to the dorsal column nuclei. These corticonuclear projections are directed principally to the deeper parts of the cuneate and gracile nuclei (see Section 2.5) and presumably damage to this system disrupts descending control of afferent input from the moving limb. In this respect it is interesting that section of the dorsal columns at C2 has been shown to interfere with both the target-reaching and food-taking movement (Alstermark *et al.* 1986).

In their review of 1975, Heffner and Masterton attributed a higher index of digital dexterity to rodents (index: 3) than to cats and dogs (index: 2). Several studies have shown that the manipulative capacity of rodents is affected by pyramidotomy. Barron (1934) first reported permanent effects on digital usage in the rat after unilateral pyramidal tract section. The effect of bilateral section was systematically investigated by Castro (1972) using a device which specifically tested the ability of rats to retrieve small food pellets with their digits. The lesioned animals showed long-lasting deficits in both the number of attempts and the percentage of successful attempts to retrieve food. Reaching was accurate and essentially normal, but rats were unable to flex their digits properly round the food pellets. Locomotion across a wire mesh was disturbed, possibly due to the inability to grip the mesh appropriately. Once again, the degree of deficit was related to the proportion of the tract damaged, although unfortunately 100 per cent lesions were always accompanied by damage to adjoining structures such as the medial lemniscus and inferior olive. Kalil and Schneider (1975) reported a permanent loss of precise manipulation in the pyramidotomized hamster. Other effects on locomotion disappeared within a few weeks after the lesion (cf. Kennedy and Humphrey 1987). Even in a marsupial, the brush-tailed possum, with a primitive pattern of corticospinal organization (Group 1, see Section 2.9) bilateral section of the pyramidal tracts, without significant damage to other structures, disturbed the precise control of the movements of the forelimb when used for reaching and grasping (Hore *et al.* 1973).

3.6 SUMMARY

In general the most striking deficits seen after pyramidal tract section are those seen in the extremities. The effects are always much more severe after bilateral lesions and recovery is better after incomplete or after unilateral lesions. But it is difficult to believe that the entire pyramidal tract only subserves the organization of relatively independent finger movements. Paillard (1978) has pointed out that animals which are lowly ranked on a scale of digital dexterity may be highly ranked on postural tests (for instance, the performing seal), and that the concentration on the links between pyramidal tract structure and hand function may have obscured its role in the control of postural and stabilizing mechanisms that are essential for the successful execution of hand movements. This argument is set out elsewhere (Chapter 8). We should also not forget the multiplicity of cortical origins of the tract, and its different regions of termination within the spinal grey matter.

Should the opportunity arise to re-investigate these problems, it will be important to look at both the planning and the performance of complex tasks. Planning has not been tested at all, despite the fact that we know that a significant proportion of the tract is derived from areas concerned in the planning and preparation for voluntary movement. It could be important also to investigate the pyramidal tract contribution to the precise integration of motor and sensory systems seen during tactile exploration, or during the adaptation of grip force to the prevailing frictional conditions (Johansson and Westling 1984). Could these tasks be affected by the level at which the pyramidal tract section is made? Detailed quantitative kinematic studies will be required to determine whether or not reaching and manipulatory performances have been disturbed in subtle ways not easily discernible to the naked eye. It would be interesting to observe whether motor responses are more stereotyped after pyramidotomy (Tower 1940), suggesting a loss of variability in the motor strategies used to solve a given problem (Lemon 1990). The plasticity of the corticospinal system, particularly in the young animal, is such a potent source of new connectivity and function that permanent lesions are likely to be less revealing than reversible ones.

Pyramidotomy undoubtedly produces more severe disturbances in monkeys than in subprimates, particularly as far as control of the digits is concerned. This probably reflects the increased importance of the direct cortico-motoneuronal connections for individual digit control, and this is supported by the parallel development of these connections and digital skill in the young animal, although a more precise chronology of this development is needed before a causal link can be established firmly. The observation that digital control is impaired by pyramidotomy in animals such as the cat, rat and hamster in which cortico-motoneuronal connections are few or absent, suggests that the effects seen in primates do not involve the cortico-motoneuronal projections alone.

4

Corticospinal influences on the spinal cord machinery for movement

This chapter will address one of the fundamental concerns of this book, namely the impact of the corticospinal system upon the activity of target motoneurones within the spinal cord. This will include a description of the basic organization of the motoneurone pools, and of the reflex synaptic mechanisms with which descending corticospinal impulses interact during voluntary movement. It will also describe how these various inputs are transmitted at individual synapses on the motoneuronal membrane. We will describe the detailed intraspinal morphology of the cortico-motoneuronal system, as revealed by intra-axonal staining techniques, and will then examine the use of spike-triggered averaging and other technical innovations that provide new information about the functional organization of cortico-motoneuronal inputs to motoneurones in conscious animals. We shall also consider the importance of corticospinal inhibition, and the possible functions of the cortico-fusimotor projection. We shall begin with a description of the motoneurone pools.

4.1 MOTONEURONES

The populations of motoneurones which innervate particular muscles have their somata aggregated within longitudinal columns, each distributed through several segments of the spinal cord. In general, the columns of motoneurone somata which contribute axons to distally acting musculature are aggregated in the most lateral regions of the anterior horn, in both the cervical and lumbar enlargements, with flexor motoneurones usually more dorsally situated than extensor motoneurones. Descriptions of the arrangements of these 'motor nuclei' were obtained in earlier work by plotting the cells in which chromatolytic changes followed the section of particular motor nerves (Sherrington 1898; Romanes 1951; Sterling and Kuypers 1967). The more recent introduction of methods employing the retrograde transport of substances which can be identified histochemically, after they have been accumulated in the somata of neurones whose axons or terminals have been exposed to them, has greatly facilitated the descriptions of motor columns. The extent of a motoneurone column is indicated for the cervical cord of the monkey in the findings of Jenny and Inukai (1983) (see Fig. 4.1). The central zone of the anterior horn is occupied by the columns of somata of motoneurones innervating more proximally acting musculature, while the most medial motoneurones innervate axial muscles.

Even though the somata of the motoneurones supplying a given muscle are so organized into cigar-shaped columns, having a transverse diameter of only a few hundred microns, dendritic processes extend from each of the somata for a millimeter or more to occupy much more extensive zones, which can extend through the whole of the anterior grey matter. Figure 4.2 plots the spread of motoneurone dendrites of a single motoneurone ramifying through the anterior horn of a representative cervical segment of the spinal cord of a monkey. Such a cell could be impaled with an HRP-filled microelectrode, HRP injected into the cell by iontophoresis, and the structure of the motoneurone later revealed by reconstruction from

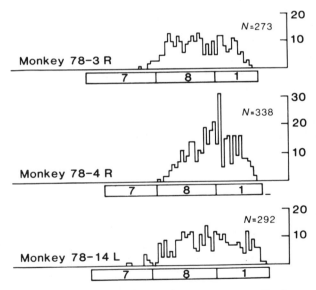

FIG 4.1 This figure documents, for three monkeys, the distribution, mostly within segments C8 and T1, of the somata of motoneurones innervating the extensor digitorum communis muscle. The numbers of somata, labelled by the retrograde transport of HRP from the muscle nerve in the forearm, are plotted per 250 μm rostrocaudally through this region of the spinal cord. For each monkey, *N* indicates the total number of labelled motoneurones revealed following injection of HRP into the muscle nerve. (From Jenny and Inukai (1983). Copyright © 1983. Reprinted by permission of Wiley-Liss, a division of John Wiley and Sons Inc.)

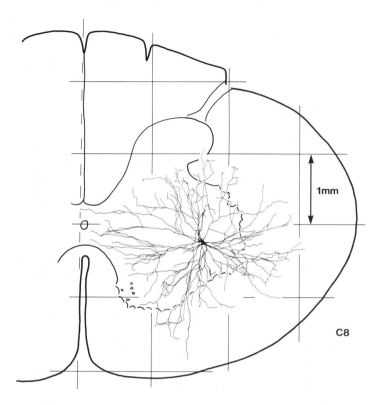

1mm

C8

FIG 4.2   A schematic diagram of a representative section through the C8 level of the spinal cord of a macaque monkey. On this diagram has been superimposed a two dimensional drawing of a camera lucida reconstruction of an HRP-filled motoneurone. Although the soma of the motoneurone is located within a thin longitudinal column which, in cross section, appears as the nucleus of the motor nerve innervating a given muscle, the extensive dendritic tree of this motoneurone, and of its neighbours, spreads through a much larger spinal territory and beyond the anterior horn. Some dendrites extend into the white matter. Synaptic boutons, even in regions remote from the motor nucleus, could conceivably contact these extended dendritic branches.

superimposition of a large number of transverse sections through the spinal cord, stained using the diamino-benzidine reaction to reveal the presence of HRP (see Brown and Fyffe 1978; Brown 1981; Lawrence *et al.* 1985). It will be clear that the dendritic surface of a motoneurone on which synaptic impacts may be brought to bear has an enormous distribution. There are major practical consequences of this extensive spread of the dendritic surface and it will be evident immediately that the anatomical locations of identified synaptic boutons from a particular source will have to be related to the widespread enmeshed dendritic surfaces within their vicinity, not just to the obvious somata that are located in an equivalent region and that may be revealed by conventional histological methods for staining cell bodies, e.g. Nissl.

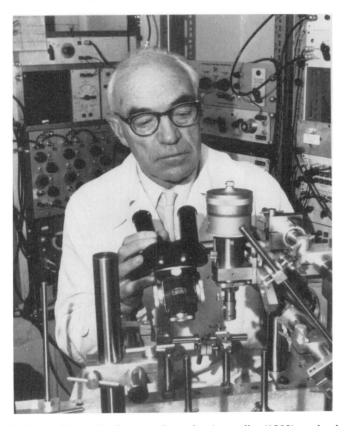

FIG 4.3   Sir John Carew Eccles was born in Australia (1903) and educated at Melbourne University and at Magdalen College, Oxford. He was Rhodes Scholar for Victoria (1925) and worked with Sherrington to obtain his D. Phil. He moved, in 1937, from a Fellowship at Magdalen College to be Director of the Kanematsu Institute of Pathology in Sydney. He was then appointed Professor of Physiology at the University of Otago in New Zealand (1944), before moving to The John Curtin School of Medical Research in the Australian National University as that institute's foundation Professor of Physiology (1951). He received the Nobel Prize for Physiology and Medicine in 1963 for his work, mostly conducted within The John Curtin School of Medical Research, which revealed the mechanisms of excitation and inhibition, and the details of the reflex control, of motoneurones in the spinal cord of the cat. This photograph was taken in his laboratory in The John Curtin School of Medical Research.

4.2 INTRACELLULAR RECORDINGS OF SYNAPTIC EVENTS

The introduction of electrolyte-filled capillary microelectrodes into mammalian spinal cord neurophysiology by Brock *et al.* (1952), Woodbury and Patton (1952), Frank and Fuortes (1955), and Eccles (1957) (see Fig. 4.3), among others, provided the opportunity to make intracellular recordings in individual spinal motoneurones, to identify the muscle innervated by this motoneurone (by registration of an antidromic action potential in it following electrical stimulation of a particular muscle nerve) and to make observations on the subthreshold events generated by activity in nervous elements which were presynaptic to the motoneurone under study. By this means the synaptic influences exerted on motoneurones and evoked by activation of a variety of afferent pathways, and the detailed organization of these effects, could be studied. The sign or direction (excitatory or

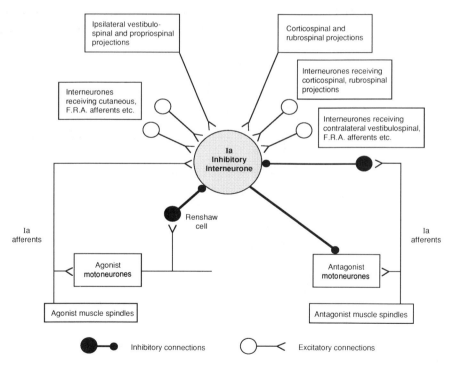

FIG 4.4   A diagrammatic representation summarizing some of the excitatory and inhibitory connections converging upon the Ia inhibitory interneurone which serves to direct reciprocal inhibitory influences to the motoneurones of antagonist muscles when the muscle spindles of agonist muscles are stretched in eliciting a tendon jerk reflex (from Lundberg 1979).

inhibitory) of the synaptic actions revealed in these records could be regarded as the basic machinery for the reflex responses that had been described earlier (Liddell and Sherrington 1925; Lloyd 1941, 1946). Most of our knowledge concerning the detail and the pattern of the interconnections between neurones in the mammalian spinal cord has been obtained by recording from cells in the lumbosacral spinal cord of the cat (Eccles and Lundberg 1958; Burke 1968). From this work the general principles of connectivity, of recurrent inhibition, and of reciprocal innervation have been confirmed. The rules governing connectivity of particular afferent fibres with a synergic motoneurone population have also been established. These have been summarized in Chapter 1.

In addition, a wealth of specialized and detailed information has been accumulated which documents the particular connections that are made by identified afferents whose receptor organs may be selectively activated (Jack 1978). The degree of convergence which may be demonstrated on particular interneurones interposed within defined reflex circuits has also been determined (see Jankowska 1992 for a review). The common Ia interneurone and the autogenic Ib inhibitory interneurone have been examined

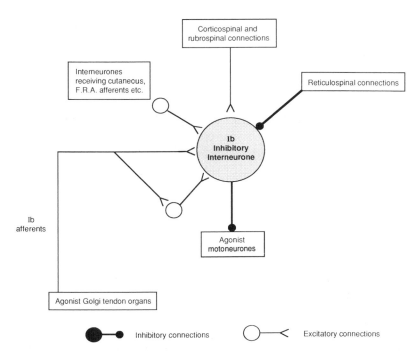

FIG 4.5 A diagrammatic summary of the convergence of influences upon the Ib inhibitory interneurone which is engaged by afferents from Golgi tendon organs and causes reflex inhibition of agonist motoneurones (from Lundberg, 1979).

using these approaches. Figure 4.4 summarizes Lundberg's account of the circuit diagram derived from the studies of Lindstrom (1973) and involving some of the identified connections made with the common Ia inhibitory interneurone in the cat. Figure 4.5 illustrates convergence on the Ib inhibitory pathway to motoneurones. Evidence, derived from facilitation of the disynaptic inhibitory response recorded in a motoneurone when stimuli were delivered to two of these convergent pathways, allowed the general proposition to be made that the particular variety of peripheral and descending connections illustrated in this figure exerted their influence via the same interneurones (Lundberg *et al.* 1977a, b; 1978).

4.3 PATTERN OF GROUP Ia INNERVATION OF HINDLIMB MOTONEURONES

A major conclusion derived from the studies of cat hindlimb innervation was, of course, that the afferents from the primary endings in the muscle spindle (group Ia afferents with rapidly conducting axons) made mono-synaptic connections with alpha motoneurones of the receptor-bearing or homonymous muscle (Fig. 1.12). Together these comprised a myotatic unit. In addition, the motoneurones of mechanical or functional synergists (heteronymous motoneurones) received monosynaptic excitatory synaptic connection from branches of the same afferent fibres (Eccles *et al.* 1957; Eccles and Lundberg 1958; Mendell and Henneman 1971). Hongo *et al.* (1984) provided a description of the pattern of Ia innervation of the lumbar spinal cord of the monkey. In addition to the linkage of Ia afferents with synergic motoneurones of muscles acting about a single joint, the same afferent fibres may contribute excitatory connections to groups of moto-neurones innervating muscles acting about other joints. This, together with the pattern of reciprocal inhibition of functionally antagonistic moto-neurones, was regarded earlier by Lloyd (1946) as part of the 'integrative' system for movement control by the spinal cord.

4.4 Ia INNERVATION OF FORELIMB MOTONEURONES

Since our interest in this volume is voluntary movement, and since in most studies this has been investigated in the forelimb, the organization of the cervical spinal cord is of more direct interest to us than that of the lumbar. There is much less information concerning the pattern of organization of peripheral afferent inputs to the cervical spinal cord, but the information already gathered does suggest that the generalizations made above for the hindlimb may be of only limited applicability to the forelimb (Willis *et al.* 1966; Clough *et al.* 1968).

Fritz *et al.* (1989) have provided a detailed examination of the pattern of Ia connections between primary spindle afferents from groups of fore-limb muscles in the cat and the motoneurones supplying these and related muscles. The pattern of connectivity was found to be much more com-plicated than for the hindlimb, and the motoneurones of a given muscle were shown to be in receipt of monosynaptic projections from the group Ia fibres of many associated muscles. The connections indicated that the same motoneurones could be conceived, under different conditions, to be serving as components of a number of quite separate synergic groups of muscles, interconnected by common Ia innervation, but with different func-tional relationships to a forelimb movement, especially at the wrist. It was pointed out 'that the synergistic–antagonistic relations between the forelimb muscles are not constant but change according to the intended movements . . . patterns of heteronymous Ia connections have developed which support the organization of these changing synergies. This suggests that the central organization of the many different synergies which are necessary for the large repertoire of movements indeed are matched by corresponding patterns of Ia connections'. (Fritz *et al.* 1989). In the monkey, widespread connections of afferents amongst motoneurone pools of wrist extensor and flexor motoneurones were shown by Flament *et al.* (1992a), and a similar complexity of Ia convergence on to forelimb motoneurones also exists in man (ter Haar Romeny *et al.* 1984; Pierrot-Deseilligny 1989).

Interestingly, some of the most distally acting muscles controlling move-ments at the wrist and digits have rather poorly developed Ia connections, and no obvious patterns are detectable (Marsden *et al.* 1972; Matthews 1984; Fritz *et al.* 1989). In the cat, this arrangement is also apparent in the organization of the recurrent (Renshaw) feedback, in that motoneurones of distal muscles lack recurrent collaterals of their axons (Cullheim and Kellerth 1978). Electrophysiological data suggest that they neither generate, nor receive, recurrent inhibition. Since one of the proposed functions of such inhibition within reciprocally organized groups of muscles is to control the activity of the Ia inhibitory interneurones, which in turn influence the antagonistic patterns of activity in such muscles, the lack of such an organization amongst the motoneurone pools of distally acting muscles suggests the possibility of highly flexible relationships between them (Hörner *et al.* 1990).

4.5 PROPRIOSPINAL NEURONES

In the cat, supraspinal influences from the cerebral cortex do not impinge directly on motoneurones. Rather, as Lloyd illustrated in 1941, impulses set up by electrical stimulation of the pyramidal tract are indirectly transmitted to motoneurones via interneurones (see detailed account of those observations in Phillips and Porter 1977, pp. 124–135). Gelfan (1964) has estimated that, on average, connections between Ia afferents and lumbar motoneurones in the dog make up only 0.5–1 per cent of the motoneurone's total synaptic input. It was suggested that the synaptic influences of bulbospinal and other supraspinal pathways which make more direct connections with motoneurones will be served also by a comparably small proportion of the total connections (i.e., a few per cent). Therefore the dominating synaptic input to motoneurones must be derived from spinal interneurones. Labelling of last order interneurones projecting to a specific group of motoneurones may be provided by retrograde transneuronal transport of WGA-HRP after an injection into a muscle nerve (Harrison *et al.* 1984). Transneuronally labelled last-order interneurones were found to extend from rostral C1 to caudal T5 and then, after a gap, a few more were seen between L3 and the border of L4/5 following an injection into the nerves to deltoid. In these experiments, either dorsal roots or the spinal cord were sectioned to prevent anterograde transport of the WGA-HRP. The findings of Alstermark and Kümmel (1990a) suggest that a single motor nucleus made up of about 300 motoneurones receives projections from at least 4500 to 6000 last-order interneurones. Some of these will be excitatory and some inhibitory; there is some debate as to whether these interneurones are preferentially labelled by WGA/HRP transneuronal labelling (Alstermark and Kümmel 1990b). Moreover, the power of the synaptic effects produced by different groups of afferents to the motoneurone must be studied. There may be very great differences in the synaptic efficacy of different pathways (Jankowska and Roberts 1972; Brink *et al.* 1983a).

As with other aspects of spinal neuroanatomy, most of what we know about last-order interneurones has been derived from studies of the lumbar spinal cord. Last-order interneurones are found in large numbers ipsilaterally in laminae V to IX, while contralaterally, they appear to be restricted to lamina VIII. As has been indicated above, both excitatory and inhibitory interneurones would be expected to be identified by this transneuronal retrograde transport, and these may be separately classified into a number of different interneuronal populations:

(1) ipsilaterally, the interneurones in lamina V and VI mediate non-reciprocal inhibition from group I afferents (Brink *et al.* 1983b);

(2) in lamina VI–VII of the midlumbar segments, they contribute excitation and inhibition from group II muscle afferents (Cavallari *et al.* 1987);

(3) in lamina VII, they produce reciprocal inhibition from group Ia afferents (Jankowska and Roberts 1972; Hultborn and Udo 1972);

(4) in lamina VIII, they mediate effects from vestibulo- and reticulo-spinal fibres (Kozhanov and Shapovalov 1977), but not from corticospinal axons. Some have projections which cross the midline;

(5) in the ventromedial part of lamina VII are located the cells involved in recurrent inhibition (Eccles *et al.* 1954; van Keulen 1979; Brink *et al.* 1983b; Fyffe 1991).

Groups (1)–(3) all receive monosynaptic excitation from the pyramidal tract, and hence provide a pathway for disynaptic inhibition (1), (2), and (3) or disynaptic excitation (2) of motoneurones.

Illert *et al.* (1976a, b; 1977, 1978) recorded from cells in the upper segments of the cervical spinal cord (C3–C4) of the cat which served to relay corticospinal, and also rubro-, reticulo-, and tecto-spinal, influences to forelimb motoneurones. These propriospinal neurones make monosynaptic contacts with motoneurones and Ia inhibitory interneurones in the

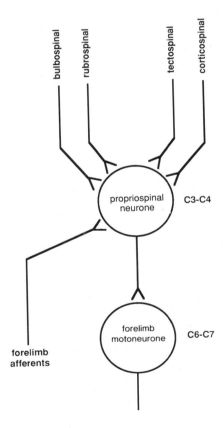

FIG 4.6   A diagram to indicate the role of propriospinal neurones at the C3–C4 level of the spinal cord in relaying convergent influences from descending pathways (cortico-, tecto-, rubro-, and bulbo-spinal) to forelimb motoneurones situated at lower cervical levels of the spinal cord and controlling forelimb muscles of the cat. (Adapted from Baldiserra *et al.* (1981).)

forelimb segments (C_6–T_1) of the spinal cord (Illert *et al.* 1977). While a proportion of the propriospinal cells has been shown to receive excitatory and inhibitory inputs from muscle spindle and cutaneous afferents from the forelimb (Alstermark *et al.* 1984), they are all in receipt of descending connections, including powerful corticospinal influences, and can presumably respond by selecting the motor nuclei which must be recruited to the specific motor task. Figure 4.6 summarizes the schema which relates the C3–4 propriospinal neurones to forelimb movements in the cat (after Baldiserra *et al.* 1981). Lundberg (1979) states 'the convergence on common propriospinal neurones suggests that several higher motor centres may participate in activation of motoneurones via these premotoneurones'. This convergence is certainly one way in which the simultaneous activity known to occur in several motor centres during performance of the same motor act could be integrated to influence motoneuronal discharge.

Alstermark *et al.* (1991) examined C3–C4 propriospinal neurones in the cat by intracellular recording of their responses to a variety of stimuli and then by morphological study of the cellular geometry revealed by intracellular injection of HRP. Propriospinal neurones projected to the motor nuclei of the digits, wrist, elbow, shoulder, and the axial muscles as well as to other parts of the grey matter. Frequently a given propriospinal neurone delivered terminations within several motor nuclei which could innervate muscles acting at different joints. For different groups of propriospinal cells, terminations were found in relation to motoneurones, to both motoneurones and Ia inhibitory interneurones or purely in association with Ia inhibitory interneurones. The axons of propriospinal neurones bifurcate to provide, in addition to their influence on spinal motor nuclei, ascending projections to the lateral reticular nucleus in the brainstem and hence they are in a position to inform the cerebellum about activity within this population of premotor interneurones and the integrated input to them from peripheral afferents and from descending pathways (Alstermark *et al.* 1990b).

A group of these C3–C4 propriospinal neurones with descending axons has been implicated by Alstermark and his colleagues in the behavioural responses of the cat when reaching for a target with the forelimb (see Section 3.5). Alstermark and Kümmel (1990b) examined the transneuronal transport of WGA-HRP within the propriospinal system. The efficiency of this transport is considered to be influenced by the degree of activity in the pathways labelled (Jankowska 1985). Alstermark and Kümmel (1990b) contrasted the transneuronal labelling of last-order interneurones from the deltoid muscle when this muscle was involved either in unrestricted walking or in target-reaching. Labelled, presumed last-order interneurones were found from the C2 to the T1 segment. Most of the interneurones were located in the C5–T1 segments, and these cells were labelled during both types of movement, although many more were labelled in walking than in target-reaching. In reaching, a population of interneurones was labelled in the C3–C4 segments that was not found during walking; this is in keeping with the role of this population of propriospinal neurones in mediating the descending command for target-reaching with the forelimb.

4.6 STUDIES IN HUMAN SUBJECTS

Using the methods briefly referred to in Chapter 1 (Section 1.19), it is possible to obtain information in human subjects about the reflex connections of populations of peripheral afferents, by their influence on stimulus related changes in probability of the firing of a single motor unit recorded from a selected muscle. While the subject maintains a given level of background activity in the motor unit, afferent volleys may be injected into the central nervous system by stimulation of a peripheral nerve. Changes in the firing probability of the motoneurone will be produced by the synaptic influence impinging on that motoneurone as a result of the imposed stimulus. These changes can be revealed by the poststimulus time histogram (PSTH) of the motor unit discharges for a large number of repetitions of the stimulus. Only those motor unit discharges which are time-locked, in their probability of occurrence, to the stimulus, will sum in the preferred temporal domain of the resultant histogram. All other events, which are randomly associated with the timing of the stimulus, will be evenly distributed through the total analysis period (Stephens *et al.* 1976; Ashby and Zilm 1982a, b). By using such methods, the pattern of synaptic connectivity influencing upper and lower limb muscles have been analyzed. The interpretation of the results has been based very much on the spinal reflex connectivity established in animal experiments.

Ashby and Zilm (1982b), for example, delivered weak electrical stimuli, just below threshold for the motor axons, to the motor nerve (lateral peroneal nerve) of the tibialis anterior muscle from which they recorded single motor units. Figure 4.7 illustrates the PSTHs which define the alterations in firing probability of three tibialis anterior motoneurones produced by weak stimuli delivered to the nerve. In each case, a brief period of increased probability of firing was followed by a period of decreased probability. These changes in probability could be matched by simulating a stimulus induced excitatory postsynaptic potential (EPSP) causing depolarization of the motoneurone (Ashby and Zilm 1982a). This EPSP had the characteristics of the composite, group I evoked monosynaptic potential that can be recorded intracellularly from motoneurones in experimental animals. It occurred with the appropriate latency, also consistent with the H-reflex latency in these subjects, and it was not produced by stimulation of the muscle nerve supplying antagonist muscles or by stimulation of the skin.

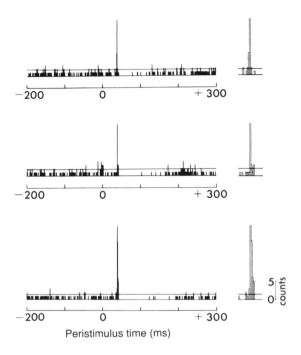

FIG 4.7   For each of three human tibialis anterior motor units, the diagram plots
the changes in probability of firing associated with the delivery of a weak electrical
stimulus, below threshold for the motor axons to the muscle nerve, at time O. There
is a period of increased firing probability (expanded in the diagrams on the right)
lasting 2 to 5 ms, followed by a period of decreased firing probability. Each cross-
correlogram was constructed for approximately 100 repetitions of the stimulus and
sums approximately 500 discharges of the motor unit. The mean firing probability,
plus two standard deviations, derived from the occurrences during the 200 ms
prestimulus period, is indicated by the horizontal line. (Reproduced with permission
from Ashby and Zilm (1982a).)

Ashby and Zilm (1982a) have also shown that the period of decreased
probability following the initial increase is related to the size of the increase,
and this is best explained by the phenomenon of the after-hyperpolarization
of the motoneurone, which dictates the minimum interval after which a
discharged motoneurone can normally fire again. These authors agreed
that any EPSP which was strong enough to discharge a motoneurone on
a large number of trials (e.g., a large compound EPSP excited by a volley
of excitatory inputs of either peripheral or central origin) would always
produce a post-facilitatory pause. This was much less likely for very weak
inputs, which have a very low probability of causing the motoneurone to

discharge. This point will be taken up again in the section on spike-triggered averages (STA) and cross-correlation techniques (Section 4.11).

The shape of the cross-correlogram peak is determined approximately by the first derivative of the EPSP waveform (Knox and Poppele 1977; Kirkwood 1979). Indications of the rise time and the magnitude of the underlying EPSP can also be derived from the temporal profile of the cross-correlogram, and the effects of other synaptic influences simultaneously affecting the motoneurone in the form of synaptic 'noise' can also be assessed (Kirkwood 1979; Fetz and Gustafsson 1983; Ashby and Zilm 1982a; Cope *et al.* 1987; Midroni and Ashby 1989). The method has widespread applicability to the analysis of neuronal connectivity underlying mechanisms for voluntary movement performance, and we shall return on a number of occasions to the results of cross-correlation studies in one or other of its forms.

Stephens and his colleagues have exploited this approach to demonstrate the influence of both cutaneous and muscular inputs upon the discharge of motoneurones supplying the intrinsic muscles of the hand (Buller *et al.* 1980; Garnett and Stephens 1980). The method has revealed distributed projections of these afferents with relatively strong effects on the muscles acting on the stimulated digit, as well as weaker effects from neighbouring digits. Both the single unit and the EMG data suggest a complex cutaneomuscular reflex with successive excitatory and inhibitory effects (termed E1, I1, and E2 by Stephens). The earlier components are thought to be spinal in origin, while the E2 component is probably transcortical (see Section 6.5).

Pierrot-Deseilligny (1989) has examined human subjects for evidence which could implicate a propriospinal system in man, available for activation in association with conscious, voluntary movement. Interneurones are, in this account, divided into two populations—the first involved in reflex functions and the second, among which are the C3–C4 propriospinal cells just considered, concerned with the transmission of descending motor commands from supraspinal centres. These projection interneurones also receive inputs from peripheral receptors, which could provide an anatomical substrate for modification of the descending commands by afferent activity influenced by the state of the limb, and could perform this modification at a 'pre-motoneuronal' level (see Fig. 4.6; Jankowska and Lundberg 1981). Pierrot-Deseilligny used a modified PSTH method (Fournier *et al.* 1986) to look for evidence of non-monosynaptic excitatory influences on spinal motoneurones produced by weak stimulation of peripheral nerves. This was achieved by delivering each weak stimulus at a fixed delay after the previous motor unit spike, chosen and adjusted so that the monosynaptic excitatory effects would arrive at a time when the motoneurone was refractory due to after-hyperpolarization, yet the influence of any later polysynaptic EPSPs would be detectable as an increase in probability of firing of the motor unit, because the after-hyperpolarization would have decayed by the time these later synaptic changes occurred.

Using these techniques, applied to the study of motor units in human forelimb muscles, a second, smaller peak in firing probability was found in 60 per cent of wrist flexor motor units when weak stimuli were provided to the median or the ulnar nerve. This late excitation was not evoked by cutaneous stimulation and because of the very weak shocks used, it was ascribed to low threshold (group I) afferents in the forelimb nerve. The central latency of these late effects was found to range from 3 to 6 ms, allowing time for interneurones to be involved, and it was proposed that the interneurones implicated in this action in man could be analogous to the C3–C4 propriospinal neurones identified in the cat's spinal cord. These, it will be recalled, all receive excitation from descending pathways.

Baldissera and Pierrot-Deseilligny (1989) examined the late conditioning, by weak stimulation of the ulnar nerve, of the monosynaptic H-reflex set up in flexor carpi ulnaris by median nerve stimulation. They made these measurements at rest and at the onset of wrist flexion to produce 20 per cent of maximal force. At the onset of contraction of the muscle the ulnar nerve volley which had produced very little facilitation of the reflex activity at rest, evoked a large reflex facilitation with a conditioning-test interval of 3 ms (Fig. 4.8). This facilitation has been ascribed to the convergence on to propriospinal neurones of both low-threshold group I afferents from the ulnar nerve and also descending excitatory commands from the cortex.

Evidence has also been obtained in experiments of this kind that, in the human upper limb, delayed inhibitory actions may be set up by afferent influences, most strongly by cutaneous afferents, and also relayed to motoneurones through 'premotoneuronal' interneurones (Fig. 4.6). Here is another set of parallel observations to those reported for C3–C4 propriospinal neurones in the cat. It is postulated that the inhibition by cutaneous afferents of the 'pre-motoneuronal' interneurones, for the existence of which this indirect evidence has been obtained in man, could play an important role in termination of a movement 'which the brain does not easily and reliably plan ahead of movement execution' (Pierrot-Deseilligny 1989). It is suggested that the exteroceptive activity resulting from, say, contact with a target (or with an unexpected obstacle) could inhibit the descending command for movement to that target at a propriospinal level and thus curtail the movement.

While accepting that the results obtained in these studies on human subjects indicate the existence of non-monosynaptic descending excitatory pathways to motoneurones, evidence for a measurable impact of such connections in the generation of EPSPs is missing in the direct recordings from motoneurones made in anaesthetized primates (Jankowska *et al.* 1975b;

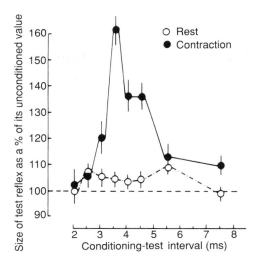

FIG 4.8 The increase in size of a test reflex (expressed as a percentage of its control value) is plotted against the conditioning-test interval when a conditioning
stimulus to the ulnar nerve (below motor threshold) precedes the test stimulus used
to evoke an H-reflex in the flexor carpi ulnaris muscle of the human forearm. If
the conditioning stimulus is delivered at the onset of a voluntary wrist flexion (filled
circles) rather than at rest (open circles), there is a marked facilitation of the reflex
response with a time-course which has been explained by convergence on to propriospinal neurones of influences from low threshold group I afferents (ulnar nerve)
and descending (voluntary) commands from the cerebral cortex. Each symbol represents the mean ± 1SE from 20 measurements. (Reproduced with permission from
Baldiserra and Pierrot-Deseilligny (1989).)

Fritz *et al.* 1985; Lemon 1990). In recordings from a sample of 76 hand
and forearm motoneurones showing clear monosynaptic excitation in
response to stimulation of the pyramidal tract, only 5 showed evidence of
di- or oligo-synaptic EPSPs (see Fig. 4.37a, b). However, since most of
these motoneurones responded with a strong IPSP following the monosynaptic EPSP, it is possible that any later EPSPs, that could have been
present, were masked. In conscious monkeys, poststimulus time histograms
of motor unit discharge in response to single stimuli applied to the motor
cortex or pyramidal tract are dominated by short-latency monosynaptic
excitation, and are generally devoid of longer-latency effects (Palmer and
Fetz 1985b; Lemon *et al.* 1987; see Figs 4.31 and 8.3). The same is true
of responses in motor units, recorded from hand and forearm muscles of
human subjects, to non-invasive brain stimulation (see Rothwell *et al.*
1991). The functional role of propriospinal pathways in natural, voluntary
movement performance in the primate clearly needs further evaluation.

4.7 SYNAPTIC EXCITATION IN THE SPINAL CORD

In an effort to better understand the precise mechanism of synaptic interaction between connected neurones and to subject this mechanism to some of the forms of analysis (for example, quantal analysis) which had been so revealing in the study of the chemically mediated neuromuscular junction of the frog (del Castillo and Katz 1954), the monosynaptic excitatory connections made by a single group Ia afferent fibre with a receiving motoneurone became the most obvious and conveniently available example in the central nervous system. From measurements of mean amplitude of synaptic potentials evoked by an impulse in a single Ia afferent fibre and the standard deviation of the mean, estimates could be made of possible quantal size of the EPSP, and of the probability of quantal release, which would explain these findings if certain theoretical conditions applied to synaptic transmission at these sites (Kuno 1964).

Many of the experimental observations employed spike-triggered averaging (STA), using simultaneous recordings from a single group Ia fibre in a dorsal root and intracellular registration of membrane potentials changes in a given motoneurone, to extract the average amplitude and time-course of a 'unit' monosynaptic EPSP i.e., the average depolarization produced in a single motoneurone by a single nerve impulse in a single Ia afferent fibre (Mendell and Henneman 1971; Burke *et al.* 1979; Jack *et al.* 1971). When this method sampled, for the same Ia afferent, many motoneurones innervating different muscles, information was gained about the extent of that afferent's distributed influence on the receiving dendritic membranes of a large number of enmeshed motoneurones. It became obvious that the influences of the one afferent fibre had different magnitudes and different time-courses of effect on separate motoneurones. These were, in part, explicable by locations of the responsible synapse on different regions of the extensively distributed dendritic trees of the motoneurones, the smaller and slower expected to be more remote from the somatic recording electrode than the larger and more rapidly rising and decaying. Jack *et al.* (1971) plotted this distribution for a large sample of monosynaptic synapses on lumbar motoneurones in the cat's spinal cord (Fig. 4.9).

In 1964, Kuno showed that individual unit EPSPs recorded in a motoneurone which followed single impulses in the same Ia fibre fluctuated in amplitude. A whole new approach to the understanding of excitatory synaptic actions on spinal motoneurones flowed from the combination of quantal analysis of these fluctuating synaptic responses with morphological reconstruction of the exact anatomical connection at which the unit EPSP was produced. The method of injecting HRP intra-axonally into axons within the spinal cord which had been electrophysiologically identified as group Ia fibres arising from primary muscle spindle endings, together with

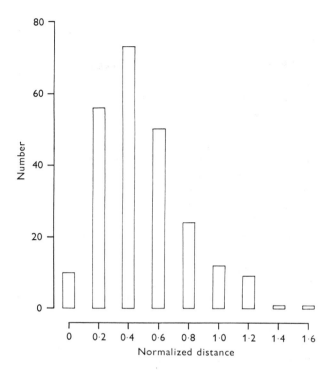

FIG 4.9 A plot of the calculated locations of the synaptic terminals responsible for the generation of unitary group Ia EPSPs by actions on the somata and dendrites of a population of spinal motoneurones in the cat. On the basis of measurements of the voltage time-courses of the EPSPs, each was assigned a distance location normalized with respect to the membrane characteristics of the receiving cell. A small proportion (about 0.5 per cent) of the 236 Ia synapses in this diagram were found to have a somatic location. Most were distributed at dendritic locations. (From Jack *et al.* (1971.))

the intracellular labelling of motoneurones with HRP to delineate their dendritic profiles in full had been exploited by Burke *et al.* (1979) and by Brown and Fyffe (1981) to reveal connectivity between Ia axons and motoneurones using the light microscope.

Redman and Walmsley (1983a, b) delivered stimuli to a single axon by passing brief currents through the intra-axonal electrode while they recorded the unit EPSP responses evoked by these stimuli in individual receiving motoneurones. The noisy records of the evoked synaptic potentials were then analysed by the deconvolution technique of Edwards *et al.* (1976a, b) and, later, by the revised method of Jack *et al.* (1981). This had the effect of subtracting the physical and physiological noise from the records to reveal the underlying individual synaptic events. These were

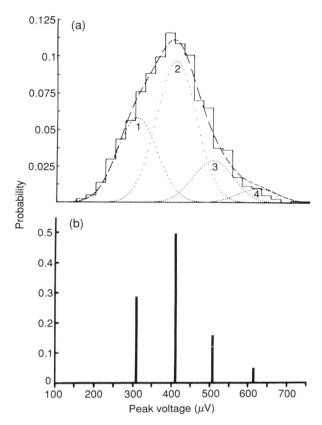

FIG 4.10   (a): The peak voltages of 800 repetitions of an evoked unitary group Ia EPSP are plotted in this histogram. The dotted lines, labelled 1 to 4, are normal distributions each with a standard deviation of 51 μV which was the standard deviation of the noise in this example. The sum of these distributions is indicated by the dashed line. (b): The sequence of discrete EPSP amplitudes and the probabilities associated with each of these for this sample of occurrences. (Reproduced with permission from Redman (1990).)

found to fluctuate between different discrete amplitudes which had different probabilities of occurrence. In general, these amplitudes for a given unit EPSP were integer multiples of the increment between adjacent amplitudes. Figure 4.10(a) illustrates a histogram of peak voltages constructed from 800 records of an evoked EPSP. Figure 4.10(b) plots the amplitudes and the frequency of occurrence of these amplitudes in the evoked EPSP, and reveals that each evoked response in this case occurred with an amplitude of either 300, 400, 500, or 600 μV, each amplitude having the probability indicated on the ordinate.

The average peak amplitude of the incremental EPSP (which Redman equated to a quantal EPSP) was found to be approximately 90 μV for unit EPSPs generated near the soma of receiving cells. This form of analysis could reveal, in some cells, a fluctuation pattern for the EPSP amplitude which included only failures or a single amplitude for all the other events. Such all-or-nothing occurrences suggested generation of the EPSP by release (or failure of release) at a single synaptic bouton. When the amplitude of the EPSP fluctuated between a number of different amplitudes separated by equal quantal increments, (as in Fig. 4.10(b)), the distribution of events could best be described by a compound binomial fit in which different probabilities of release are associated with different release sites and the probability of release at any one site is independent of whether or not release occurs at any other site.

Redman (1990, p. 174) summarized some of these results. For most single fibre evoked EPSPs, the time course of the individual component synaptic events 'associated with each discrete amplitude could be calculated by extracting and averaging records that contributed to that amplitude only. Usually the time course of the EPSP was the same for each amplitude'. This indicated that the components were generated by release sites at the same or very similar electrotonic distances from the recording electrode. 'For a few EPSPs that had an average time course of a complex nature (e.g., a rapid rising phase followed by a prolonged peak and a slow decay), the time course was not the same for each discrete amplitude. These were fortunate examples, because it was possible to show that the different discrete amplitudes had different time courses and, as a consequence, the quantal EPSPs that combined to form the different amplitudes also had different time courses'. The correlation of such recordings, indicating generation of separate components of the single fibre's EPSP at different electrotonic locations, with anatomical evidence of different locations of the synaptic boutons contributed by branches of the afferent fibre to that moto-neurone, was an important element in the development of the theory of excitatory synaptic connectivity.

Redman and Walmsley (1983b) examined the hypothesis that, for these synapses, a quantal EPSP is generated when the transmitter is released at a single bouton. The quantal content of the maximum discrete amplitude would then be equal to or less than (if, under the conditions of the experiment, some boutons did not release transmitter in response to the stimulus) the number of boutons delivered to the motoneurone's dendritic surface by that group Ia fibre. Figure 4.11 provides an example from their results obtained from a combination of reconstruction of the precise synaptic morphology revealed with light microscopy, and the analysis of fluctuation patterns of the EPSP generated in the motoneurone by impulses in the Ia fibre contributing these boutons.

In the light of the evidence from electron microscopy (Fyffe and Light

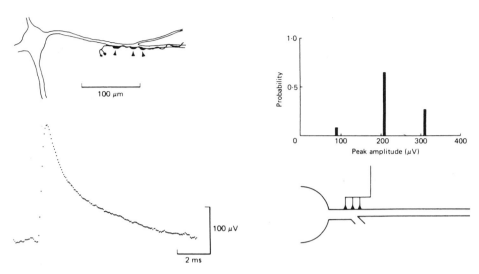

FIG 4.11   The combined intra-axonal and intracellular labelling (with HRP) of a single group Ia afferent fibre and the motoneurone from which unitary EPSPs caused by impulses in that fibre had been recorded, allowed the histological reconstruction of the synaptic contacts provided by three boutons in line and close together on the same dendrite (top left). Deconvolution analysis revealed three discrete amplitudes represented within the unitary EPSP (top right). This suggests that the separate quantal components of the single fibre EPSP derive from release at one or more of the separate boutons (bottom right). Quantal amplitude is of the order of 100 μV and the maximum unitary EPSP amplitude (of 300 μV) occurs when all three boutons release transmitter. In response to a given impulse in the Ia fibre, the probability of simultaneous release from all three sites is of the order of 0.25. (Diagram kindly provided by S. J. Redman and reproduced with permission from Redman and Walmsley (1983b).)

1984) that some group Ia boutons contacting motoneurones contain more than one release site as determined by morphological criteria, it is necessary to modify Redman and Walmsley's findings of an equivalence of numbers of boutons with numbers of quantal release sites for the excitatory EPSP. If a bouton may contain more than one release site, and if it is the number of release sites that is to be equated with the number of quanta contributing to a single Ia fibre's EPSP, it follows from the experimental observations and their analysis by these deconvolution methods that release sites, even if situated within a single terminal, must operate independently to account for the compound binomial distribution of peak amplitudes, and that a higher proportion of release sites, than was indicated by simple counting of boutons, may fail to release transmitter in response to a presynaptic impulse under the conditions of these experiments.

These refined methods of detailed analysis of connectivity have been applied to other central nervous system synapses. Walmsley *et al.* (1985) examined the connections of group I afferents with dorsal spinocerebellar tract (DSCT) neurones in the cat's spinal cord. Here, group I fibres may form, in addition to small 1 μm $\times$ 1 μm contacts, large elongated synapses up to 20 μm long which contain multiple release sites. Electrophysiological recordings demonstrate that it is possible to describe the large EPSPs generated (and their fluctuations in amplitude) if quantal EPSPs of average amplitude around 140 μV are independently released from different release sites, and with different probabilities of release (Walmsley *et al.* 1988).

4.8 MORPHOLOGICAL ANALYSIS OF OTHER CONNECTIONS IN THE SPINAL CORD

In theory, it should be possible to examine other synaptic connections between single fibres and motoneurones or interneurones using these techniques. There are, of course, experimental difficulties to be overcome when the size of the receiving neurone is small, as it may be for some interneurones, and the opportunity to maintain stable intracellular recordings for long periods is diminished. While not all presynaptic fibre elements may be clearly identifiable by electrophysiological methods, and also be accessible to intra-axonal recording and single fibre stimulation, combined with intra-axonal injection of HRP for morphological studies, a number of such systems have been approached in this way, and at least partial descriptions are available to guide our thinking about the mechanisms of synaptic interaction that can determine functional outcomes of activity in these systems. Finally, some relatively local interactions can be examined from a morphological point of view if complete filling of one cell such as a motoneurone, accompanied by complete filling of another cell, for example a Renshaw cell, enables the connections between the two to be described in microscopic detail. Fyffe (1991) successfully labelled pairs of Renshaw cells and motoneurones in the cat's spinal cord. A small number (average of three) of synaptic contacts with the proximal dendrites (not the somata, where reciprocal inhibitory synapses from Ia interneurones are located) of the receiving motoneurone were contributed by axon collaterals of a Renshaw cell. EM confirmation of these contacts as inhibitory synapses was provided.

4.9 SPINAL CORD CONNECTIONS MADE BY FIBRES OF DESCENDING MOTOR PATHWAYS

A large number of supraspinal structures are now known to influence spinal interneurones and motoneurones (Kuypers 1981; Baldiserra *et al.* 1981;

Shapovalov 1975). Kuypers' interpretation of the function of the different descending motor pathways was based principally on their different patterns of spinal termination (see Section 2.9). In this scheme, he originally distinguished two main groups of descending fibres: a dorsolateral and a ventromedial group. The dorsolateral group comprises crossed fibres in the rubrospinal and corticospinal tracts which terminate mainly upon short propriospinal interneurones located in the dorsolateral intermediate zone. These interneurones make short, local connections, principally with motoneurones supplying muscles acting about the distal joints of the extremity. In the primate, these same motoneurones receive direct connections from both rubrospinal and corticospinal fibres. In contrast, the ventromedial group of pathways comprise mostly uncrossed fibres from the lateral and medial vestibular nucleus, medial pontine and medullary reticular formation, and the interstitial nucleus of Cajal, as well as some crossed tectospinal and vestibulospinal fibres (medial longitudinal fasciculus, MLF). These fibres terminate in the ventromedial intermediate zone, to some extent bilaterally, and thereby influence long propriospinal neurones and motoneurones innervating muscles acting on the trunk and girdles. The functional consequence of this pattern of termination would be that the dorsolateral group of descending fibre systems is more concerned with movements of the extremity, including hand movements, while the ventromedial group controls locomotion, posture and reaching. The evidence for this functional dichotomy is presented in Kuypers' reviews (1978, 1981).

The fine detail of the spinal terminations made by different descending pathways has now been extensively studied by the intra-axonal HRP technique. Shinoda *et al.* (1986a) have used this technique to label single vestibulospinal axons in the spinal cord of the cat and described the appearance in the light microscope of the collateral branches and the terminal arborizations of these descending axons (Fig. 4.12).

Axons contributing to the lateral vestibulospinal tract (LVST) had multiple axon collaterals, each contributing endings within a restricted zone of the spinal cord which had a rostrocaudal extent of less than 1 mm (760 μm). These collaterals projected into lamina VIII and the medial parts of lamina VII and made apparent contacts with the cell bodies and proximal dendrites of motoneurones in the ventromedial region of the anterior horn of the spinal cord. Some terminals of these axon collaterals were contributed to the ventral parts of lamina VII and the adjacent lamina IX. It could be deduced that these descending axons contributed synapses to the motoneurones of forelimb muscles. Rubrospinal axons have also been studied in this way in the cat (Shinoda *et al.* 1982).

As we have described earlier, Kuypers and his colleagues used injections of fluorescent tracers at different levels of the spinal grey matter to estimate the degree of collateralization amongst different descending pathways in the rat, cat, and monkey (Huisman *et al.* 1981, 1982). In these

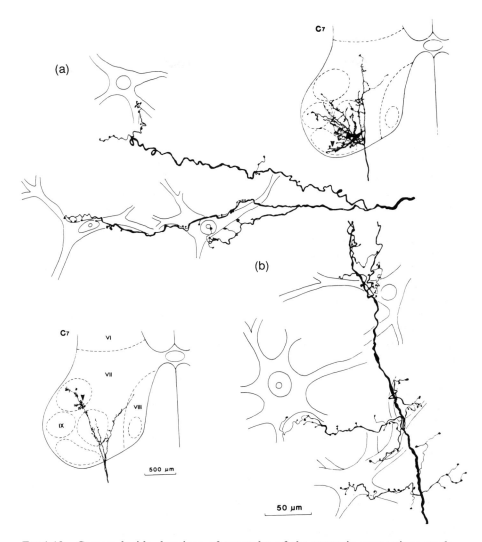

FIG 4.12   Camera lucida drawings of examples of the synaptic connections made
by lateral vestibulospinal tract axons (LVST) with motoneurones revealed in transverse sections of the cat's spinal cord at C7. (a) Terminal branches of a collateral
of the LVST axon penetrate lamina IX (inset: upper right) and form synapses on
the somata and proximal dendrites of motoneurones. (b) Another terminal collateral of an LVST axon appears to make synaptic contact with the somata of motoneurones in lamina IX (arrowhead in inset at lower left). In general, LVST axons
contacting medial motoneuronal cell groups were much more common than those
innervating the more lateral motor columns. (Reproduced with permission from
Shinoda *et al.* (1986a).)

experiments, the injection site of one fluorescent tracer was confined to the dorsal horn and intermediate zone of the grey matter between C5 and C8. After an interval, the same animals were re-operated and a different tracer injected into the spinal cord at a more caudal level, ranging from T1 to S3 in different cases. The proportions of single and double-labelled neurones in the red nucleus, nucleus raphé magnus (NRM), and pontine tegmentum were counted. A high proportion of double-labelled neurones would indicate a widely collateralized system, with neurones branching to innervate remote segments of the spinal cord. Both the raphéspinal and reticulospinal projections were considered to contain a large proportion of highly collateralized axons, since in the cat NRM, for example, 50–60 per cent of neurones were double-labelled. In contrast the rubrospinal projections were focused, with only 4 per cent of neurones double-labelled after a lumbar injection in the cat. The collateralization of the rubrospinal projections showed phylogenetic differences, being greater in the rat (20 per cent) than in the cat or monkey. Huisman *et al.* (1982) concluded that more focussed systems were essential to the control of specific motor acts, such as relatively independent finger movements. However, a highly branched connectivity within the spinal cord does not necessarily imply a lack of functional specificity. For example, Grantyn *et al.* (1987) found that individual reticulospinal neurones collateralize widely within the brainstem and upper cervical segments; but the widespread connections made by an individual neurone could be interpreted as subserving a common motor goal, such as the activation of eye, ear, and neck muscles required for an orientating response (Grantyn and Berthoz 1987).

4.10 DIVERGENCE OF CORTICO-MOTONEURONAL COLLATERALS IN THE MONKEY

A major theme of this book, as with its predecessor, *Corticospinal Neurones*, is the evaluation of relationships between structure and function of the corticospinal neurones which, in the primate, by-pass the interneuronal machinery of the spinal cord, and overtake supraspinal structures which could influence spinal mechanisms for movement, so that they come to exert direct excitatory actions monosynaptically on to motoneurones (Bernhard *et al.* 1953; Bernhard and Bohm 1954; Preston and Whitlock 1961; Landgren *et al.* 1962a). In the previous chapters we introduced the anatomical location and organization of this cortico-motoneuronal system and the morphological substrate at a supraspinal and cortico-cortical level for its activation. Here we shall concern ourselves with recent information which relates to the spinal terminations of the axonal collaterals of individual cortico-motoneuronal cells and with the impact of these cells upon particular populations of spinal motoneurones.

4.10.1 Evidence from intraspinal stimulation

The first clear evidence for the pronounced intraspinal collateralization of the corticospinal system came from experiments in which the antidromic responses of single corticospinal cells elicited by intraspinal stimulation were recorded in the cat and subsequently in the monkey (Shinoda *et al.* 1976, 1979, 1986b). These experiments adapted the technique introduced by Abzug *et al.* (1974) for mapping the distribution of vestibulospinal axons in the cat. In their most detailed study, Shinoda *et al.* (1986b) mapped the intraspinal branching of 408 cat corticospinal neurones whose cell bodies were in the motor cortex. Nearly all forelimb corticospinal neurones had three to seven collaterals at widely separated segments of the cervical and upper thoracic cord. About a third projected to the lumbar cord. For 20 neurones, the intraspinal course of each corticospinal collateral was mapped by systematic stimulation in many closely spaced penetrations. Individual intraspinal axon collaterals were slowly-conducting (as slow as $1\,\text{m.s}^{-1}$) and had an average rostrocaudal extension of 2.6 mm. Antidromic responses originating from collaterals, as opposed to spread of current leading to direct activation of the stem axon in the white matter, could be distinguished by a number of criteria, including the threshold and latency of the antidromic responses. These authors found no systematic differences in the branching patterns of the 30 fast and 19 slow cat corticospinal axons they examined in detail.

Turning now to the monkey data, Shinoda *et al.* (1979) recorded from 54 neurones which could be antidromically activated from within the motoneurone pools in the cervical cord. Thus these neurones were probably cortico-motoneuronal: 28 were activated from only one segment, and six from more than one segment. Only one neurone could be activated from motor nuclei more than three segments apart. The remaining 20 neurones were activated from both a motor nucleus and other unspecified regions of the grey matter, even though later studies (Lawrence *et al.* 1985) revealed that most of the intraspinal branches of cortico-motoneuronal collaterals were confined to the region of the motor columns in lamina IX. Therefore, more than half of the sample of cortico-motoneuronal cells studied by antidromic stimulation appeared to have axon terminals in zones outside the limits of a motor nucleus at a single segmental level. In the monkey, Shinoda *et al.* (1979) found that their presumed cortico-motoneuronal axons were somewhat less branched than were corticospinal axons which did not terminate amongst the motor nuclei. Twenty per cent of neurones terminating in the C7–8 motor nuclei were reported as branching to the thoracic cord, although this was tested with a coarse stimulating electrode at T2–3, which may have activated branches still destined to reach forelimb, and particularly hand motor nuclei in T1 (Jenny and Inukai 1983). Of a further 156 neurones which could not be classified with certainty as being activated from within the motor column, 44 (28 per cent) were activated from both the cervical grey and thoracic cord. The relatively restricted pattern of intraspinal branching of cortico-motoneuronal axons revealed by this study was subsequently confirmed by STA of cortico-motoneuronal cells facilitating monkey hand muscles (Buys *et al.* 1986; see below).

4.10.2 Evidence from intracortical microstimulation

The converse of the approach adopted by Shinoda and his colleagues is to activate single cortical cells and examine the responses in either single motoneurones (by intracellular recording) or by registration of action potentials recorded from single motor units. Alternatively, divergence to different muscles can be detected by averaging of multi-unit EMG (Cheney and Fetz 1985; Lemon *et al.* 1987; Lemon 1990). In the great majority of studies of this kind, investigators have reported the activation of multiple muscles from a single cortical site, even though the possibility of physiological synaptic spread from the cortical stimulating electrode has been minimized by using a single intracortical stimulus of low strength (typically less than 10 μA). Further evidence for divergence is provided by the observation that stimulation at a single cortical site with a single 20 μA pulse evoked monosynaptic EPSPs in 27/61 hand and forearm motoneurones (Lemon, Fritz, Illert, Muir, and Yamaguchi, unpublished; Lemon 1990). However, it is impossible to ascertain how many cortico-motoneuronal cells are excited by such stimuli, and electrical stimulation of the cortex has thus been unable to yield unequivocal results concerning the divergence of influence of single cortico-motoneuronal cells provided by the branching of an individual axon's collaterals.

4.10.3 Evidence from intra-axonal labelling

Intra-axonal injection of HRP has been employed to study the spinal collaterals of single corticospinal neurones in both the cat (Futami *et al.* 1979) and the monkey (Shinoda *et al.* 1981; Lawrence *et al.* 1985). Shinoda *et al.* (1981) demonstrated that, in the monkey, in addition to collaterals to intermediate regions of the spinal cord (laminae V, VI, & VII) major projections could be traced into lamina IX, which was unequivocally revealed by the presence within it of cell somata and proximal dendrites of motoneurones which had been labelled retrogradely with HRP transported from axons in forelimb motor nerves. Shinoda concluded that a single corticospinal axon may terminate in up to four motor nuclei and that terminals 'make apparent contacts with proximal dendrites or distal dendrites of the motoneurones'.

Lawrence *et al.* (1985) extended these observations by combining the intra-axonal injection of HRP into identified corticospinal axons issuing from pyramidal cells in the 'arm' area of the cortex, but not projecting to lower thoracic segments of the spinal cord, with intracellular injection of HRP into spinal motoneurones identified by their antidromic action potentials to be innervating intrinsic muscles of the hand through the ulnar or median nerve. These motoneurones all received monosynaptic EPSPs when cortico-motoneuronal fibres were activated by the cortical stimulus. Even though a much larger number of axons and motoneurones were studied, in only seven cases could synaptic contacts be visualized in subsequent light microscopy of parasagittal histological sections of the spinal cord. Only when the filled axon, which could be traced longitudinally for only 0.5 to 1.25 mm in the dorsolateral white matter in these studies, gave rise to an intraspinal collateral in the immediate segmental vicinity of the identified and labelled motoneurones was it possible to identify a synaptic contact between the two. In these seven cases, at least at the level of light microscopy, the contacts defined the originating axon anatomically to be a cortico-motoneuronal fibre, and the distribution of its collateral could be documented.

Figure 4.13 illustrates the branching distribution of a collateral of one such cortico-motoneuronal fibre in the cervical spinal cord of a monkey. In the central region of the C8 segment of the spinal cord (which was 4.1 mm in length), the stem axon gave rise to a main collateral, which ran approximately 0.5 mm caudally and ventromedially before entering lamina IX. Extensive branching then occurred within a cylinder about 0.5 mm in diameter and 1.5 mm in length, condensed into a single plane in the illustration of Fig. 4.13 by the compression of the camera lucida reconstructions from 14 parasagittal sections of the spinal cord, each 100 μm in thickness. Many of the branches could be followed through very fine fibres to terminations in synaptic boutons or clusters of boutons. *En passant* synapses occurred frequently along the length of the fine branches. The finest and most distant branches extended outside the major cylinder of collaterals to spread through 0.9 mm dorsoventrally, 1.4 mm mediolaterally and beyond 3.6 mm longitudinally. The longitudinal extension was achieved principally by means of two thick collaterals, which arose from proximal branches of the main collateral and ran caudally within lamina IX, giving off other branches along the way. The longest of these reached the rostral border of spinal segment T_1. It is possible that, had a longer length of stem axon been revealed by these methods, additional collateral branches from the same axon could have greatly extended the cylinders of influence and the size of the population of motoneurones contacted. This would be consistent with the findings that a single cortico-motoneuronal cell contacts most of the motor units in its target muscle (see below).

The cortico-motoneuronal fibre shown in Fig. 4.13 made synaptic contact with each of the only two ulnar motoneurones innervating intrinsic hand

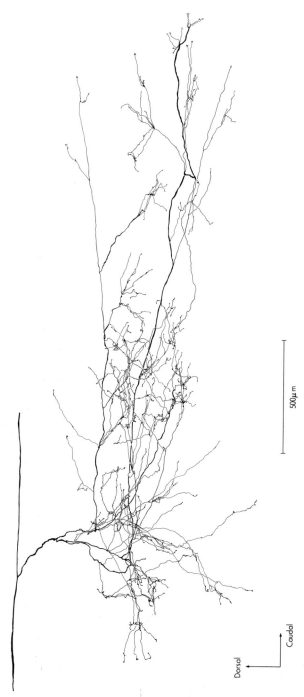

500μm

Dorsal

Caudal

FIG 4.13 Camera lucida reconstruction of the arborization of a main collateral arising from a cortico-motoneuronal axon running in the lateral funiculus of the monkey's spinal cord. This reconstruction was achieved by matching the trajectories of HRP-filled branches of the collateral which were distributed through 14 parasagittal sections, each 100 μm thick, through the C8 and T1 segments of the spinal cord. The arborization was most dense within a horizontal cylinder through 1.5 mm of the central portion of C8. Many branches, and a multitude of boutons, were located within lamina IX. Some branches extended beyond the region of the motoneurones. This reconstruction was performed by Dr D. G. Lawrence. (From Porter 1987.)

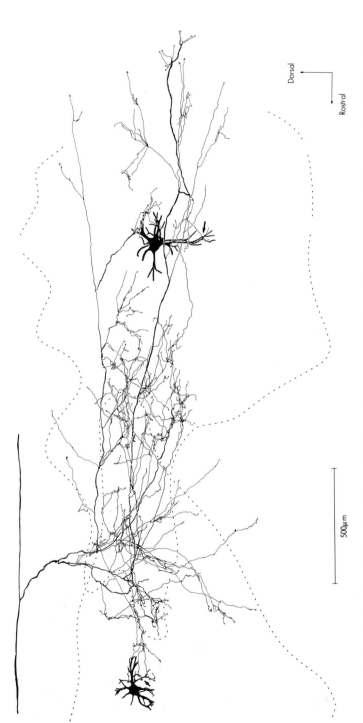

Dorsal

Rostral

500μm

FIG 4.14 The arborization of the main collateral of the cortico-motoneuronal axon illustrated in Fig. 4.13 traversed a cylinder within spinal segment C8 between two ulnar motoneurones innervating intrinsic muscles of the hand. The somata of these two motoneurones are illustrated. The dendritic trees of the two motoneurones occupied territories outlined by the interrupted lines. Each motoneurone received a synapse from a branch of the cortico-motoneuronal collateral (arrowed). (From Lawrence, Porter and Redman (1985). Copyright © 1985. Reprinted by permission of Wiley-Liss, a division of John Wiley and Sons Inc.)

muscles that were completely filled with HRP in the same segment of the spinal cord. These somata were separated by 2 mm longitudinally. Even so, part of the dendritic tree of each motoneurone overlapped with that of the other in the same region of the cord as the main collateral arborization of the cortico-motoneuronal fibre (dashed outlines enclose the dendritic territories except where exceedingly long dendritic branches extended through the gaps in these boundaries to outlying regions in Fig. 4.14). Only two synaptic contacts between this fibre and the motoneurones could be identified with light microscopy. A large *en passant* synapse was located on a dendrite 40 μm from the soma of the rostral motoneurone, and a smaller *en passant* synapse was located 200 μm from the soma of the caudal motoneurone (Fig. 4.15).

In another animal, two cortico-motoneuronal fibres provided collateral branches in the vicinity of the somata and dendrites of two stained ulnar

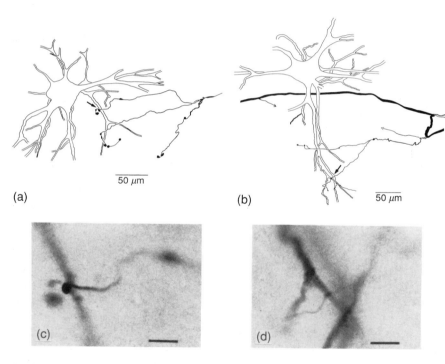

FIG 4.15   Reconstructions of the rostral (a) and caudal (b) motoneurones of Fig. 4.14 to illustrate the sites of presumed synaptic contact (arrows) between branches of the cortico-motoneuronal axon collateral and dendrites of the moto-neurones. Photomicrographs through the 100 μm thick actions illustrate the regions of synaptic contact (c) and (d). Calibration bar for photomicrographs = 10 μm. (From Lawrence *et al.* (1985). Copyright ©1985. Reprinted by permission of Wiley-Liss, a division of John Wiley and Sons Inc.)

motoneurones situated close together in the dorsal part of lamina IX in the rostral part of the first thoracic spinal segment (T_1). Five cortico-motoneuronal synapses between these elements were identified, two on one motoneurone and one on the other, from the more rostrally stained fibre, and one on each motoneurone from the more caudally identified fibre (Fig. 4.16).

This sample of cortico-motoneuronal synaptic contacts, which meet the light microscopic criteria for contacts between a bouton and a process of a motoneurone, is altogether too small to provide reliable general indications about connectivity. However, for this very small sample of fibres with proven contacts on motoneurones innervating intrinsic muscles of the hand, the individual collateral branches of which were completely filled, the few cortico-motoneuronal boutons identified and the multitude of other boutons whose terminations could not be allocated to identified cells, were mostly associated with lamina IX and motoneurones, and they were orientated longitudinally within these motoneurone columns. Contacts were made with dendrites, several of them displaced 600–750 μm from the soma along dendritic branches which were 850 μm to 1.7 mm in length. The boutons were small. They ranged in size from 0.6 μm × 3.0 μm to 2.4 μm × 3.6 μm, in these preparations, which may be compared with the range of size of Ia boutons on motoneurones of the cat, which measured from 3.0 μm × 3.5 μm to 3.5 μm × 7.0 μm (Brown and Fyffe 1978, 1981) under similar conditions.

As yet, the direct registration of spikes in a cortico-motoneuronal fibre simultaneously with the registration of the unit EPSPs caused by those spikes in a target motoneurone has not been performed. Hence the amplitude of depolarization produced in a single motoneurone by a single impulse in a cortico-motoneuronal fibre has not been measured. Nor have the deconvolution methods of Redman and Walmsley been applied to these synapses to analyze the relationship between release sites and possible quantal events at these contacts. Electron microscopy of corticospinal synapses, some of which, in the vicinity of motoneurones in lamina IX of the spinal cord, could be cortico-motoneuronal, has revealed that, among the varieties of synapse which can be described, only the S synapses of Bodian (1975) reveal signs of degeneration when the motor cortex is damaged in the monkey. Bodian makes it clear that these terminals contain spherical vesicles, are asymmetrical synapses, and must be presumed to be excitatory to the receiving dendrites. In his hands, the large (L) synaptic bulbs on motoneurone somata which were associated with subsynaptic cisterns, (C terminals of some other authors) were clearly *not* derived from either the descending systems or from posterior root afferents because they remained unaffected by spinal cord or dorsal root section. These terminals clearly derive from elements intrinsic to the spinal cord such as interneurones.

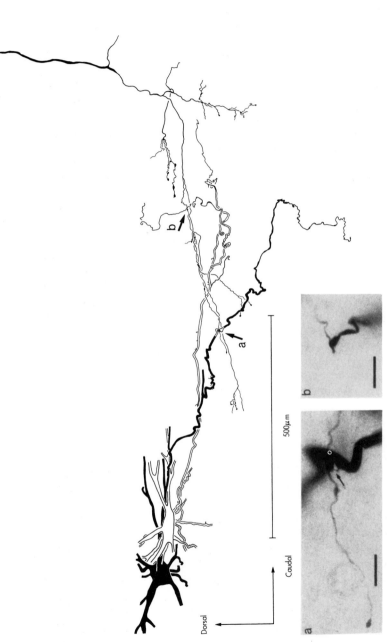

FIG 4.16 In another monkey, two ulnar motor neurones innervating intrinsic muscles of the hand, both situated close together within the spinal cord, were each in receipt of synaptic contacts from the collateral branches of both of two cortico-motoneuronal axons vizualised within the same region of the cord. One part of the collateral of one of these cortico-motoneuronal axons is here revealed contacting a distal dendrite of each of the motoneurones (at a and b). Only those parts of the collateral and of the motor neurones' dendritic trees associated with these two synapses are reproduced in the figure. Calibration bar for photomicrographs = 10 μm. Note the probable axospinous contact revealed by the arrow at a. (From Lawrence et al. (1985). Copyright © 1985. Reprinted by permission of Wiley-Liss, a division of John Wiley and Sons Inc.)

For this reason, the recent report by Ralston and Ralston (1985) requires independent confirmation before its conclusions are accepted. These authors labelled corticospinal axons with a radioactive label anterogradely transported from the precentral motor cortex of the monkey. They could then identify by autoradiography profiles in the EM sections which were associated with silver grains in the overlying photographic emulsion. There are some uncertainties attending the precision of resolution of this association at the EM level (Friedman *et al.* 1986). Ralston and Ralston (1985) indicated that all the labelled axons in the ventral horn were myelinated and $1-6\,\mu$m in diameter. They found synaptic contacts on small, medium, and large proximal dendrites as well as on cell bodies in lamina IX. Most of the contacts, as would have been expected from Bodian's studies, were of the S type. However, they also found labelling of L (or C type) synapses and labelling of presumed inhibitory boutons containing pleomorphic vesicles and in contact with cell somata. We know of no other evidence for direct inhibitory connections from corticospinal fibres, and are inclined to ascribe this last observation to distortions and errors resulting from the presence of silver grains in a different plane to that of the synaptic profile. A similar heterogeneity of terminal types has not been found for rubro-motoneuronal synapses (Ralston *et al.* 1988). In due course EM studies which examine synapses on identified (by labelling) corticospinal axons *and* labelled motoneurones will be needed to finalize this matter.

4.11 DEMONSTRATION OF CORTICO-MOTONEURONAL FACILITATION OF FORELIMB MUSCLE ACTIVITY BY SPIKE-TRIGGERED AVERAGING

4.11.1 The techniques used

Spike-triggered averaging of multi-unit EMG allows the identification, in the motor cortex of conscious monkeys, of corticospinal cells which directly influence activity in motoneurones innervating forelimb muscles. The method was introduced by Fetz *et al.* in 1976, and its principal features are illustrated in Fig. 4.17. The multi-unit EMG recorded from a limb muscle is rectified and averaged with respect to discharges of a single neurone recorded in the contralateral motor cortex. Cancellation of negative and positive-going components of the multi-unit action potentials in the EMG signal is prevented by the rectification of the EMG signal prior to correlation, although some postspike effects, particularly the stronger ones, can be detected in averages of unrectified EMG (Botteron and Cheney 1989). The duration of the average is usually chosen so as to indicate a reasonable prespike period which allows measurement of the level of EMG activity before cell discharge, and a postspike period which is long enough to detect

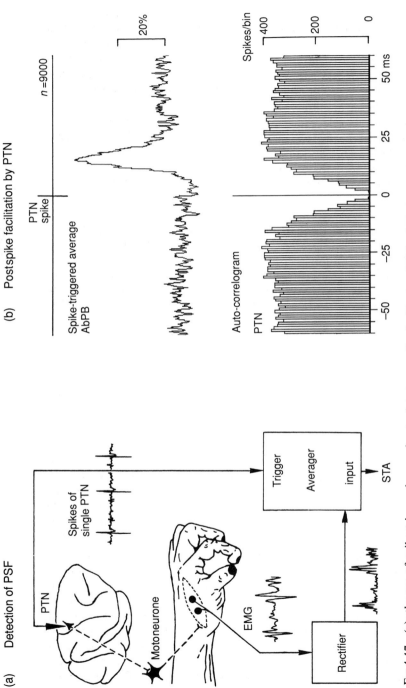

FIG 4.17 (a): the use of spike-triggered averaging to detect postspike facilitation (PSF) of EMG recorded from monkey hand muscles. The putative cortico-motoneuronal connection from a single pyramidal tract neurone (PTN) to the motoneurones of the muscle is indicated by a dashed line. EMG is rectified and averaged with respect to PTN spikes. (b): example of PSF produced in spike-triggered average (STA) of EMG from a thumb muscle (AbPB) by 9000 PTN spikes. Vertical scale indicates 20 per cent modulation of background EMG level. PTN discharge is at time zero. Auto-correlogram of the PTN spikes is shown below. (Lemon, unpublished observations.)

all short latency (< 50 ms) postspike effects. As Fig. 4.17a suggests, the discharge of a cortical neurone with excitatory synaptic influences upon motoneurones should result in an increased probability of motoneuronal discharge time-locked to the moment of cortical cell discharge. The strength of this synaptic input is undoubtedly small in relation to total synaptic drive to the target motoneurone, and therefore the probability of motoneuronal discharge being caused by the EPSP originating from the cortical cell is low; estimates are provided below (see Section 4.13). For this reason the EMG has usually to be averaged with respect to a large number of spikes before any clear excitatory response, the postspike facilitation (PSF), can be detected in the average. The probabilistic nature of the excitatory connection can be observed in the accumulating average as small, irregular increases in the PSF peak.

An example of PSF of an intrinsic hand muscle, abductor pollicis brevis (AbPB) by a PTN is shown in Fig. 4.17b. It commences at about 10 ms after PTN discharge and the principal peak of the facilitation lasts for about 12 ms. The peak of the PSF represents a 40 per cent modulation of the background EMG activity. The autocorrelogram of the PTN is also shown. Note the absence of any periodicity in its discharge; this argues against the PSF being the result of synchrony of the triggering CM cell with other unidentified units (see below).

4.11.2 The cortico-motoneuronal origin of postspike facilitation

There is a substantial body of evidence to suggest that these strong PSF effects are mediated by the direct cortico-motoneuronal projections. This evidence concerns the latency, duration, and amplitude of PSF, and the general lack of postspike facilitation from neurones lacking direct, monosynaptic connections.

The *latency* of PSF is consistent with the estimated conduction time over the cortico-motoneuronal pathway (Fetz and Cheney 1980; Lemon *et al.* 1986); the latency data for PSF produced by cortical cells in muscles of the monkey's hand and forearm is shown in Table 4.1. The clearest demonstration of the monosynaptic origin of these effects has been demonstrated directly by use of the cross-correlation technique (see Kirkwood 1979) to look for the influence of discharges from a single cortico-motoneuronal cell upon activity of a single motor unit recorded from an intrinsic hand muscle during performance of a precision grip task between the thumb and index finger (see Lemon *et al.* 1986). In most cases, as will be described below, the cross-correlogram peaks generated were brief (< 2.5 ms half-width) and suggestive of a monosynaptic rather than an oligosynaptic influence. Moreover, the onset latency found in the cross-correlations of 16 single cortico-motoneuronal cells with single motor units was slightly longer than that produced in the same motor unit by weak stimulation of the medullary

TABLE 4.1 Characteristics of cortico-motoneuronal facilitation in macaque monkey.

Muscle group	No. PSFs	Latency		Rise time (ms)	Duration (ms)	Amplitude (% mod.)
		Onset (ms)	Peak (ms)			
Precision grip task* n = 91 'fast' CM cells, 5 monkeys						
Intrinsic hand	168	11.3	16.1	4.8	15.3	12.3
Forearm	35	9.5	14.2	4.7	14.0	9.1
Wrist flexion–extension task† n = 49 CM cells						
Forearm	134	6.3	8.6	2.3	5.2	7.0

Sources: * Lemon *et al.* 1986, 1991 † Kasser and Cheney 1985

pyramidal tract, which is known to produce monosynaptic EPSPs in every hand motoneurone in the monkey (Fritz *et al.* 1985; Lemon 1990). It is therefore reasonable to suggest that the earliest peak in the poststimulus time histogram for pyramidal tract stimulation is derived from activation of cortico-motoneuronal synapses. The mean difference in latency between these peaks and those seen in the CM cell-motor unit cross-correlograms was 1.12 ms $\pm$ 0.53 ($n = 33$ CM cell-motor unit pairs), and in most cases (24/33) this extra delay was exactly equal to the conduction time from cortex to medulla for the PTN in question (antidromic latencies were typically 0.6–1.4 ms for most PTNs in this study) (Lemon, Werner and Mantel, unpublished observations). The results are shown in Fig. 4.18. Further evidence has been provided by non-invasive magnetic stimulation of the motor cortex in the conscious monkey, a procedure which is known to directly excite corticospinal neurones at the level of the cortex. Responses elicited by this technique were identical in latency to those found in STA from cortico-motoneuronal cells recorded in the same monkey (Edgley *et al.* 1990).

Further evidence comes from the observation that PTNs with rapidly conducting axons generate PSF with shorter latencies than do those with slow axons, as might be predicted from the longer central conduction time for the slow PTNs (see Fig. 4.22). In two monkeys investigated by Lemon *et al.* (1991), PSF onset latency in the intrinsic hand muscles was 11.6 ms (SD $\pm$ 1.6 ms), compared to 15.1 ms (SD $\pm$ 2.1 ms) for the slow PTNs. As might be expected, a given CM cell generates PSF in forearm muscles at shorter latencies than in the more distal intrinsic hand muscles (Table 4.1 and Fig. 4.19; see Lemon *et al.* 1986).

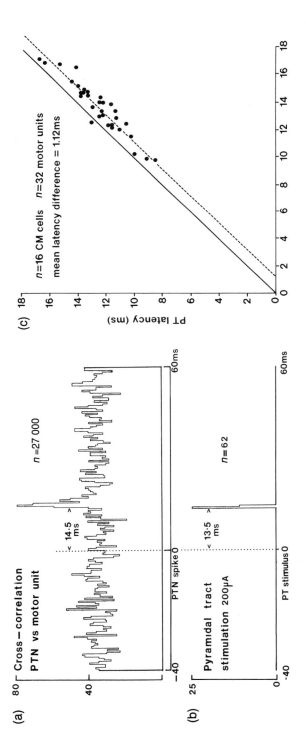

FIG 4.18 Evidence for the cortico-motoneuronal origin of postspike effects of PTN activity on discharges from single motor units recorded from hand and forearm muscles during performance of a precision grip task in the monkey. (a): Cross-correlation of activity in a single motor unit referenced to 27 000 spontaneous discharges from a PTN, which discharged at time zero. After correction for trigger pulse delays, the onset latency for the postspike peak was 14.5 ms. This represents the conduction delay from cortex to motor unit. (b): Response of the same motor unit to stimulation of the pyramidal tract at time zero (single pulse of duration 0.2 ms and strength 200 μA). Since all hand motoneurones receive a CM–EPSP from the pyramid, it is likely that the latency of this response (13.5 ms) is a reliable measure of the minimum conduction delay in the cortico-motoneuronal pathway from pyramid to motor unit. The difference (14.5–13.5 = 1.0 ms) is exactly equal to the conduction time from cortex to pyramid for this PTN; this was determined from the antidromic latency of this PTN. (c): Plot of cross-correlogram onset latency (abscissa) versus PT latency (ordinate) for 32 CM cell–motor unit pairs investigated in this way. The mean latency difference was 1.12 ms (indicated by dotted line). (Lemon, Werner, and Mantel, unpublished observations.)

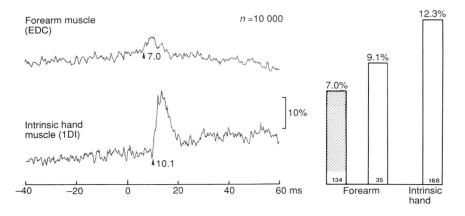

FIG 4.19   Postspike facilitation of EMG recorded from a long forearm muscle (extensor digitorum communis, EDC) and from an intrinsic hand muscle (1st dorsal interosseous, 1DI) by the same CM cell. Note the longer latency (arrowed) and larger peak amplitude of the PSF in 1DI. Scale indicates 10 per cent peak modulation of background EMG for both averages (Bennett and Lemon, unpublished). The bars on the right indicate the mean peak amplitude of PSF in forearm and intrinsic hand muscles for CM cells sampled during the precision grip task (open bars; Lemon *et al.* 1986, 1991) and during a wrist flexion/extension task (hatched bar; Kasser and Cheney 1985). Amplitude expressed as percentage modulation of background EMG. Numbers within bars indicate numbers of STAs upon which these data are based. (see also Table 4.1.)

The *amplitude and duration* of PSF is also consistent with what is now known about the unitary EPSPs at the cortico-motoneuronal synapse. This point will be taken up again later (see Section 4.13). Finally, in experiments in which PTNs can be identified unequivocally by antidromic invasion from correctly positioned stimulating electrodes in the pyramidal tract, it is rare to find any postspike effects from unidentified neurones, i.e. from presumed 'non PTNs'. Of 62 postcentral neurones recorded in areas 3a, 3b, 1, and 2, some of which may have been corticospinal, only one area 3a neurone produced a PSF (Widener and Cheney 1988 and personal communication), a finding consistent with the anatomical evidence that few postcentral PTNs terminate in the ventral horn (Kuypers 1981; Ralston and Ralston 1985). Postspike facilitation of forelimb muscle activity by motor cortex PTNs has not been observed in the cat (Armstrong and Drew 1984b), where cortico-motoneuronal connections are sparse or absent (see Section 2.9).

We can conclude that the fast-rising component of the PSF peak does result from cortico-motoneuronal excitation. The term 'cortico-motoneuronal' has thus been used to describe cortical cells which produce

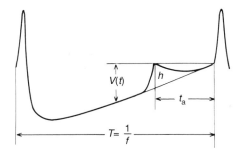

First-order correlation: $P_1(M|C)=f(EPSP)$

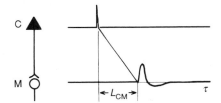

Second-order correlation: $P_2(M|C)=P_1(M|A) \otimes P_1(A|C)$

Serial   Collateral

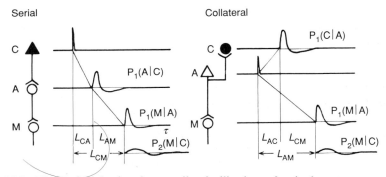

FIG 4.20 Theoretical basis of postspike facilitation of spinal motoneurones by cortico-motoneuronal cells. Top: schematic representation of EPSP superimposed on membrane potential of active motoneurone. T, interval between action potentials; $V(t)$, difference between membrane potential and threshold; h, height of EPSP peak; t_a time during which EPSP may trigger motoneurone action potential. Bottom: connections between cells which could potentially contribute to correlations between a cortical cell C, and a motoneurone, M. The first-order correlation, produced by a direct CM connection, is indicated as a peak occurring at latency L_{CM} after the cortical spike. Second-order correlations are mediated by a third neurone, A, which contacts the motoneurone and receives input from C (serial circuit) or sends a collateral to C (collateral circuit). Diagrams at right illustrate expected first- and second-order correlation peaks and their relative onset latencies. (Reproduced with permission from Fetz and Cheney (1980).)

brief PSF at an appropriate latency. This convention will also be used in this book; it is, of course, used in a correlative rather than in a neuro-anatomical sense.

Some postspike effects are not monosynaptic in origin, and these include the postspike suppression (PSS) of EMG activity, which has a longer latency than PSF and which is presumed to be disynaptic in the monkey (Cheney *et al.* 1985; Jankowska *et al.* 1976; see Section 4.17). PSF has been obtained in wrist and digit muscles by Mewes and Cheney (1990) from thalamic neurones. As indicated in Fig. 4.20, the second-order correlation, whether by way of serial or collateral connections, is much weaker than for a monosynaptic connection. In these cases, one must suppose that the inherent weakness of the second-order correlation (i.e. the requirement for successive discharges along the chain of connected neurones) is outweighed by other factors, such as the divergence of the first-order neurone (see Fetz and Cheney 1980). Thus PSS might be readily detectable in an average because the triggering PTN made contact with inhibitory interneurones with widespread inhibitory connections within the motoneuronal pool of the muscle whose activity was suppressed.

Some PSFs show two clear components, a brief, principal component and a broader 'skirt' on either side of the principal peak. These components have also been recognized in other descending systems. In the cat, Davies *et al.* (1985) cross-correlated activity in inspiratory bulbospinal neurones with that of inspiratory motoneurones. They described both 'narrow' peaks (<1.1 ms half-width) and broader, 'medium-width' peaks (2–5 ms half-width). The narrow peaks were all consistent with monosynaptic bulbospinal action, while some of the broader peaks, which had latencies too short to be consistent with the conduction time in the bulbospinal axon, were best explained by synchrony between a number of bulbospinal neurones. Thus the 'skirt' in the STA of forelimb muscles probably reflects the presence of synchrony between the triggering cortico-motoneuronal cell and other cortical neurones, including other cortico-motoneuronal cells (Smith and Fetz 1989; see Section 2.1). Although the unrealistically early onset of some PSFs can be explained in this way, the strength of synchrony between spontaneously discharging cortical pyramidal tract neurones is relatively weak, as shown by direct cross-correlation of neighbouring neurones (see Section 2.1) and theoretical calculations show that it would require a large population of cortical neurones to show short-term synchrony with each other for this to produce the effects observed in the broader STAs (Abeles 1991, pp. 109). Hence synchrony does not contribute substantially to the main PSF peak generated by cortico-motoneuronal cells. A clear example of this is shown in Fig. 4.21, which demonstrates that synchrony between two neurones does not lead necessarily to postspike effects from both cells. Synchrony between cortical cells, including that associated with low-frequency oscillation, does not therefore question PSF

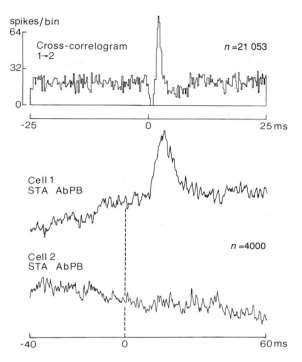

FIG 4.21   Test for the significance of synchronization between motor cortex neurones on the production of PSF. Records were made from two motor cortex neurones via the same microelectrode; one of them (Cell 1) was identified as a PTN (see also Fig. 2.5, p. 46). The cross-correlogram indicates a peak in the activity of Cell 2 1–2 ms after discharge of Cell 1 at time zero. When 4000 spikes had been averaged, Cell 1 showed a clear PSF in the STA of AbPB. But despite the strong synchronization between the two cells, no PSF was observed in AbPB with Cell 2. (Reproduced with permission from Lemon (1990).)

as a genuine spike-related event (Smith and Fetz 1989; Lemon 1990). Widespread synchrony might be expected to increase greatly the probability of recording from neurones exerting postspike effects. But in fact the yield is low (see below).

The signal-to-noise ratio of the PSF is dependent on the numbers of cortical spike events used to generate the average, and this improves in relation to the square root of the spike event count. Unequivocal postspike facilitation of muscles by cortico-motoneuronal cells can be observed with as few as 50 spike events (Bennett and Lemon, unpublished), but generally a minimum of 2000 spike events has been adopted. Much larger numbers have been sampled to prove that *no* postspike modulation of the EMG is present. The reproducibility of the PSF can be established by showing that it is present throughout the period of recording of a cell/muscle pair. This is done by dividing the total data available into different epochs of 2000–4000 spikes and averaging the STAs from each epoch (Lemon *et al.* 1986).

It is important to stress the causal nature of the PSF; this method can establish that a cortico-motoneuronal cell actually generates activity in the target muscles. This is quite different to methods of analysis which allow one to establish the close temporal association between the discharge of a cortical cell with movement performance or EMG activity, but do not infer a causal relationship between them (Fetz *et al.* 1989; Lemon 1990; Houk *et al.* 1987). However, both approaches are required to establish the synaptic linkage between a cortico-motoneuronal cell and the functional employment of this linkage during movement performance.

4.11.3 The proportion of motor cortex neurones producing postspike effects

In the initial studies the proportion of cortical neurones producing these effects was extremely difficult to estimate because of the selective nature of the sampling of discharges of neurones. Fetz and Cheney (1980) examined 370 motor cortex neurones discharging during a wrist flexion-extension task; 27 per cent of these cells produced clear PSF in at least one of the wrist flexor or extensor muscles studied. But the yield from neurones identified as PTNs was substantially higher at 55 per cent.

In their study, Lemon *et al.* (1986) attempted to increase the yield of such neurones by selecting neurones to examine for STA on the basis of four criteria. These were:

(1) location: within the hand region of area 4, often deep within the rostral bank of the central sulcus;

(2) microstimulation: neurones were selected if they were found at loci which yielded movements of the digits with low ICMS currents ($< 10\,\mu$A);

(3) Pyramidal tract neurones (PTNs): most selected neurones were fast PTNs (antidromic latency from the pyramid 0.7–2.0 ms, conduction velocity estimated at 30–100 ms^{-1});

(4) Task relationship: neurones were selected if their activity was deeply modulated during the precision grip task which was performed by the monkeys.

The yield of neurones showing clear PSFs was much higher when all criteria were satisfied (44/60 PTNs or 73 per cent) than for unselected neurones (14/45 or 31 per cent). In a more recent study (Bennett, Flament and Lemon, unpublished) area 4 of both hemispheres in a M. nemestrina monkey was studied. 143 PTNs were recorded for which it was possible to construct STAs of EMG from 6 to 8 hand and forearm muscles with a minimum of 2000 PTN spikes. Of these 143 PTNs, 106 were fast PTNs (antidromic latency <2.0 ms) and of these 56 (53 per cent) were positively identified as cortico-motoneuronal cells.

We can conclude that the proportion of cortical output neurones which are cortico-motoneuronal cells is small. Sampling difficulties preclude an accurate estimate. Although approximately half of the fast PTNs, and a smaller proportion of slow PTNs (see below), may be cortico-motoneuronal cells, the PTNs themselves probably represent only about 10–20 per cent of the layer V output neurones (see Section 2.1). Against this it must be remembered that their discharge probably results from activity in many thousands of other neurones, both locally and including those located in the cerebellum, basal ganglia, and other cortical areas without direct projections to the spinal cord. The significance of these PTNs and cortico-motoneuronal cells in relation to the activation of specific motor units in the movement task is therefore probably out of all proportion to their modest number.

4.11.4 Postspike facilitation from both slow and fast PTNs

In 1953, Bishop *et al.* first distinguished 'fast' and 'slow' PTNs, with rapidly and slowly conducting axons. There is strong evidence for important functional differences between these classes of PTN (see Chapter 5). In general, the suggestion has been that since animals, such as the rat, with only slowly conducting corticospinal fibres, possess few, if any, CM contacts, then 'slow' PTNs in the primate will also lack this type of connection (see Section 2.9). In the primate, electrophysiological evidence for slowly conducting corticospinal fibres giving rise to monosynaptic inputs to motoneurones is difficult to obtain because it is impossible to assess the segmental delay of such effects. In the case of the large fibres, a monosynaptic action of volleys excited in the corticospinal tract by cortical or pyramidal tract stimulation could be determined by measuring the delay between the arrival of the *earliest* volley at the spinal segment in which the motoneurone is located and the onset of the EPSP, recorded intracellularly from the moto-neurone (Phillips and Porter 1977, p. 144–147). This approach is impracticable for the slower fibres for three reasons:

(1) the dispersion of their action potentials (due to variation in their conduction velocities) makes it difficult to detect any synchronous volley representative of such a fibre population within the corticospinal tract;

(2) the resultant temporal dispersion of postsynaptic action means that no late, compound EPSP can be detected in the motoneuronal record;

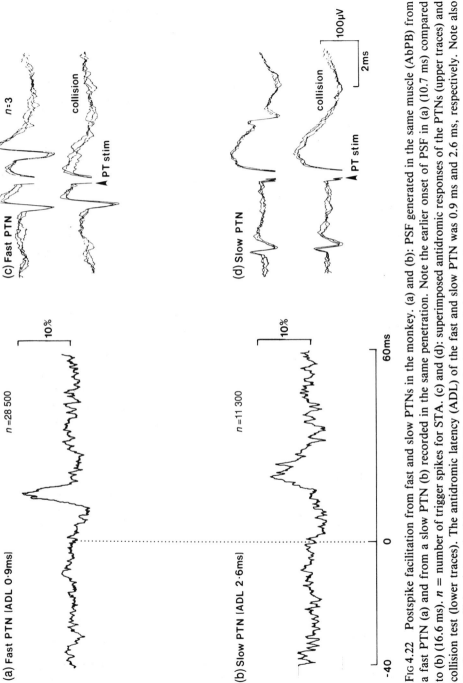

FIG 4.22 Postspike facilitation from fast and slow PTNs in the monkey. (a) and (b): PSF generated in the same muscle (AbPB) from a fast PTN (a) and from a slow PTN (b) recorded in the same penetration. Note the earlier onset of PSF in (a) (10.7 ms) compared to (b) (16.6 ms). $n =$ number of trigger spikes for STA. (c) and (d): superimposed antidromic responses of the PTNs (upper traces) and collision test (lower traces). The antidromic latency (ADL) of the fast and slow PTN was 0.9 ms and 2.6 ms, respectively. Note also the longer collision interval of the slow PTN. (Reproduced with permission from Lemon et al. (1991).)

(3) these late EPSPs may be masked by the earlier EPSPs and IPSPs originating in the faster fibres.

One solution to this problem is the application of spike-triggered averaging to the population of 'slow' PTNs. Fetz and Cheney (1980) and Lemon *et al.* (1986) both reported that slow PTNs gave rise to postspike facilitation. Lemon *et al.* (1991, 1993) re-investigated this problem making STAs from both slow and fast PTNs located within the hand region of area 4. The frequency of occurrence of PSF from fast and slow PTNs was compared. PTNs were categorized as 'fast' or 'slow' on the basis of their antidromic latency from the rostral part of the medullary pyramid. 'Fast' and 'slow' PTNs had latencies of shorter or longer than 2.0 ms, respectively. This boundary value corresponds approximately to an axonal conduction velocity of $30 \, \text{m.s}^{-1}$ (Lemon *et al.* 1986). PSF produced by a fast and by a slow PTN recorded in the same microelectrode penetration upon the same target muscle (AbPB) is shown in Fig. 4.22. The fast PTN had an antidromic latency of 0.9 ms from the medullary pyramid (Fig. 4.22(c)), compared to 2.6 ms for the slow PTN (Fig. 4.22(d)). The PSF amplitude is about the same in each case. Note the later onset and longer duration of the PSF produced by the slow PTN.

The results from 270 fast and slow PTNs recorded in three monkeys are shown in Table 4.2. In all three monkeys, PSF generated by fast PTNs was more common (mean 54 per cent) than for slow PTNs (30 per cent). No differences were found in the proportion of sampled muscles facilitated by the two types of PTN. Table 4.2 also gives the mean peak amplitude of the PSF in the muscle receiving the strongest facilitation from each PTN and shows that fast PTNs exert stronger facilitation than do slow (13.3 vs 6.9 per cent). In conclusion, slow PTNs do produce postspike facilitation,

TABLE 4.2 Postspike facilitation from fast and slow PTNs.

	Fast			Slow		
	PTNs	CM	PSF size	PTNs	CM	PSF size
Monkey T20	44	35(80%)	12.8% (±6.9)	8	2(25%)	8.0%
Monkey E23	66	25(38%)	10.6% (±8.7)	9	3(33%)	7.0%
Monkey D24	106	56(53%)	14.7% (±10.6)	37	11(30%)	6.7% (±3.9)
Totals	216	116(54%)	13.3% (±8.7)	54	16(30%)	6.9% (±3.9)

PTN: pyramidal tract neurone; CM: cortico-motoneuronal cell (data from Lemon *et al.* (1993)

and some of these neurones should be considered as part of the cortico-motoneuronal system.

4.12 EVIDENCE FROM SPIKE-TRIGGERED AVERAGING FOR
DIVERGENCE OF CORTICO-MOTONEURONAL COLLATERALS IN
THE MONKEY

4.12.1 Postspike facilitation of multiple muscles: muscle fields of CM cells

One of the most important contributions of the STA technique has been to demonstrate that single cortico-motoneuronal cells can excite moto-neurones supplying different groups of muscles. The divergence of axon collaterals within the spinal grey matter, described in section 4.10 above, is the most likely explanation for this phenomenon. The STA technique allowed Fetz and Cheney (1980) to define, as the 'muscle field' of a cor-ticospinal projection neurone, the group of muscles facilitated by a single cortico-motoneuronal cell. They studied 100 cortico-motoneuronal cells, selected on the basis of their discharge during either wrist flexion or exten-sion, which showed moderate to strong PSF of wrist flexor or extensor muscles, respectively. After exclusion of any redundant EMG recordings (those in which there was evidence for significant cross-talk from one pair of electrodes to another), they found that 67 per cent of their cortico-motoneuronal cells contacted more than 2 of the 5–6 different muscles sampled, and that the mean number of muscles facilitated per cortico-motoneuronal cell was 2.4. The divergence was greater for extensor related cortico-motoneuronal cells which facilitated a mean of 2.5 muscles (of the 5–6 sampled); the flexor related cells facilitated a mean of 2.1 muscles.

In a subsequent study employing the same task, Kasser and Cheney (1985) found a rather similar value of 3.0 muscles per cortico-motoneuronal cell, this representing half of the six flexor or six extensor muscles sampled

TABLE 4.3 Macaque CM cell branching: patterns of facilitation of different muscles.

Mean no. of muscles/CM cell	% of recorded muscles showing PSF
Precision grip task*	
1.9	27.5
Wrist flexion–extension task[+]	
3.0	50.0

* 80 CM cells, 151 PSFs, mean 7.2 muscles sampled with each cell, Lemon *et al.* (1991).
[+] 49 CM cells, 134 PSFs, Kasser and Cheney (1985)

in their experiments (Table 4.3). The proportion of task-related cortico-motoneuronal cells showing clear PSF in flexor and extensor muscles is shown in Fig. 4.23 from Fetz *et al.* (1989). The majority of CM neurones (59 per cent) produced pure facilitation of either an agonist or antagonist, and cofacilitation of both was extremely rare. The second most common pattern (30 per cent of CM cells) was facilitation of agonists and postspike suppression of antagonists.

The branching of those cortico-motoneuronal axons which facilitate the intrinsic hand muscles appears to be somewhat less than of those producing PSF in forearm muscles. Lemon *et al.* (1991) studied a population of 80 cortico-motoneuronal cells which were active during the performance of the precision grip task. This task involved the co-operation of a large number of hand and forearm muscles, but the activity of each of the cortico-motoneuronal cells tested was co-activated with each of the muscles sampled during at least one phase of the task. The distribution of PSF from three different cortico-motoneuronal cells is illustrated for a range of hand

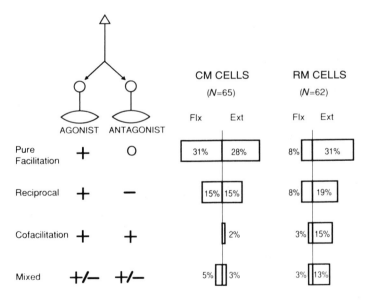

FIG 4.23 Projection of cortico-motoneuronal (CM) and rubro-motoneuronal (RM) cells in the monkey. The postspike effects on co-activated agonist wrist muscles and their antagonists include facilitation (+), suppression (−), or no effect (0). The mixed category includes cells which facilitated and suppressed agonist muscles, and some 'pure suppression' cells. Note almost complete absence of CM cells which cofacilitate antagonists. The proportions of each type of projection pattern are given separately for cells which facilitated forearm flexor and extensor muscles. (Reproduced with permission from Fetz *et al.* (1989).)

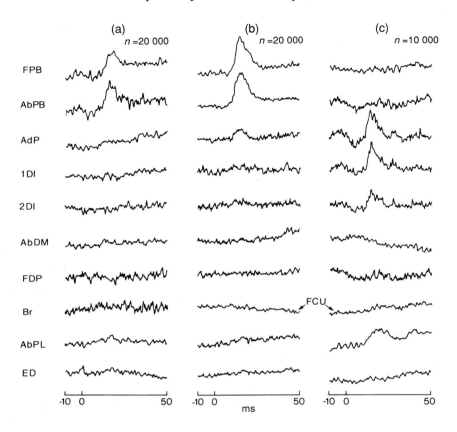

FIG 4.24 Distribution of PSF in STAs of ten different muscles recorded concurrently with three CM neurones, a, b, and c, during performance of precision grip in the monkey. Time zero in the STAs corresponds with the rising edge of the spike in the neurone. n = number of spike events used to construct the average; FPB, flexor pollicis brevis; AbPB, abductor pollicis brevis; AdP, adductor pollicis; 1DI, 2DI, 1st and 2nd dorsal interosseous; AbDM, abductor digiti minimi; FDP, flexor digitorum profundus; Br, brachioradialis; AbPL, abductor pollicis longus; EDC, extensor digitorum communis; FCU, flexor carpi ulnaris. Cell a produced PSF in 2/10, cell b in 3/10 and cell c in 4/10 sampled muscles. (Reproduced with permission from Buys *et al.* (1986).)

and forearm muscles co-operating in the task in Fig. 4.24. The 80 neurones were recorded with a sample of at least five hand and forearm muscles, the average being 7.2 (SD ± 1.8) muscles/cell. The majority of the recordings were from the intrinsic hand muscles (see Fig. 4.25).

Fig. 4.25(a) shows that for this population, each CM cell facilitated 20 per cent of the muscles with which it was sampled. This is the median value;

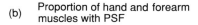

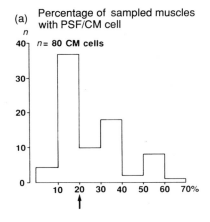

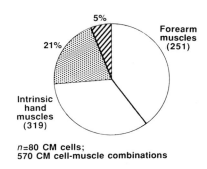

FIG 4.25   Branching of cortico-motoneuronal cells as indicated by the distribution of postspike effects amongst different forelimb muscles in the monkey. (a): Percentage of muscles sampled with a CM cell which showed clear PSF. Number of muscles in the sample varied from 5 to 10. For 80 CM cells the mean proportion of sampled muscles showing PSF was 27.5 per cent. The median value was 20 per cent (arrow) (b): proportion of the 570 CM cell-muscle STAs which showed PSF. Heavy dots indicate PSF in intrinsic hand muscles (319 STAs with 121 PSFs, 21 per cent of total) and hatching shows PSF in forearm muscles (251 STAs with 30 PSFs, 5 per cent of total). (Adapted from Lemon *et al.* (1991.))

the mean was 27.5 per cent (SD ± 15.4 per cent). The average number of muscles with PSF was 1.9 muscles/cell (Table 4.3). The range was from 10 per cent (1 of 10 muscles sampled) to 67 per cent (6 of 9). Only 9 cells (11 per cent) facilitated more than half the sampled muscles. Nineteen facilitated less than 15 per cent (PSF in one muscle only), and in 16 cases this muscle was an intrinsic hand muscle. Of the 14 most 'focused' cells, which facilitated only 1 of the 8 to 10 sampled muscles, 12 produced PSF in a single intrinsic hand muscle, and 6 of these were in a thumb muscle, suggesting a highly selective control of this important digit. As shown in Fig. 4.25(b), for this population of cells, PSF was much more common amongst the intrinsic hand muscles (121 of the 151 PSF effects seen, or 80 per cent) and was found more often than would have been expected from the proportion of CM cell-muscle pairs contributed by these muscles (319 of the 570 CM cell-muscle pairs investigated, or 56 per cent).

4.12.2 Branching within the motoneurone pool

The PSF peak in an average of a multi-unit EMG is contributed by the increased probability of discharge, in response to the arrival of the CM cell impulse, of different motor units within the target muscle (Lemon *et al.* 1986). A more precise picture of the branching of a single CM axon within the column of motoneurones supplying a single muscle can be assessed by performing a cross-correlation of activity in a CM cell and each of a number of different single motor units, recorded concurrently. Lemon *et al.* (1990) developed a technique for recording such units from hand muscles during precision grip. In most cases where a strong PSF effect was present in the multi-unit, surface recorded EMG of a muscle (as detected by STA, see Fig. 4.31), it was possible to detect clear peaks in the CM cell-motor unit correlograms. Most of these motor units were of the tonic or phasic-tonic type (Palmer and Fetz 1985a), and must have had quite low force thresholds, since the isometric forces exerted by the monkey's thumb and finger was generally less than 1 N. The distribution of effects was investigated for 13 cortico-motoneuronal (CM) cells recorded with a total of 44 discriminable motor units, with each cortical cell recorded with 2 to 7 different motor units. For 10 cells, all of the motor units tested showed a positive correlogram peak, and this included one CM cell which facilitated all 7 motor units recorded within the thumb muscle, AbPB (Lemon, Werner and Mantel, unpublished observations).

These findings suggest that CM cell axons branch to innervate many (if not all) motor units within the motor nucleus of its target muscle. This distributed pattern of organization probably reflects the rostrocaudal orientation of the CM axon collaterals described above (Lawrence *et al.* 1985), which would be ideally suited for contacting each of the motoneurones for a given muscle, since these motoneurones are organized in long narrow columns which may extend over two or three spinal segments (Sherrington 1898; Jenny and Inukai 1985; see Fig. 4.1). The finding is also consistent with the high probability of synaptic contact being made with all motoneurones exerting a defined distal action which must be deduced for a cortico-motoneuronal fibre which engages one of these motoneurones. Such a situation would explain the findings of Lawrence *et al.* (1985) in their small sample of cortico-motoneuronal contacts with intrinsic hand motoneurones referred to above.

The relative sizes of different motor units recorded simultaneously from the target muscle was assessed in these experiments by inspection of the motor unit-triggered average (MU-TA; Lemon *et al.* 1990). No consistent relationship was found between motor unit size assessed in this way and amplitude of the correlation peaks produced by a given CM cell, although there was a tendency for the smallest, tonically firing units to receive the strongest facilitation (Lemon, Werner, and Mantel, unpublished observations).

4.12.3 Functional significance of collateralization of CM axons

The widespread synaptic impacts made within the motor nucleus of a single muscle would allow a single CM cell to exert a facilitatory influence over many different motoneurones, and therefore to contribute to motoneuronal activity over a range of EMG and force levels. A similar distributed system of synaptic connections has also been observed for muscle spindle afferents (Mendell and Hennemann 1971).

The facilitation by a CM cell of different target muscles is potentially of great significance. In the monkey there are 29 muscles acting on the digits. Most of these are active during the precision grip task, and many are recruited in a highly fractionated fashion during the movement phase of the task (Muir 1985). Most CM cells facilitate a relatively restricted group of these muscles, and it seems quite possible that this focused pattern of facilitation contributes to the fractionation of muscle activity during precision finger movements. Because it has not been possible to sample all the muscles moving the fingers, we can only estimate the real proportion that would be facilitated by a single cortico-motoneuronal cell. In this respect it is interesting that Buys *et al.* (1986) found that the number of facilitated muscles rose together with the number of sampled muscles (suggesting facilitation of a relatively constant proportion of those sampled) until ten muscles were sampled, when the proportion fell. This effect was due to the increasing proportion of forearm muscles in the sample: compared to intrinsic hand muscles, PSF in forearm muscles is a relatively infrequent phenomenon for this population of CM cells (see Fig. 4.25(b)). This result suggested that sampling a greater number of muscles would not yield more facilitated muscles, and confirmed the relatively focused output of the CM cell population.

However, CM cells which facilitate single muscles are very much in the minority. We can conclude that the fundamental organizing principle of the cortico-motoneuronal output is one of influence over activity in multiple muscles. The low probability of occurrence of PSF makes it very difficult, on the basis of the samples obtained to date, to attribute any statistical significance to the frequency with which specific combinations of target muscles are found to be facilitated. Although the great majority of CM cells reported by Cheney *et al.* (1991) facilitated either flexors or extensors, they did not find evidence for CM cells facilitating any particular combinations of muscles within these agonist groups. Buys *et al.* (1986) found some interesting functional combinations in the muscle fields of their CM cells. Some of these combinations reflected the anatomical and functional relationship between the target muscles. For example, some cells influenced both first dorsal interosseous (1DI) and extensor digitorum communis (EDC) (Fig. 4.26(f)); both muscles are involved in extension of the

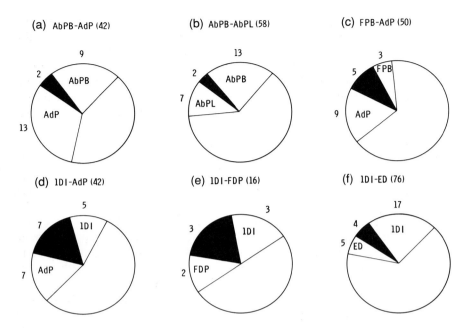

FIG 4.26   Distribution of PSF from monkey cortico-motoneuronal cells amongst different combinations ((a)–(f)) of hand and forearm muscles. The area of each circle indicates the total number of group CM neurones (numbers in parentheses) recorded concurrently with the pair of muscles indicated. The labelled segments show the proportion of these cells that produced PSF in each of these muscles, and the shaded area indicates the proportion producing facilitation in *both* muscles, which could be either anatomical synergists (e.g., FPB and AdP) or functional synergists (e.g. 1DI and AdP). Numbers of cells in each category are given adjacent to the appropriate segment. For abbreviations see legend Fig. 4.24. (Reproduced with permission from Buys *et al.* (1986).)

interphalangeal joints. Other CM cells had fields which reflected task-related synergies, such as the facilitation of both the 1DI and the thumb adductor, AdP. These muscles are two of the 'prime movers' within the intrinsic group of hand muscles employed in the production of precision grip. However, once again the small number of observations available means that only the combinations in Fig. 4.26(c), (d) are statistically significant, that is, they occur with a frequency greater than that predicted by a random connectivity of CM cells within the motoneurone pools of the sampled muscles.

What is the functional significance of the muscle field during movement? Bennett and Lemon (1991) demonstrated that for 6 CM cells which each facilitated two or more intrinsic hand muscles, CM cell activity paralleled the fractionation of activity amongst these muscles during the precision grip task. Most of the cells were preferentially active during periods when one target muscle was much more active than the other. For 5/6 cells, this preferential coupling to one of the cell's target muscles was with the muscle which received the strongest PSF from the cell. This muscle was also shown to receive an enhanced facilitation from the CM cell during these periods of fractionated activity. The specific recruitment of the CM cell during these periods suggests that the pattern of synaptic influence detected by the STA technique is of real significance for determining the relative levels of activity in different intrinsic hand muscles (Bennett 1992). If functional muscle synergies are expressed in terms of the synaptic weightings of CM cells, this might represent one means of reducing the very large number of possible muscle combinations with which the motor control system has to deal.

In man, Stephens and his colleagues have made extensive use of the cross-correlation technique to reveal synchronization of motor units in different limb muscles. They have collected a considerable amount of evidence to suggest that these synchronized units indicate the presence of branched inputs that are common to a given pair of motor units, and that an important source of these synchronized inputs is the corticospinal tract. Datta and Stephens (1990) found that, for the 1DI muscle, correlation of discharges recorded from pairs of motor units showed a narrow central peak of 1–6 ms for most pairs (see Fig. 4.27). Motor unit synchronization is common in muscles moving the fingers (Bremner *et al.* 1991a) although its amplitude shows considerable variation across subjects and across motor unit pairs, with the largest degree of synchrony observed between motor units having similar force thresholds. Datta and Stephens (1990) showed that the time course and amplitude of motor unit synchrony can be matched very precisely by a model which assumes simultaneous arrival of joint EPSPs from branched last-order inputs to the motoneurones supplying the synchronized motor units, as originally proposed by Sears and Stagg (1976). Depending on the average size of these unitary EPSPs, one can calculate the proportion of active inputs to motoneurones which are common to the motor unit pair, and the proportion will be greater for smaller EPSPs (50–100 per cent of inputs for a mean $50\,\mu\text{V}$ EPSP and 20–50 per cent for $100\,\mu\text{V}$ EPSP). Bremner *et al.* (1991a, b) showed that synchrony was also present between motor units recorded in different finger muscles, although it was generally weaker than that between units within the same muscle. Strength of synchrony fell off with distance between the digits moved by the respective motor units of the pair, being twice as strong for ring–middle finger pairs than for ring–index finger pairs. There were also consistent differences in the strength of synchrony between different functional 'compartments', for muscles abducting, extending, and flexing the index finger; flexor muscles showed the least synchrony. Assuming joint EPSPs of mean amplitude $100\,\mu\text{V}$, Bremner *et al.* (1991b) calculated that common inputs

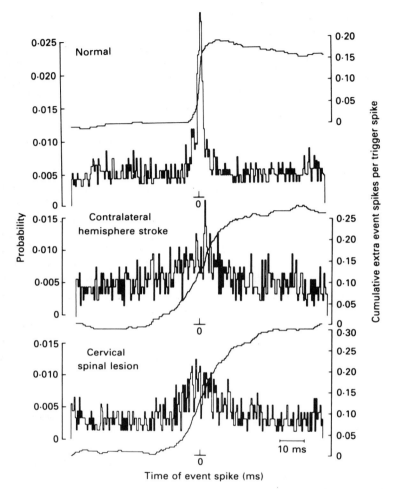

FIG 4.27 Synchronization of motor unit firing in human 1DI. Cross-correlogram of activity from a motor unit in 1DI with reference to 1000 discharges of a second unit recorded simultaneously from the same muscle during weak steady voluntary isometric abduction of the right index finger. Bin width 391 μs. Corresponding cumulative sum (CUSUM) analyses are also shown (scale on right). In all three panels, the reference or trigger motor unit was discharged at a steady discharge rate of 10 impulses per second by the subject. The top panel is from a normal subject, the middle panel from a patient with a contralateral cerebral hemisphere infarction, and the lower panel from a patient with a C7-T1 partial spinal lesion. Strength of synchronization is given by the height of the CUSUM between inflexions for the duration of synchronization and was 0.184, 0.250, and 0.2292 extra event (or sample) unit spikes per reference (or trigger) spikes for the top, middle, and lower panels, respectively. Note the replacement of the narrow short-term synchrony peak in the normal case with a much broader type of synchrony in the two pathological cases. (Reproduced with permission from Datta *et al.* (1991).)

to motor units in different muscles would account for between 8 and 52 per cent of the excitatory synaptic drive.

There are a large number of possible sources of common input to spinal motoneurones, including segmental afferent inputs from muscle spindles and other peripheral receptors. However, several lines of evidence suggest that, at least for hand muscle motoneurones, much of the short-term synchrony has a corticospinal origin. First, the observation that short-term synchrony is stronger in the intrinsic hand muscles than in more proximal limb muscles is incompatible with a synchrony having a peripheral afferent origin from muscle spindles, since spindles generally exert more powerful effects upon their homonymous motoneurones for proximal than for distal muscles (Datta *et al.* 1991). Second, synchrony was still observed in the hand muscles of a patient who was completely deafferented (Baker *et al.* 1988). Third, short-term synchrony is absent in the affected hand of patients with stroke or suffering spinal damage. Datta *et al.* (1991) found that the narrow central peaks in a sample of normal patients (mean duration 11.3 ms for 1DI motor unit pairs) were replaced by a broader peak in stroke patients (mean duration 35.4 ms). Finally, in a patient showing mirror movements associated with the Klippel–Feil syndrome, and in whom magnetic stimulation suggested that corticospinal axons branch to innervate motoneurones of homologous muscles on both sides, short-term synchrony was present between motor units recorded from the 1DI on both sides, a phenomenon never observed in normal subjects (Farmer *et al.* 1990; see Fig. 4.28).

4.13 THE POWER OF INDIVIDUAL CORTICO-MOTONEURONAL SYNAPSES

Cortico-motoneuronal synapses transmit information from the motor cortex to a large number of target motoneurones. Information about the excitatory strength of an individual CM synapse is essential to our understanding of how the spatial and temporal coding of activity within the CM system influences a given motoneurone. Two considerations which will be addressed later in this chapter are (1) the importance of convergence from many CM cells, which together make up the cortico-motoneuronal 'colony' of Phillips and Porter (1977, p. 155), upon a single motoneurone (Section 4.15), and (2) the transmission of precise patterns of impulse discharge activity from a CM cell to a target motoneurone (Section 4.16).

4.13.1 Evidence from Spike-triggered Averaging

If each cortico-motoneuronal axon establishes only one or a few synaptic contacts with each of the motoneurones to which its influence is directed, as the findings with intra-axonal HRP suggest for the motoneurones of

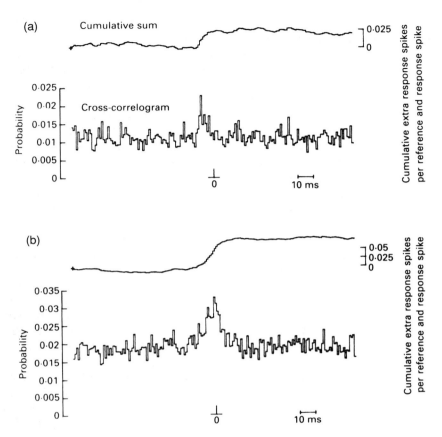

FIG 4.28   (a): Cross-correlogram and cumulative sum (CUSUM) constructed from motor unit recordings in a patient with Klippel–Feil syndrome and congenital mirror movements affecting the hands. Cross-correlation between the firing of two motor units recorded within the left 1DI muscle during a steady voluntary contraction. (b): One motor unit recorded from the right 1DI, the other from the left 1DI during steady voluntary contractions of both muscles. This type of correlation between activity in the two hands was never found in normal subjects. Number of reference spikes was 3614 in (a) and 4769 in (b). Bin width, 1 ms. (Reproduced with permission from Farmer *et al.* (1990b).)

the intrinsic muscles of the hand, the unitary synaptic contributions made by each cortico-motoneuronal fibre could be small (Lawrence *et al.* 1985). Asanuma *et al.* (1979) used STA of intracellularly recorded responses in monkey lumbar motoneurones, to seek the influences on them of the discharge of single pyramidal cells in the motor cortex which could be activated antidromically by very weak stimuli (5 μA or less) delivered in the vicinity of the motoneurone pool. They state (p. 83) that: 'Unitary EPSPs were evoked in one or two motoneurones by each of 5 PT neurones'. This again indicated divergence of CM influence within a motoneurone pool. They provide details for only two unitary EPSPs, resulting from spike-triggered averages of membrane potential changes following the discharge of a single PT neurone: these had average amplitudes of 25 μV and 120 μV. These findings are consistent with the fact that the majority of minimal cortico-motoneuronal EPSPs, evoked in lumbar motoneurones of the monkey by electrical stimulation of the cortex, were less than 200 μV in amplitude and their size ranged from 30 μV to 1.2 mV. Some of these EPSPs could have been due to the activation of a single CM axon (Porter and Hore 1969; Jankowska *et al.* 1975b). If the smaller EPSP reported by Asanuma *et al.* (1979), and the smaller values of the minimal EPSPs recorded by Porter and Hore, resulted from averaging of responses in which a proportion of failures of release occurred, the inference could be drawn that unit cortico-motoneuronal EPSPs, at least in anaesthetized monkeys, could have amplitudes similar in size to quantal Ia EPSPs in cat moto-neurones, producing about 100 μV at peak depolarization.

Spike-triggered averages of multi-unit EMG suggest that the discharges of a single CM cell can have a significant influence on motor unit activity. In the STA, all correlated discharges of the motor units which contribute to the EMG are summed within the average, although there may be some cancellation effects of their individual action potentials at the recording electrodes (Lemon *et al.* 1986). Two measurements of this modulation have been adopted. Either the peak of the PSF, or the area under it, is expressed as a percentage of the background level of EMG (Fig. 4.29). Both are measures of the strength of the PSF *relative* to the background EMG. A CUSUM of the average can be very useful for detecting weak postspike effects; a measure of the *absolute* size of the PSF can be given by the trough-to-peak height of the CUSUM (Bennett 1992).

There are some difficulties with making these measurements with any degree of precision. For instance, the estimate of background level can be complicated by the inherent 'noise' in the STA, and by non-stationarities in the average, which usually reflect task-related co-activation of both CM cell and motor unit (see Lemon *et al.* 1986, their Fig. 6). If the STA is made from spikes of a rapidly discharging cell with interspike intervals of 100 ms, the CM cell will contribute facilitation both to the PSF peak *and* the background, and for strong PSF, this may substantially affect the level of background, leading to a significant underestimate of the PSF peak amplitude (Lemon and Mantel 1989). A clear indication of this effect is the dip in the average that usually precedes a strong PSF (see Fig. 4.31, for example); this probably reflects the autocorrelogram of the triggering cell and results from the disfacilitation of the target motoneurones during the period between the trigger spike and the preceding spike from the same cell (Lemon and Mantel 1989).

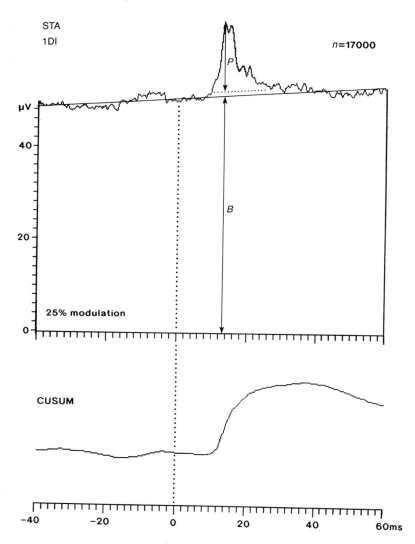

FIG 4.29 Measurement of the relative and absolute amplitude of postspike facilitation of rectified EMG activity by a monkey cortico-motoneuronal cell during precision grip. Above: STA of EMG recorded from the 1DI muscle with respect to all CM cell spikes (n = 17 000) recorded over a period of about 10 min. Cell discharge at time zero and dotted line. The average is scaled so as to include the baseline (zero volts) so as to give a true impression of the size of the PSF peak relative to background EMG. Peak ampitude (*P*) is measured to the mean background (*B*) voltage (full line) underneath the peak minus 1 SE of *B* (short dotted line). Percentage modulation = (*P/B*) × 100 per cent. Below: the cumulative sum (CUSUM) derived from the STA above. The amplitude of the CUSUM can be used as a measured of the absolute size of the PSF. (Bennett and Lemon, unpublished observations).

A further complication is that the amplitude of PSF in an average varies according to the level of EMG activity in the target muscle. Figure 4.30 shows an example of the changing size of PSF from STAs constructed from data recorded during the steady hold period of the precision grip task. Separate STAs were constructed from data selected according to the level of EMG activity: high, medium, and low. Both the relative and absolute size of the PSF varied with EMG level (Bennett 1992). Of 43 CM cell–muscle combinations tested, in 23/42 (55 per cent) of cases the relative size of PSF increased with EMG level. It decreased in 6/42 (14 per cent) cases and remained unchanged in 13 (31 per cent) cases. In a few instances no PSF could be detected at the lowest EMG level tested. These variations may reflect the different strength of synaptic connections made by a CM cell with different motoneurones recruited at different force levels (see Section 4.12).

Despite these uncertainties, the relative amplitude of the PSF can be a useful measure, because it does allow comparison of the postspike effects of the same cell upon different muscles. Most CM cells exert different strengths of facilitation upon the muscles constituting their muscle field (Fetz and Cheney 1980; Buys *et al.* 1986; Cheney *et al.* 1991; Lemon *et al.* 1991). For example, a single CM cell can exert effects ranging from 4 per cent to 54 per cent on different intrinsic hand muscles. Table 4.1 shows that, on average, CM cells sampled during the precision grip task produced larger PSF in intrinsic hand than in forearm muscles (mean peak amplitude of PSF was 12.3 per cent and 9.1 per cent, respectively). A comparison is shown in Fig. 4.19. In Table 4.1, the ten largest PSFs in the intrinsic hand muscles ranged from 20 per cent to 42 per cent, and the mean amplitude of these PSFs (27.6 per cent) was twice as large as that for the ten largest PSFs in the forearm muscles (13.5 per cent, range 9 to 21 per cent). The mean size of PSF in forearm muscles (9.1 per cent) is similar to the value of 7.0 per cent given by Cheney *et al.* (1991) for PSF produced in wrist and digit muscles for CM neurones active during the wrist flexion/extension task.

For a given group of muscles, fast PTNs produce consistently larger PSF than do slow PTNs (Table 4.2). The mean amplitudes given are for the largest PSF effect observed for each PTN in the sample. Despite the number of fast PTNs in the sample, there was a large standard deviation for the amplitude of PSF produced by these PTNs, which results from the wide range of effects observed (4–54 per cent), whereas only a small range of weak effects was seen with the slow PTNs (4–15 per cent). Shinoda *et al.* (1986b) found no difference in the extent of branching of slow versus fast PTNs in the cat.

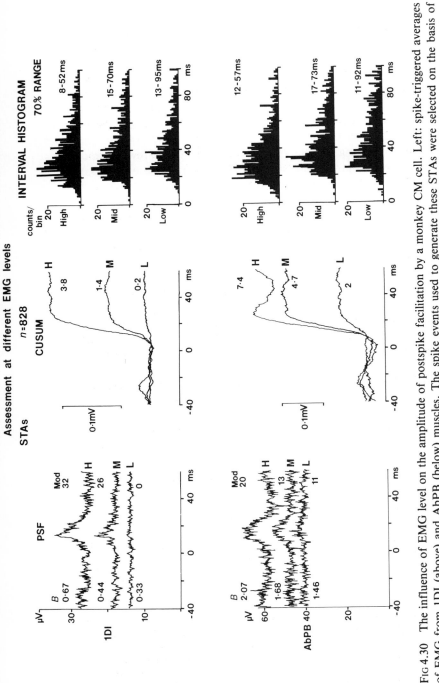

FIG 4.30 The influence of EMG level on the amplitude of postspike facilitation by a monkey CM cell. Left: spike-triggered averages of EMG from 1DI (above) and AbPB (below) muscles. The spike events used to generate these STAs were selected on the basis of the amplitude of the ongoing EMG level, recorded from each muscle during maintenance of a steady precision grip by the monkey. Spikes were divided into three groups: those associated with low (L), mid (M) and high (H) levels of EMG. The same number (828) of spikes contributed to each STA. In both muscles, the background EMG level in the STA (*B*) and the percentage modulation of the PSF (Mod) increased with EMG level. Values of *B* are given as a percentage of the peak recorded EMG. Middle: cumulative sums (CUSUMs) derived from the STA at each EMG level. The amplitude of the CUSUM increased with EMG. Right: interval histograms of CM cell activity. The range of intervals covering 70 per cent of the spikes in the histogram is given at the extreme right. Shorter

4.13.2 Evidence from cross-correlations between CM cells and single motor units

The amplitude of the individual EPSP generated by a CM cell in a single target motoneurone can be much more readily assessed from a cross-correlation than from an STA. Examples of correlograms are shown in Figs. 4.18 and 4.31 (Lemon, Werner, and Mantel, unpublished observations).

The correlation in Fig. 4.31 is between a fast PTN and a motor unit recorded from the contralateral thumb muscle, AbPB. Note the much higher discharge frequency of the PTN compared to its target motoneurone (modal interspike interval 27 ms and 68 ms, respectively). Most of the correlation peaks had narrow half-widths (<2.5 ms for 43/63 peaks; see Table 4.4), and their latency was consistent with monosynaptic activation by the CM cell (see Section 4.11). Nearly all of the motor units were recorded from intrinsic hand muscles, and most were in AbPB.

Table 4.4 summarizes the properties of the cross-correlation peaks. Three different measures of correlation peak amplitude are given: k, which measures the size of the single largest bin relative to the background firing rate of motor unit discharge; k', which compares the area of the whole peak to the background rate; and MPI (mean percentage increase) which averages the extra motor unit discharges in each of the bins above the background level and gives the average increase as a percentage of that level (Cope *et al.* 1987). The background level of motor discharge was assessed from periods of the correlogram remote from the postspike peak (e.g. the first 25 and last 25 ms of the correlogram shown in Fig. 4.31).

In keeping with the findings for PSF of multi-unit EMG activity, different CM cell–motor unit combinations exhibit a wide variation in efficiency of transmission. As shown in Table 4.4, the MPI in motor unit firing rate can vary between 8 per cent and 257 per cent of the background rate.

TABLE 4.4   The influence of CM cells on activity of single motor units.

Duration (half-width)	Correlation peak amplitude			Firing probability peak area ($\times 10^3$)
	k	k'	MPI	
2.6 ± 1.8 ms	2.3 ± 0.9	1.7 ± 0.5	64 ± 47%	89.4 ± 59.1
(0.5–8.6)	(1.3–4.7)	(1.1–3.6)	(8–257)	(16–218)
$n = 63$	$n = 63$	$n = 63$	$n = 63$	$n = 10$

All values are means ± SD, range given in brackets. Data from 4 monkeys, 27 CM cells, 52 single motor units (mostly in AbPB), 63 positive cross-correlations. Half-width: duration of correlation peak at half its peak amplitude; k, k', and MPI (mean % increase) are defined in the text. Peak area defines the number of additional motor unit discharges that occur per CM cell spike (data from Lemon, Werner, and Mantel, unpublished observations)

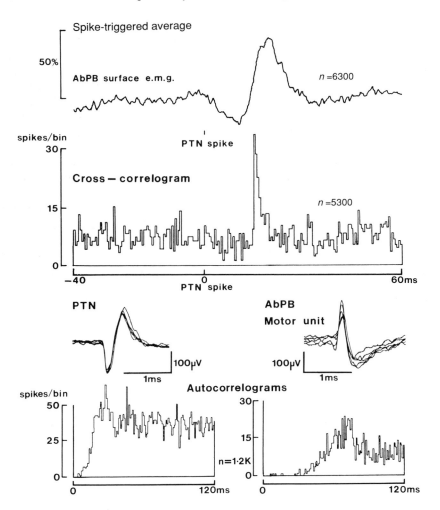

FIG 4.31 Direct facilitation of an intrinsic hand muscle motor unit by a PTN in the monkey. Top: Large PSF (>50 per cent) produced by a PTN in the STA of surface recorded EMG from the thumb abductor (AbPB). 6300 trigger spikes, PTN discharge at time zero. Middle: cross-correlogram of activity recorded from a single AbPB motor with respect to 5300 trigger spikes from the PTN, discharge again at time zero. Bin-width 0.5 ms. Note brief cross-correlation peak. Below: super-imposed plots of action potentials recorded from the PTN and motor unit, together with their respective auto-correlograms. Note the much higher firing rate in the PTN. All data recorded during precision grip. (From Lemon and Mantel, unpublished observations.)

However, for a given CM cell, the variation in its postspike effects upon each of its different target motoneurones was much smaller.

The measure k is identical to that used to measure the peak percentage modulation of postspike facilitation in an STA. For situations in which several motor units were recorded from the same muscle, the mean k value can be calculated to give an indication of the strength of the CM cell over the motoneurone pool as a whole. As shown in Fig. 4.32, there is generally a good agreement between this mean k value and the percentage modulation of the PSF, derived from the STA of surface recorded, multi-unit EMG from the same muscle. This indicates that larger PSF of multi-unit EMG generally reflects more powerful synaptic effects of the CM cell upon each target motoneurone.

The work of Fetz and Gustaffson (1983), Gustaffson and McCrea (1984) and Cope *et al.* (1987) has investigated the influence of individual EPSPs on motoneuronal firing rate in cat spinal motoneurones. This work has made it possible to estimate the size of the cortico-motoneuronal EPSP which underlies the effects observed in CM cell–motor unit cross-correlations. Assuming that the values derived by Cope *et al.* (1987) are indeed applicable for CM inputs to monkey motoneurones, the range of

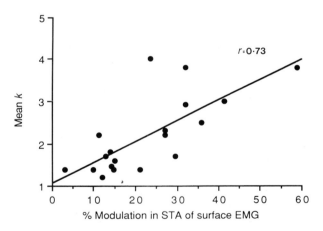

FIG 4.32 Relationship between strength of facilitation of single motor unit and of multi-unit EMG activity by single CM cells in the monkey. The strength of single motor unit facilitation was measured from the peak-to-baseline ratio (k) of the CM cell-motor unit cross correlation peaks for 19 CM cells, each recorded with 2 to 7 different motor units from the same muscle. The mean value of k for these different units was calculated and plotted (ordinate) against the percentage modulation of the PSF peak in the STA (abscissa) of surface EMG recorded from the muscle in which these units were located (AbPB, AdP, and 1DI). The regression line indicates that large PSFs are probably the reflection of large CM influences on each individual motor unit. (From Lemon, Werner, and Mantel, unpublished observations.)

MPI values shown in Table 4.4 would be produced by individual CM EPSPs ranging from 27 μV to 857 μV. The mean value would be 213 μV (MPI 64 per cent), and the ten largest effects would have been produced by a mean EPSP of 500 μV (MPI 150 per cent). These values are not inconsistent with the values referred to above which have been derived by other techniques. They also resemble the known values for unitary EPSPs produced in motoneurones by other segmental afferent and descending systems (Kirkwood and Sears 1978, 1982; Redman 1990).

The efficiency of transmission at the CM synapse can be calculated from the proportion of cortical spikes which give rise to discharge of the target motoneurone within the correlation peak (the 'peak area' of Cope *et al.* 1987). These data (see Table 4.4) were derived for 10 CM cell–motor unit pairs for which correlograms were constructed to exclude any periods in which the cell and the motor unit were not co-activated. The values given suggest that 1000 CM cell spikes will result in between 16 and 218 additional discharges of a steadily firing target motoneurone.

Cross-correlation of CM cell and motor unit activity has thus provided important clues regarding transmission at individual CM synapses, and confirms that some CM cells can exert a very powerful influence over their target motoneurones. It should be borne in mind that the data given in Table 4.4 are not fixed values for a given CM synapse. They represent the mean strength of correlation under the conditions prevailing at the time of the experiment. There is evidence to suggest that the size of the correlation peak will be affected by the firing rate of both the CM cell and its target motoneurone (Ellaway and Murphy 1985; Lemon and Mantel 1989). At present, these represent the best available data for CM transmission estimates with the firing rates of cells observed in the fully conscious animal.

4.14 CONVERGENCE OF CORTICO-MOTONEURONAL INFLUENCES ON TO SPINAL MOTONEURONES

4.14.1 Convergence upon monkey and baboon motoneurones

When a population of cortico-motoneuronal fibres is activated simultaneously, their unitary EPSPs sum in a receiving motoneurone to produce a compound cortico-motoneuronal EPSP akin to that produced in the motoneurone by electrical stimulation of group I afferents in its muscle nerve (Preston and Whitlock 1961; Landgren *et al.* 1962a). Such compound EPSPs could be graded in amplitude, but not significantly in latency or time-course, by modifying the strength of a single cortical shock to recruit different numbers of CM elements to this projection. The CM colony, all projecting unit cortico-motoneuronal EPSPs to the one motoneurone, was usually spread through a large territory on the cerebral cortex (Landgren *et al.* 1962b; Andersen *et al.* 1975; Jankowska *et al.* 1975a; see Chapter 8). All the members of the colony, in favourable circumstances, may be activated simultaneously by a maximal stimulus to the cerebral cortex or by stimulation of all the fibres in the pyramidal tract at the level of the medulla.

Such experiments revealed that not all motoneurones received the same maximal convergent compound EPSPs. For the baboon's forelimb, larger influences were exerted on motoneurones whose muscles acted about distal joints of the limb (Phillips and Porter 1964). Indeed, about half of the motoneurones supplying a proximally acting muscle like triceps brachii received no measurable monosynaptic excitation, even when large stimuli were applied to the cortex: some of these stimuli produced inhibitory potentials in the triceps motoneurones. Meanwhile, all motoneurones with axons supplying intrinsic muscles of the hand through the median nerve received cortico-motoneuronal EPSPs.

Clough *et al.* (1968) measured the maximal cortico-motoneuronal EPSPs in a large number of motoneurones identified by antidromic stimulation of forelimb nerves. The largest responses (of up to 5 mV of depolarization) were recorded in motoneurones supplying the intrinsic hand muscles and the long extensor of the fingers, extensor digitorum communis. Fritz *et al.* (1985) and Lemon (1990) confirmed these observations for 358 motoneurones identified as supplying different hand and arm muscles of the monkey. These authors measured the sizes of monosynaptic EPSPs in these motoneurones when they were produced by direct stimulation of the fibres passing through the pyramidal tract. In the latter case, the stimulating electrode tip was carefully positioned within the tract at the mid-medullary level so as to evoke a large volley in the rapidly conducting fibres in the dorsolateral funiculus. In these experiments the electrode was positioned so that this volley was maximal with a stimulating current of 200 μA. Control experiments revealed that no volleys, and no motoneuronal EPSPs, were evoked by delivering shocks of similar strength with the electrode tip positioned just dorsal to the pyramidal tract. A summary of the findings on the differential distribution of convergent cortico-motoneuronal connections is provided in Fig. 4.33. The mean amplitude of the monosynaptic EPSPs evoked by maximal pyramidal tract stimuli in these anaesthetized preparations was larger in motoneurones supplying the hand muscles (3.15 mV) than in those innervating forearm muscles supplied by the median (1.90 mV), ulnar (1.30 mV), and deep radial nerves (1.55 mV). The largest compound EPSP was in a second dorsal interosseous motoneurone and measured 7.5 mV. However, it was noticeable that a small number of intrinsic hand motoneurones received very small compound EPSPs (<500 μV). Biceps and triceps motoneurones received either a weak EPSP (<1 mV) or none at all.

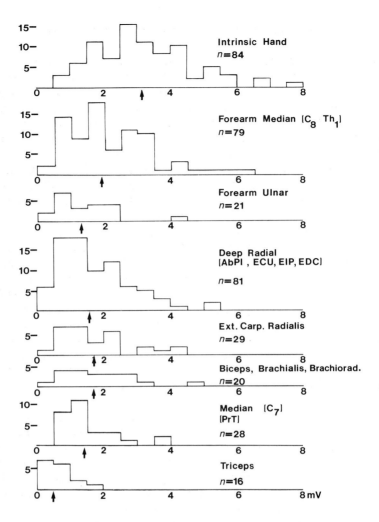

Monosynaptic EPSP Amplitude

[Pyr 200μA]

Fig 4.33 Amplitudes of monosynaptic cortico-motoneuronal EPSPs in different motoneurones in the lower cervical spinal cord of the monkey. EPSPs were evoked by a single stimulus delivered to the contralateral medullary pyramidal (Pyr) tract. The shock strength was 200 μA, which produced a near maximal fast descending volley in the lateral corticospinal tract. Monkeys were anaesthetised with chloralose and small doses of barbiturate. Recordings were made with citrate-filled glass micropipettes from motoneurones exhibiting antidromic potentials of at least 55 mV in amplitude. All motoneurones were identified antidromically from the nerves shown. Arrows indicate the mean CM EPSP amplitude for each group. Muscle abbreviations: AbPL, abductor pollicis longus; ECU, extensor carpi ulnaris; EIP, extensor indicis; EDC, extensor digitorum communis; PrT, pronator teres. (From work by Fritz, Illert, Kolb, Lemon, Muir, Weidemann, and Yamaguchi, and appearing in Lemon (1990). Reproduced with permission.)

Jankowska *et al.* (1975b) investigated the action of stimulating the leg area of the macaque motor cortex on PSPs recorded from leg and foot motoneurones. They found monosynaptic EPSPs in all motoneuronal groups investigated, supplying flexors and extensors and proximal as well as distal muscles. However, failure to evoke these EPSPs occurred much more often for motoneurones of proximal muscles (acting at the knee and hip) than for more distally acting muscles. These authors measured the amplitude of EPSPs in different motoneurones in response to a 0.5 mA surface anodal stimulating pulse. The largest EPSPs (mean 700 μV) were in motoneurones innervating intrinsic foot muscles, indicating a more extensive projection to these than to more proximal muscles.

All of the above refers only to the monosynaptic EPSPs recorded in response to the fastest component of the monkey's corticospinal tract, with a maximum conduction velocity of 60–72 m.s^{-1} (Phillips and Porter 1964; 1977, pp. 269–269; Edgley *et al.* 1990). As pointed out above (see Section 4.11), intracellular recording of compound responses to stimulation of large numbers of corticospinal fibres cannot be used to identify any cortico-motoneuronal action of slowly conducting fibres. In most of the recordings made by Fritz *et al.* (1985), the response to pyramidal stimulation was dominated by the monosynaptic EPSP and the large and long-lasting disynaptic IPSP that followed it. Even in motoneurones with no pronounced IPSPs, disynaptic EPSPs were rarely observed (see Fig. 4.37 and Section 4.6).

Although estimates of the magnitude of cortico-motoneuronal effects deduced from the size of postspike facilitation of EMG records in conscious animal experiments must be treated with caution, it is interesting to note that the variation in size of these postspike effects produced by single CM cells is generally consistent with the pattern described above: the largest PSF effects are detected in intrinsic hand muscles and PSF in wrist extensor muscles is stronger than that found in wrist flexors (Fetz and Cheney 1980). Finally, a brief report by Belhaj Saif *et al.* (1990) suggests that CM effects in biceps and triceps muscles is small (1–5 per cent modulation) or absent. It must be implied that the larger compound CM EPSPs that can be recorded in intrinsic hand motoneurones compared to forearm motor neurones may result from a combination of the larger colony (more CM cells) converging on a given motoneurone, and the stronger mean facilitation exerted by individual members of the colony (see Section 4.13).

Relatively few studies have addressed the important question of the convergence on to motoneurones of different sizes. In the cat, both fast and slow motoneurones are influenced by both fast and slow corticospinal inputs, and there is no correlation between the conduction velocity of a motoneurone's axon and the latency of the disynaptic corticospinal EPSP in it (Araki *et al.* 1976; Pellmar and Somjen 1977). Alstermark and Sasaki (1986) have shown that disynaptic pyramidal EPSPs in cat cervical

motoneurones were smaller in fast motoneurones than in slow motoneurones. A similar tendency was found for EDC motoneurones in the
baboon by Clough *et al.* (1968). More recently, Palmer and Fetz (1985a, b)
found that monkey forearm motor units of different response types
(phasic–tonic, tonic, ramp, etc.) could all be excited by single-pulse ICMS
in the motor cortex, but no clear evidence for a relationship between
response amplitude and motor unit type or size was found.

4.14.2 Convergence upon motoneurones in man

There is a parallel between these observations on the power of convergent
excitation from cortico-motoneuronal cells on to motoneurones in the
baboon and monkey and observations made in man using non-invasive
magnetic and electric stimulation of the brain to excite corticospinal
pathways. These studies have also clearly demonstrated a stronger facilitation of distal than of more proximal muscles. Motor units in hand
muscles typically respond at short-latency with a brief and powerful facilitation. It has been demonstrated that the first motor unit recruited voluntarily
is also the first unit to respond when the intensity of magnetic stimulation
is increased (Hess *et al.* 1987; Bawa and Lemon 1993). The earliest phase
of the facilitation occurs at latencies consistent with CM conduction (Day
et al. 1989). In theory, then, it should be possible to use non-invasive
stimulation to assess the convergence of CM input in man and to do this
in the absence of any synaptic depression that might be caused by the
anaesthetic agents employed in studies of the monkey and baboon.
However, there are technical problems that must be borne in mind when
interpreting results obtained with these new and exciting techniques. First,
both electrical and magnetic stimulation produce multiple repetitive
discharge of corticospinal neurones (Kernell and Wu 1967; Day *et al.* 1987,
1989; Edgley *et al.* 1990, 1992; Burke *et al.* 1990). These repetitive volleys
are sufficient to produce multiple firing of hand motoneurones and maximal motor twitches in hand muscles. In single motor unit studies it has proved possible to identify increased periods of motoneuronal discharge probability in association with the waves of descending discharge (Day
et al. 1989; Boniface *et al.* 1991). These appear as discernable subpeaks
within the short latency response peak revealed in a PSTH of a spontaneously firing motoneurone. But in studies of whole EMG the existence
of bursts of multiple corticospinal discharges makes it difficult to assess
the compound EPSP resulting from a single corticospinal volley. A second
problem is that it is difficult to be certain that the stimuli are exciting the
entire corticospinal output to a given muscle or motor unit, or that outputs
to different muscles are being equally well excited. With these considerations in mind, we shall review the evidence that has been accumulated
to date.

Palmer and Ashby (1992) examined the effects of magnetic stimulation on the poststimulus time histograms of repetitively discharging single motor units recorded from a number of upper limb muscles. In each of the subjects they investigated, they recorded the PSTH for at least one motor unit in the 1DI muscle in response to magnetic stimulation of the contralateral hemisphere. They calculated the number of additional discharges evoked by 1000 successive stimuli at an intensity which was just below that required to produce a clear twitch in the 1DI muscle. Responses of motor units recorded from other muscles to exactly the same stimulus intensity were normalized to the 1DI responses. Their results are summarized in Fig. 4.34. Responses in EDC were, on average, slightly smaller than in 1DI, whereas responsive biceps motor unit effects were only 37 per cent as strong as those in 1DI. Triceps and deltoid motor units tended to be rather unresponsive to magnetic stimulation (13/29 and 10/20, respectively), and some were inhibited, especially those motor units located in the long and lateral heads of triceps. For responses in 1DI motor units, the amplitude of the underlying, presumed cortico-motoneuronal EPSP was estimated at

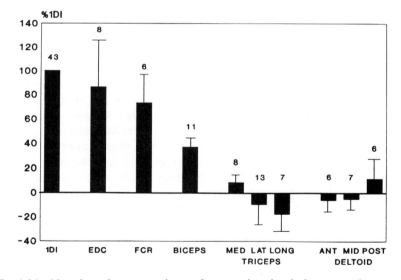

FIG 4.34 Net short latency actions of magnetic stimulation over the cortex on motoneurones of various upper limb muscles in man. The changes in firing probability (in extra or fewer counts per 1000 stimuli) have been normalized to the response obtained for motor units recorded in the 1DI muscle of the same subject and with the same intensity of stimulation. The means of these values are shown with the standard error of the mean. 1DI, EDC, and FCR received the strongest net facilitation. Short latency facilitation of motoneurones of more proximal muscles (such as biceps) was weaker. Motoneurones of some proximal muscles received no net facilitation. The number of motor units investigated is indicated at the top of each column. (Reproduced with permission from Palmer and Ashby (1992).)

2.9 mV (Palmer and Ashby 1992). However, this is probably an under-estimate, since it is unlikely that all of the CM colony converging on to the investigated motoneurone was excited in this experiment. Brouwer and Ashby (1990) showed that, even in relaxed subjects, strong magnetic stimuli can elicit responses in 1DI and EDC that had amplitudes around 25 per cent of the M wave elicited in the same muscles by direct stimulation of its nerve. Responses in biceps were small (1–2 per cent of M wave) and absent in triceps.

An important contribution of non-invasive studies in man has been the demonstration of corticospinal influence over muscle groups which have received little attention in the animal literature (see Rothwell *et al.* 1991). Thus, following brain stimulation, clear-cut facilitation of shoulder and intercostal muscles, of the diaphragm, and even of the large anal sphincter have been demonstrated (Merton *et al.* 1982; Gandevia and Rothwell 1987; Gandevia and Plassman 1988; Colebatch *et al.* 1990b). Evidence for the existence of connections which could provide an increasing influence of the corticospinal system in man, beyond that evident in monkeys, with control over proximal limb and trunk muscles, is also available from anatomical studies (see Section 2.9).

The comparative size of corticospinal influences over different muscles is certainly of very great interest. The approach used by Palmer and Ashby (1992), described above, investigated the effect of a submaximal volley on motor units of different muscles. But a proper comparison is difficult unless the entire corticospinal output to each different muscle can be excited. Day *et al.* (1989) and Colebatch *et al.* (1990b) applied strong electrical or magnetic stimuli and observed the discharge of motor units in a hand muscle (1DI), or in deltoid or in pectoralis major. Their results suggested equally powerful cortico-motoneuronal projections for 1DI and deltoid motoneurones. When subjects discharged a motor unit voluntarily at around 10 per second, then the PSTH revealed that both deltoid and 1DI motor units tended to respond at short-latency (at about 13 and 22 ms, respectively with anodal electrical stimuli) and with a very brief duration response peak (1–2 ms), which is strongly suggestive of monosynaptic action elicited by a single, highly synchronized corticospinal volley. As the stimulus was increased, the response probability of motor units in both muscles increased and then tended to saturate at around 50–55 per cent of stimuli. i.e., on average, the motor unit responded to every other stimulus. Following Ashby and Zilm (1982a), they assumed a membrane potential excursion of 10 mV between successive action potentials that returned linearly to threshold. With these assumptions, it can be calculated that the EPSP underlying the response probabilities of deltoid units must be 5.5 mV ($P = 0.55$) and 2.2 mV for pectoralis units ($P = 0.22$). These values compare with estimates of 3–5 mV for 1DI units recorded in previous studies (Day *et al.* 1989). All these estimates are based on the discharge probability of all the subpeaks within the short-latency response of the motoneurones.

Although the apparent saturation of effects certainly suggest that the entire cortico-motoneuronal projection to the motor units investigated was being excited, in practice it is difficult to be sure of this since at high stimulation strengths the large contraction evoked usually interferes with reliable recording of an individual motor unit. Indeed, in a more recent study, Bawa and Lemon (1993) demonstrated that the earliest subpeak in the post-stimulus response to magnetic stimulation of 1DI motor units could have probabilities of up to 0.61 and that of the whole peak, up to 1.0. It is unfortunate that Colebatch *et al.* (1990b) did not record hand and shoulder muscle motor units in the same subjects and with the same stimulus intensity. Their results suggest an equally powerful influence over motor units in both muscles and this does not agree with the results obtained with magnetic stimulation for both single units and whole muscle EMG by Ashby and his colleagues (Brouwer and Ashby 1990; Palmer and Ashby 1992). The results of these other workers have clearly suggested a stronger CM influence on the motoneurones innervating more distal muscles. This conflict remains to be resolved by further study, although the explanation for it may derive partly from differences in the action of the two types of non-invasive stimuli (see Rothwell *et al.* 1991), and partly from differences in the sampling of motor units.

4.15 FUNCTIONAL CONSEQUENCES OF DIVERGENCE AND CONVERGENCE OF SMALL-AMPLITUDE CORTICO-MOTONEURONAL SYNAPTIC ACTIONS

From all the observations that have been reported, it is clear that each cortico-motoneuronal axon is capable of delivering synapses to a very large number of motoneurones, each of which may receive only one or a few boutons from a single collateral of that fibre. Each bouton may be capable of producing a quantal EPSP of only $100 \mu V$ or so in amplitude, if the measurements made on group Ia synapses provide relevant indications of quantal amplitude (Redman 1990). But this relatively weak contribution from individual CM cells must be outweighed by the large number of CM fibres that converge upon the motoneurones innervating muscles acting about the distal joints of the forelimb. If we assume a value of 5 mV for a large compound CM EPSP in a hand muscle motoneurone, and estimate that each of the individual CM cells generates a $200 \mu V$ EPSP or less (see Table 4.4). If these individual CM effects are independent and do not shunt one another significantly, the number of contacts involved in the compound EPSP production must be at least 25 and may be in the order of 50 to 100. This set of cortico-motoneuronal collaterals projects from the cortical colony, and each collateral provides one or a few synapses to the single motoneurone. If a given CM axon contributes several intraspinal collaterals to a single motoneurone (which would seem necessary to explain the size of some of the larger single CM EPSPs), then the number of CM cells in a colony would be proportionately smaller. However, if the CM synapses behave in a manner similar to that shown for the Ia input (Redman 1990), the probability of release of transmitter and generation of a quantal EPSP at many of these release sites may be low, with a high proportion of 'failures' in the statistical distribution of EPSP amplitudes. If so, it is more likely that the number of CM cells in a motoneurone's colony could be larger than 100. Such a speculative estimate is in keeping with the yield of monkey cortical cells that can be shown by the STA method to facilitate a given motor nucleus.

Even if the divergence of a single cortico-motoneuronal axon is so wide as to be capable of influencing a very large number of motoneurones, it will be as a consequence of activity generated in this axon along with a selected combination of a large number of other residents of that motoneurone's colony that a particular motoneurone will be brought to firing level and the motor unit become activated. The small size of the contribution that a given cortico-motoneuronal synapse makes to the overall depolarization may allow very fine grading of the responsiveness of motoneurones and aid in the selection of particular motor units to the motor task and in the fractionation of muscle action. Some idea of the significance of the colony's input for motoneuronal activity was given by Cheney *et al.* (1991), who combined the currently available estimates of compound EPSPs in wrist extensor motoneurones with known firing rates of CM cells during maintenance of wrist position against an intermediate external load of 0.1 Nm; a compound EPSP size of 2.0 mV was assumed (see Fig. 4.33). For CM cells that facilitated wrist extensor muscles and which had a mean firing rate of 62 Hz during steady holding, they calculated that these CM cells could produce an increment in the firing rate of wrist extensor motoneurones by up to 12.4 Hz, which is around 60 per cent of the firing rate which these motoneurones actually show at 0.1 Nm. Of course, these calculations also serve to remind us of the importance of other excitatory inputs, including those from interneurones, which are needed to make the motoneurones fire at the observed rates. The precise contribution of any one CM cell to the firing rate of its target motoneurones will also depend on its own pattern of activity. Such patterns of discharge vary widely between CM cells and it has been suggested that these patterns represent different types of control mechanism for motoneurone activity (Fetz *et al.* 1989; see Chapter 5).

It is possible that the appropriate co-operative activity in a large number of CM neurones provides the structural basis for the refined control of skill and precision of motor performance at the distal joints of the limb and the capacity, through selection of motor units, to fractionate the use of distally acting muscles. These functions are clearly dependent on corticospinal actions. It remains to be established that a special contribution comes from cortico-motoneuronal synapses and to investigate further the mechanism by which these actions are produced. We have, as yet, little information about the orchestrated and co-ordinated impulse activity which is projected through a whole ensemble of corticospinal fibres in association with even a simple movement of the fingers. Approaches to the study of this are, however, feasible and will be taken up in later sections of this book.

4.16 TEMPORAL FACILITATION OF CORTICO-MOTONEURONAL EXCITATION

Intracellular records of the EPSPs produced in spinal motoneurones by repetitive activation of corticospinal projections reveal that the amplitudes of the successive waves of depolarization increase following the later volleys in the train. Initially this property was considered to be due to the increasing potency of synaptic transmissions at cortico-motoneuronal synapses because no evidence was obtained of increases in the amplitude of the descending corticospinal volleys (Landgren *et al.* 1962a). Although populations of local interneurones or propriospinal neurones may also have been caused to discharge by the actions of repetitive corticospinal volleys, little evidence for delayed synaptic impacts from these sources was obtained from intracellular records (see above). The phenomenon of temporal facilitation of cortico-motoneuronal EPSPs recorded in motoneurones of the monkey's spinal cord has been studied and the time course of the facilitation has been measured (Porter and Hore 1969; Porter 1970; Muir and Porter 1973; see Phillips and Porter 1977, pp. 65–77). It has also been observed following repetitive stimulation of pyramidal tract fibres (Jankowska *et al.* 1975a; Shapovalov 1975; Fritz *et al.* 1985). The latter studies found that the most distal hand motoneurones received a relatively weak degree of temporal facilitation compared to that evoked in motoneurones innervating muscles acting at the wrist and elbow. Fritz *et al.* (1985) found that, in intrinsic hand muscle motoneurones, the mean amplitude of the third EPSP generated by a train of three 200 μA pyramidal shocks was only 1.5 times larger than that of the first EPSP, compared to 2.5 times for extensor carpi radialis motoneurones and 2.1 times for elbow flexor motoneurones. When motoneurones receive repetitive bombardment from cortico-motoneuronal fibres, this difference may partly compensate for the smaller CM EPSPs in wrist as compared to hand motoneurones (see Section 4.14 and Fig. 4.33).

Phillips and Porter (1964; 1977, pp. 65–77) suggested that temporal

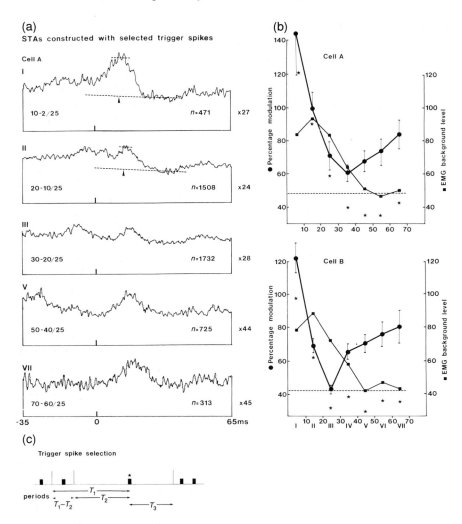

FIG 4.35 Influence of discharge pattern on the production of PSF by monkey CM cells. (a): STAs of EMG from flexor pollicis brevis (FPB) constructed with groups of CM cell trigger spikes selected as shown in (c). The trigger spike (asterisk) was selected on the basis of both the preceding (T_2) and succeeding (T_3) interspike interval. T_1, maximal preceding interspike interval; T_2; minimal preceding interspike interval; T_3, minimal interspike interval succeeding the selected trigger spike. No additional spikes were allowed to fall in the periods T_2 and T_3. Trigger-spike selection criteria are indicated as T_1-T_2/T_3, e.g., the STA labelled VII was triggered by a group of spikes with a preceding interval of 70–60 ms and a succeeding interval of not less than 25 ms. STAs labelled I to VII are triggered by spikes with successively longer interspike intervals. All STAs have been rescaled, such that the

facilitation in cortico-motoneuronal pathways may have functional significance in relation to the voluntary management of muscle contraction and that the facilitation is, indeed, a property of cortico-motoneuronal synapses. That it is not dependent on recruitment to synchronous discharge of additional elements at a cortical or spinal level is indicated, however, by the degree of postspike facilitation of muscle activity which follows the discharges of a single, identified cortico-motoneuronal cell when long or short intervals between impulses are used in the construction of the correlogram. Fetz and Cheney (1980) found, in one case of an injured CM cell, that pairs of impulses separated by brief interspike intervals were particularly effective in generating postspike facilitation of target muscles in conscious monkeys carrying out a movement task. This phenomenon was investigated in more detail for naturally firing CM cells by Lemon and Mantel (1989). These authors selected, as triggers for an STA, spike events which were preceded by a particular interspike interval. This approach allowed the relative amplitude of postspike facilitation (the percentage modulation) to be measured for intervals varying from 2 ms to 70 ms. Controls were carried out to show that these changes were not attributable to the different levels of EMG activity associated with different interspike intervals (i.e. high and low EMG levels associated with short and long intervals, respectively). For all CM cells studied ($n = 17$) three clear phases of facilitation could be identified. Spikes preceded by very short intervals (<10 ms) elicited large PSF (see Fig. 4.35); this was shown to be partly a result of temporal *summation* of the response of the motoneurone pool to the pretrigger and trigger spikes respectively, and partly due to temporal *facilitation* of individual motoneurones, as described by Phillips and Porter

---

background EMG levels just after the PSF have the same amplitude, to allow for direct comparison of the facilitation effects; the scaling factor ($\times$ 24, $\times$ 27, etc.) is shown on right. Trigger spikes occur at time zero. Dashed lines in I and II indicate the estimates of the PSF peak and background EMG level; arrows indicate the point at which these were measured. Note that the effects for group V and VII are stronger and earlier than for group III. (b): Upper panel, changes in percentage modulation (●) of PSF with interspike intervals for cell A (same cell as in part (a) of this figure). Duration of interval preceding trigger spike shown on abscissa. The absolute amplitude (*) of the PSF and the background EMG (■) level were measured in the same arbitrary units (right ordinate). The background level peaked for the group II spikes and then fell steadily, as did the size of the PSF. In contrast, the percentage modulation of the PSF fell over group I to IV and then increased again with the longer intervals. Vertical bars approximate the possible measurement errors involved and are equal to ±25 per cent of the maximum noise level in the STA. The horizontal dashed line indicates the percentage modulation found for this cell–muscle combination in the STA constructed with all (unselected) spikes. Lower panel, a similar plot for a different CM cell. (Reproduced with permission from Lemon and Mantel (1989).)

Interval—selected spikes

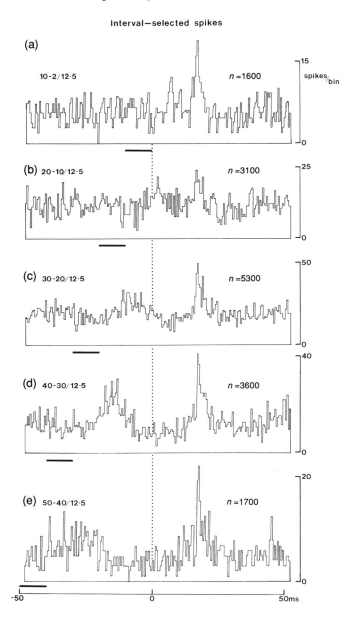

FIG 4.36 Effect of variation in CM interspike interval on discharges from an AbPB motor unit facilitated by the cell. The cross-correlation of motor unit discharges with all (unselected) spikes is shown in (f). (a)–(e) show the cross-correlograms of motor unit activity with CM spikes selected according to firing interval (for criteria see Fig. 4.35). The duration of the interval in which the preceding spike was allowed to fall is shown by thick horizontal lines. Trigger spike at time zero. Bin width: 0.5 ms. The shortest interval spikes (a) produced the most

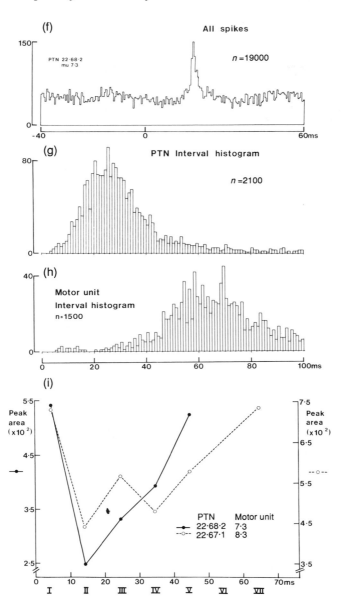

pronounced correlogram peak; there was then a marked fall for the interval group 20–10 ms (b); the strength of correlation then increased steadily towards the longer intervals. The results for this unit (●) are plotted in (j), which shows the strength of the correlation in terms of peak area ($\times 10^2$) (see text for definition). Time-interval histograms of the PTN and motor unit discharges shown in (g) and (h), respectively. Results from a second CM cell-motor unit combination are also shown in (j) (○). (Reproduced with permission from Lemon and Mantel (1989).)

(1964). This latter phenomenon was clearly shown by comparing the responses of single motor units to CM spikes preceded by different intervals (see Fig. 4.36a).

Spikes preceded by interspike intervals of 20–40 ms produced substantially less facilitation than was seen for shorter interspike intervals. This should probably be thought of as the baseline level of excitation that is substantially augmented by the short-interval spikes. Long-interval spikes (50–60 ms) also produced an unexpectedly strong facilitation. This may be because long-interval spikes occur mainly during low-level EMG activity, where it is likely that the discharge rate of target motoneurones is also low, making them more susceptible to discharge by incoming CM EPSPs (see Ellaway and Murphy 1985). Interestingly, the short-term synchrony that exists between single motor units recorded from human hand muscles, some of which is likely to be of corticospinal origin (see Section 4.12), has been shown to be particularly influenced by presynaptic sources discharging at frequencies in the 1–12 Hz and 16–32 Hz range (Farmer *et al.* 1990a). The latter frequency range would include the long interspike intervals shown by Lemon and Mantel (1989) to be very effective during low levels of EMG activity.

These results make it possible to suggest that the temporal profile of impulses in cortico-motoneuronal fibres may be particularly important in selecting those motoneurones which will be brought to discharge. Temporal features of natural cortico-motoneuronal discharge will be considered Chapter 5.

4.17 CORTICAL INHIBITION OF MOTONEURONES

In the Rede Lecture, *The brain and its mechanism*, given in Cambridge in 1933, Sherrington emphasized the role of inhibition in the following terms: 'The brain seems a thoroughfare for nerve-action passing on its way to the motor animal. It has been remarked that Life's aim is an act, not a thought. Today the dictum must be modified to admit that, often, to refrain from an act is no less an act than to commit one, because inhibition is co-equally with excitation a nervous activity.' As far as is known, all cortico-motoneuronal effects are excitatory. But the intracellular recordings of synaptic potentials evoked in the spinal motoneurones of the monkey and the baboon by stimulation of the corticospinal tract revealed inhibitory postsynaptic potentials (IPSPs) with latencies 1.2 ms to 1.4 ms longer than those of the monosynaptic EPSPs (Preston and Whitlock 1960; Landgren *et al.* 1962a). Preston and Whitlock's results revealed that excitation followed by inhibition was the commonest result of stimulating large numbers of corticospinal fibres.

In man, Cowan *et al.* (1986) reported that non-invasive brain stimulation

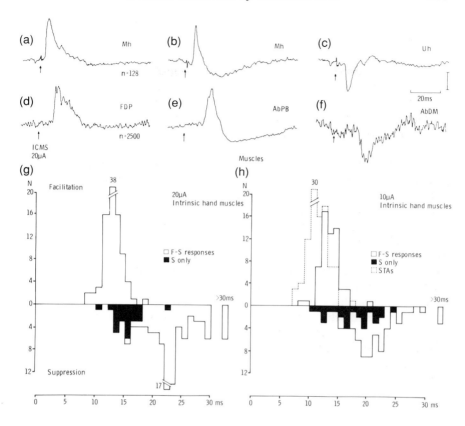

Fɪɢ 4.37 Effects of single pulses of intracortical stimuli on monkey hand muscles and motoneurones. (a)–(f): Comparison of responses produced by single pulse ICMS in stimulus-triggered averages of membrane potentials recorded intracellularly from three different hand motoneurones ((a)–(c)) in an anaesthetized monkey and of EMG recorded from three muscles (d)–(f) in a conscious monkey. Stimulus strength was 20 μA in all cases; 128 and 2500 stimulus events were used for the upper and lower averages respectively. (a),(b) hand motoneurones antidromically excited from the median nerve at the wrist (MNh), and (c) from the ulnar nerve (UNh). Stimulus onset at arrow. Calibration: 300 μV (a), 150 μV (b) and 75 μV (c). (g) and (h): Onset latencies of facilitation and suppression in ICMS-triggered averages of EMG from intrinsic hand muscles. Responses showing 'pure' suppression (filled columns) had consistently shorter latencies than mixed responses of facilitation (f) followed by suppression (S). Number (N) of observations plotted on ordinate. Onset latencies of post*spike* facilitation in STAs of hand muscle EMG have been plotted in (h) (dashed lines). Note earlier latency of postspike effects. (Reproduced with permission from Lemon *et al.* (1987).)

could produce inhibitory effects on H-reflex excitability of various muscles at a latency only 1–2 ms longer than that of the early excitation. Inhibition of motoneuronal discharge by electrical and magnetic stimulation of the motor cortex has been observed for deltoid and triceps in the upper limb (Palmer and Ashby 1992) and in soleus in the lower limb (Cowan *et al.* 1986; Iles and Pisini 1992).

In the conscious monkey, Lemon *et al.* (1987) found that weak, single-shock intracortical microstimulation often produced poststimulus suppression of EMG activity in forelimb muscles. The suppression either followed an initial period of facilitation (Fig. 4.37(c), (e)) or was produced without any preceding facilitation (Fig. 4.37(d)). These results appeared to reflect the EPSP–IPSP sequence produced in spinal motoneurones of anaesthetized monkeys by identical intracortical stimuli (Lemon *et al.* 1987). 'Pure' suppression of EMG was relatively rare, but its existence shows that it is possible to excite cortical outputs with a net inhibitory action on a target motoneurone pool.

The inhibitory effects on motoneurones and the suppression of EMG activity in muscles had latencies consistent with the interpolation of an interneurone in the inhibitory pathway. It has been conclusively demonstrated by Jankowska *et al.* (1976) that it is the Ia inhibitory interneurone that is interposed between the lateral corticospinal axons and the motoneurones. Convergence of peripherally generated and descending influences was demonstrated by the spatial facilitation technique: the simultaneous arrival at the spinal segment of a volley in group I fibres from an antagonist muscle, and of a volley in the corticospinal tract, could together generate an IPSP in an agonist motoneurone, while neither volley alone was effective. The identification of the responsible interneurone was further assisted, in the cat, by the demonstration that the recurrent axon collaterals of motoneurones were able to inhibit selected common Ia inhibitory interneurones via Renshaw cells (see Fig. 1.13, p. 28). The ability, therefore, for antidromic volleys delivered to appropriate ventral roots to suppress the IPSP's produced by corticospinal and antagonist group Ia volleys, secured the identification of the responsible interneurone (see Baldiserra *et al.* 1981).

Evidence gained from spike-triggered averaging suggests that some of the corticospinal input to the Ia inhibitory interneurones originates from collaterals of CM axons, and that this arrangement underpins the reciprocal facilitation and suppression of EMG in antagonistic pairs of forelimb muscles. In the studies of Cheney *et al.* (1982) and Kasser and Cheney (1985), monkeys performed an alternating flexion–extension task with controlled movements at the wrist joint and reciprocal activity of flexor and extensor muscle groups. CM neurones were selected because of consistent co-variation of their discharge with either flexion or extension. Because, in general, these cells were silent during movement in the opposite direction,

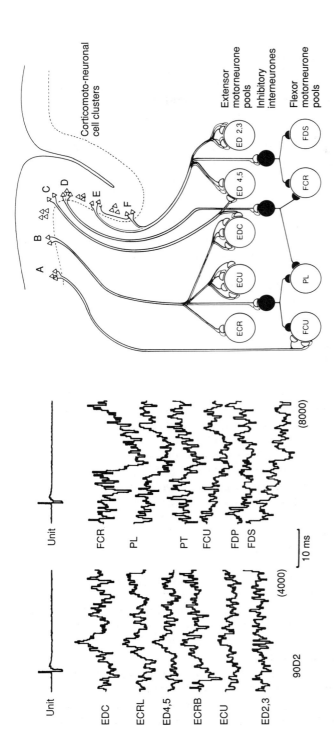

FIG 4.38 Organization of cortico-motoneuronal control of wrist extensor and flexor muscles in the monkey. Left: spike-triggered averages for a reciprocally organized CM cell. This cell produced clear PSF in several extensor muscles (STAs in left column) and clear postspike suppression in several flexor muscles (STAs in right column). (Reproduced with permission from Cheney et al. (1991). Right: diagram of simplest circuits that may mediate the three basic patterns of cortical cell influence of wrist flexor and extensor motorneurones. Correlational evidence indicates that cells may facilitate agonist muscles with no effect on antagonist muscles (A, C); facilitate agonist muscles and simultaneously suppress antagonist muscles through a reciprocal inhibitory pathway (B, E, and F); and suppress certain muscles with no effect on their antagonists (D). Clustering and interconnection of cells with common targets is also suggested by these experiments. (Reproduced with permission from Cheney et al. (1985).)

it was necessary to activate them artificially during their naturally silent phase. Glutamate was ejected from the second barrel of a double-barrelled intracortical electrode. It was then possible to investigate the influence of these chemically initiated additional spikes, occurring in the normally silent period, on the 'antagonist' muscles: this test revealed the reciprocal suppression of such antagonist muscles following the discharge of the one CM cell (Fig. 4.38; Cheney *et al.* 1982; Kasser and Cheney 1985). In another study, Fetz and Cheney (1987) demonstrated that CM cells with these reciprocal actions on agonist and antagonist motoneurones, showed a clearly decreased firing rate when the monkey transferred to a power grip task characterized by a co-contracted, rather than a reciprocal pattern of muscle activity. These results suggest that co-contraction of antagonistic muscles may exclude activation of such reciprocal cells, thus providing a disfacilitation of the Ia interneurones which would normally inhibit the antagonist motoneurones.

Examination of Fig. 4.23 from Fetz *et al.* (1989) shows that CM cells producing this pattern of reciprocal effects accounted for about one third of the 65 CM cells investigated. Cells with pure facilitation were generally more common, and CM cells eliciting only 'pure suppression' were rare. Postspike suppression is generally weaker than PSF and requires a greater number of spike events for it to be revealed. Both of these properties are consistent with its production over a pathway involving more than one synapse (Kasser and Cheney 1985; see Section 4.11). In wrist muscle EMG, the mean latency of postspike suppression is, however, about 3 ms longer than PSF, which is longer than expected for a disynaptic pathway involving the Ia inhibitory interneurone. During performance of the precision grip task, Lemon *et al.* (1986, 1987) found only a few cases of postspike suppression of EMG activity in intrinsic hand muscles. In contrast, suppression following intracortical microstimulation was found from most cortical sites tested. Reliable activation of interneuronal inhibitory pathways was presumably more common when a number of different corticospinal outputs were activated by intracortical microstimulation than when the influence of a single CM cell was tested (see Fig. 4.37). Lemon *et al.* (1987) also found that the latency of poststimulus suppression of EMG in intrinsic hand muscles was longer than that of facilitation (see Fig. 4.37), the mean difference being 4.2 ms. Note that the postspike facilitation always had an *earlier* latency than poststimulus facilitation (mean difference 1.7 ms with a single 10 μA intracortical stimulus); this phenomenon is probably due to the indirect, trans-synaptic activation of CM cells by ICMS (Bennett *et al.* 1989; see Section 8.2).

Apart from its potential functional role in integration and co-ordination of the motor output of the spinal cord, in response to descending influences from the cerebral cortex, inhibition, controlled by such corticospinal connections, could be of the greatest importance in the initiation of voluntary movement. In fast voluntary movements, prior inhibition of antagonist motoneurones is determined by the central 'command' that initiates movement, and this allows inhibition of the pre-existing posture and movement away from it (see Phillips and Porter 1977, p. 337–340). It may be that the Ia inhibitory interneurones are the major, or even the exclusive, contributors to this inhibitory influence. Increasing excitability of the agonist motoneurones is also brought about at the onset of movement, both directly and also by enhanced transmission in segmental reflex pathways. For instance, Hultborn *et al.* (1987) demonstrated that presynaptic inhibition of Ia activity from soleus or quadriceps motoneurones was released during the early part of voluntary isometric contractions. Interestingly, this release of presynaptic inhibition is particularly strong before movements requiring co-contraction of antagonist muscles (Nielsen and Kagamihara 1992).

A further important role for inhibition would be in the focusing of a specific group of muscles recruited for a particular voluntary movement. Given the fact that most CM cells appear to facilitate activity in several muscles, such inhibition would appear to be essential for the recruitment of an individual muscle without any concurrent activity in its functional or anatomical synergists.

Loss of control of these inhibitory elements may underlie the development of spasticity following cortical damage or interruption of corticospinal connections by denying the brain access to the inhibitory machinery for unlocking the spinal cord's innervation of contracting postural muscles. Attempts have been made to detect levels of activation of the common Ia inhibitory interneurones on the normal and on the affected side in patients with injury to the descending corticospinal system and evidence of spasticity. Ashby and Wiens (1989) have found some evidence to suggest that Ia induced reciprocal inhibition of motoneurones is augmented in spasticity, suggesting that Ia inhibitory interneurones are more excitable after spinal lesions. It is clear that other populations of inhibitory interneurones, influenced by corticospinal axons but not accessible to the kinds of testing used by Ashby and Wiens, may also be important in the control of tone and in relation to spasticity.

4.18 POTENTIAL ENLARGEMENT OF THE FIELD OF CORTICO-MOTONEURONAL INFLUENCE BY COLLATERAL ACTION ON FUSIMOTOR NEURONES

A large number of animal studies have found evidence for activation of γ-motoneurones and spindle afferents by electrical stimulation of the motor cortex (Granit and Kaada 1952; see review by Hulliger 1984). Pyramidotomy is also known to depress muscle spindle activity in gastrocnemius (Gilman *et al.* 1971). Monosynaptic effects on fusimotor neurones have been recorded in the cervical spinal cord of the baboon (Clough *et al.* 1971; Koeze *et al.* 1968) and in the lumbar spinal cord of the monkey (Grigg and Preston 1971; Koeze 1973) following cortical stimulation, although most of the responses recorded by Clough *et al.* (1971) had too long a latency to have been activated monosynaptically by the fastest D-wave in the corticospinal tract. Further, many distal forelimb γ-motoneurones could not be activated by corticospinal volleys. Both these properties are in distinct contrast to the responses of α-motoneurones innervating the most distal muscles.

A recent study by Rothwell *et al.* (1990) investigated the effects of non-invasive brain stimulation on the responses of muscle spindle afferents recorded by microneuronography from motor fascicles of the ulnar or radial nerves in human volunteers. Their objective was to use these responses to detect signs of cortico-fusimotor activation. They could find no evidence of such activation in relaxed subjects, even when the stimulus was strong enough to produce a clear twitch of the receptor-bearing muscle. For 26 single spindle afferents, the stimuli were delivered during a voluntary contraction of the receptor-bearing muscle; once again the effects were rather weak, and none of the afferents' discharges could be modulated by stimuli that were subthreshold for activation of α-motoneurones, as evidenced by intramuscular EMG recordings. Twelve of the 26 endings were influenced by stimuli above α threshold, and three of these responded at latencies which were early enough to suggest that they originated from activation of β-motoneurones. But all of these findings depend critically on just how sensitive the spindle afferents would be to the discharge of one, or at most a few additional fusimotor impulses elicited by brain stimulation.

It is still not clear whether corticospinal action on fusimotor neurones is conveyed by a separate population of corticofusimotor elements or by collaterals of other corticospinal or cortico-motoneuronal cells (see Phillips and Porter 1977, pp. 150–151). Whether or not independent corticospinal elements are involved, the potential exists, both through intracortical collateral projections (see Section 2.1) and potentially through the widespread arborization of intraspinal collaterals of cortico-motoneuronal axons (Fig. 4.13) for linkages between appropriate alpha and gamma motoneurones to result from corticospinal actions.

Such linkages might underlie the patterns of α–γ co-activation that have been reported in many studies (see Vallbo *et al.* 1979). But although both animal and human studies have shown that a large variety of voluntary movements are accompanied by an increase in spindle discharge, the role of the corticospinal system in this is not yet clearly established, and it must be remembered that in most studies using cortical stimulation other descending pathways were intact, including those from brainstem areas known to exert strong modulation of fusimotor discharge (Hulliger 1984). Neither have the relative effects of corticospinal discharge on γ-static and γ-dynamic fusimotor neurones been explored. Although theories of α–γ coactivation have been a dominant influence in recent years, there is evidence for more flexible patterns of activation of both γ-static and γ-dynamic motoneurones which, under some behavioural conditions, can be independent of α activity (Prochazka and Wand 1981; Hulliger 1984; Ribot *et al.* 1986; Prochazka 1989).

4.19 PRESYNAPTIC INHIBITION FROM CORTICOSPINAL FIBRES

While most of our attention has been given to the descending influences which are produced at synapses on the somata and dendrites of receiving neurones (motoneurones and interneurones) in the spinal cord, axo-axonic synapses also exist and some of the presynaptic elements apposed to boutons in the spinal cord could arise from corticospinal fibres. Physiological evidence exists to implicate these axo-axonic connections in presynaptic inhibition (Rudomin 1990). This will reduce the effectiveness of the particular synaptic boutons receiving the axo-axonic synapses, while leaving unaffected the responsiveness of the second-order neurones to other inputs not in receipt of the same axo-axonic controls. Corticospinal volleys have been found to modulate the degree of presynaptic inhibition of transmission through synapses interposed in a number of reflex pathways, including those involving group Ia, Ib, and II spindle afferents, and the largest afferents from the skin (see Baldiserra *et al.* 1981; Rudomin, 1990). As pointed out above, an important feature of descending corticospinal and rubrospinal activity may be the relief from presynaptic inhibition of Ia terminals upon homonymous and synergist motoneurones; in the cat this action is exerted by corticospinal inhibition of the first-order interneurones mediating presynaptic inhibition of the Ia fibres (see Rudomin 1990). Little is known about the role of presynaptic inhibition upon corticospinal terminals themselves, although this might be an important contributory mechanism to the modulation of corticospinal transmission that has been observed in both human and animal studies.

4.20 COMPARISON OF CORTICO-MOTONEURONAL INPUT WITH OTHER SOURCES OF INPUT TO FORELIMB MOTONEURONES

Fetz, Cheney, and their colleagues have used the STA technique to identify three important sources of input to spinal motoneurones innervating wrist and digit muscles in the monkey: from the motor cortex (CM cells), from the red nucleus (rubro-motoneuronal; RM cells), and from the dorsal root ganglia (DRG; Cheney *et al.* 1991; Flament *et al.* 1992a). All these effects were recorded under identical behavioural conditions, during the performance of a step-tracking wrist flexion/extension task. Postspike effects from dorsal root ganglia were generated by 68 afferent units recorded from the C8 and T1 dorsal root ganglia. Many of these units were probably spindle afferents, but could not be identified conclusively as such. Surprisingly, many of these afferents discharged prior to movement onset. The latency of postspike effects from the DRG (5.8 ms) was actually rather similar to that from the red nucleus (5.6 ms) or motor cortex (6.3 ms). The authors suggest that this may result partly from the inclusion of some longer-latency oligosynaptic effects in the mean value for DRG afferents and partly from an underestimate of postspike facilitation from CM and RM cells caused by synchrony (see Section 4.12 above).

Both RM and DRG units produced, on average, weaker PSF than CM cells, while the percentage of muscles facilitated by all three groups of inputs was similar, at 40–50 per cent, suggesting a similar degree of axonal branching for these different inputs. The facilitated muscles were always agonists or synergists contributing to either flexion or extension torques. PSF from CM cells was more common, and had a larger amplitude in some muscles (such as EDC) than in others, indicating a preferential distribution of CM effects (see Section 4.14 above); in contrast, the distribution of DRG effects seemed to be determined by the relative distance between the DRG input and the target motoneurone pools (cf. Lüscher and Vardar 1989).

4.21 SUMMARY

Motoneurones destined to provide innervation of a particular muscle are assembled longitudinally in a cigar-shaped column within the anterior horn of the spinal cord. Each column consists of a few hundred motoneurones and spreads through a few segments of the cord in a characteristic location. Evidence has been presented which describes the convergence of neuronal influences on to such motoneurones from peripheral receptors capable of generating reflex activities, from local segmental interneurones, including inhibitory interneurones, from propriospinal neurones, and from long descending pathways, including those making up the corticospinal system.

The methods by which the influences exerted by any of these inputs may be studied for particular motor nuclei have been introduced. These include intracellular recordings of synaptic actions on single motoneurones, which can be analyzed in anaesthetized animals to seek to understand the fundamental mechanisms of synaptic transmission at these locations, and the study of electrical responses recorded from individual muscles or single motor units in conscious, co-operating animals, including man. When the powerful techniques of spike-triggered averaging and cross-correlation analysis are then applied to these recordings, the relationships between simultaneously recorded events can be studied and the effectiveness, during normal movement performance, of the synaptic influences that are exerted by even a single corticospinal neurone can be estimated.

While providing a general account of the place of reflex actions and of interneurones in influencing motoneurone function, and while recognizing that a major, significant role for propriospinal neurones in guiding particular movements has been demonstrated, our account has concentrated on corticospinal influences on motoneurones and, in particular, on the detailed information which gives the cortico-motoneuronal components of the corticospinal system a special significance in movements performed by conscious primates, including man.

Both refined histological and electro-anatomical observations on single cortico-motoneuronal fibres in the monkey indicate significant divergence of the intraspinal collaterals of these fibres to impact on a large number of motoneurones. It is possible that, for some muscles acting about the distal joints of the limb, most or all of the motoneurones are engaged by synapses from each cortico-motoneuronal fibre which includes that muscle within its muscle field. The synaptic boutons that generate the cortico-motoneuronal synapses are small in size and only one or a few boutons are contributed to the motoneurone's dendritic surface by each cortico-motoneuronal collateral. The contribution to the synaptic excitation of a motoneurone that is made by any one cortico-motoneuronal fibre is small. However, because of the high degree of convergence of intraspinal collaterals from a large colony of cortico-motoneuronal neurones on to each motoneurone of a distally acting muscle, this synaptic influence could allow fine grading of the depolarization of the motoneurone, contribute to the selective activation of motor units during voluntary movement and be critically effective in the fractionation of muscle usage during different motor tasks.

It has been found that pyramidal tract neurones (PTNs) with both slow- and fast-conducting axons make cortico-motoneuronal connections and are capable of contributing to the refined management of muscles used in skilled voluntary movements. The influence of a single cortico-motoneuronal cell is demonstrable as postspike facilitation (PSF) of EMG activity of several muscles during a natural movement task. The magnitude of the excitatory effect produced by a given cortico-motoneuronal cell appears to be different for different muscles and it may be modified according to the nature of the task in which the motor unit is engaged. In general, however, the largest effects are detected in the intrinsic muscles of the hand and in the extensors of the wrist, while weak or no facilitatory effects can be detected in proximal muscles of the monkey's forelimb. It may be that, in man, the increased importance of cortico-motoneuronal influence is reflected in the fact that even proximal muscles receive strong cortico-motoneuronal excitation.

5

Output functions of the motor cortex

5.1 RECORDING FROM NEURONES IN THE MOTOR CORTEX

We have already documented the contributions which recordings from the cells of origin of individual cortico-motoneuronal elements have contributed to our understanding of convergence and divergence of their influences and to measurement of the effects which they are capable of producing on the machinery for movement which is located within the spinal cord.

The availability of methods which allowed the direct registration of the discharges of single neurones in the motor cortex of cats (Armstrong and Drew 1984a), monkeys (Jasper *et al.* 1958; Evarts 1965; Fetz and Cheney 1978; Lemon 1984), and of conscious human subjects (Li 1959; Goldring and Ratcheson 1972) during the performance of motor tasks, provided for the evaluation of functional associations of particular cellular elements in the brain with aspects of the movement being performed. As a result of such studies, an involvement of the discharges of neurones from a number of regions of the brain in measured aspects of movement performance has been evaluated. In addition, the responses of these neurones to a variety of inputs generated by activation of peripheral receptors or by stimulation of other relevant brain structures has been assessed. The functional significance for movement, of inputs to motor areas of the brain, will be taken up in the next chapter. Here we intend to describe the general observations that have been made on neurones in the precentral motor area of the cerebral cortex and then to examine the specific relationships which have been shown to exist between cortical elements, identified according to the targets of their projecting axons, and the management of the muscles which generate movement. We shall concentrate on those parts of such recent studies which have most significance for the theme of this book. The major contributions to general understanding of the role of the motor cortex as it was examined by Evarts and others is fully documented in Phillips and Porter (1977) (Chapter 7) and will not be repeated in full here. Several extensive reviews of this subject are available (Evarts 1981, 1986; Hepp-Reymond 1988; Cheney *et al.* 1991; Humphrey and Tanji 1991).

Many studies have examined the neuronal activity in different cortical areas that is associated with natural self-initiated movements or with constrained, learned tasks. However, the overall impression from all these studies is that neurones whose activity is related to a particular aspect of movement are found in many different cortical and sub-cortical regions. This is true, for example, of neurones whose activity appears to encode the force produced in a voluntary movement. Conversely, in any one cortical region, although there may be a majority of cells related to one particular parameter of movement, it is possible to find some neurones whose activity is related to other aspects of the same movement. Only those experiments which test the encoding of a number of different possible movement parameters have revealed this phenomenon. Finally, although 'task related' neurones are not difficult to find in the precentral motor cortex, there are many neurones in the motor areas of the cerebral cortex which do not appear to modulate their activity in association with the movement or movements performed by the experimental animal within a specific paradigm (see Thach 1978; Crutcher and Alexander 1990; Fetz 1992).

Recordings in a particular area of the cerebral cortex, theoretically, could have been derived from local intracortical interneurones, which comprise about one third of the cortical population, or from pyramidal cells with axons projecting to any one of a large variety of targets (see Section 2.1), including corticospinal (pyramidal tract) neurones, of which some, in the monkey, make up the cortico-motoneuronal projection system. The fact that this last population is only one synapse removed from the motoneurones which cause muscle contraction allows us considerable confidence in describing its functions.

The identification of neuronal discharges associated with movement performance as being generated within a particular area of the cerebral cortex has provided a general indication of functional associations of that area with movement. Yet only part of that associated discharge, occurring with movement, could be regarded as relevant to the direct management of muscles for movement performance. This is the part of the total neuronal activity projected via the pyramidal tract to engage the spinal neuronal machinery already described in Chapter 4, and the part which projects indirectly from cortex to spinal cord via the subcorticospinal systems which it engages. The elements making up the corticospinal component can be isolated by selecting only those neurones which are activated by antidromic impulses set up by pyramidal tract stimuli, an approach pioneered in the studies of Ed Evarts (Fig. 5.1). It is possible also to select out for special study those neurones within the same area of cortex whose discharge is associated with movement performance and whose connectivity serves to inform other subcortical structures, such as the pontine nuclei or the striatum, about activities in that area of cortex. And, as we have already demonstrated, it is feasible to use cross-correlation methods to identify the particular connections of cortical elements with their next target neurones,

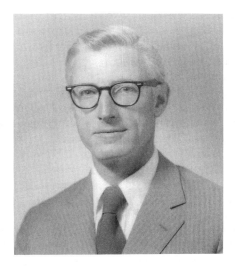

F_{IG} 5.1 Edward (Ed) Vaughn Evarts was born in New York City in 1926. He graduated from Harvard Medical School and began his research career in neuroscience in Karl Lashley's laboratory. In 1953 he joined the National Institute of Mental Health. His early studies combined his training in psychiatry and experimental psychology, and focused on the metabolism of psychoactive drugs. This work led him to research in sleep, and to developing the techniques essential to studying neurones in the sleep-waking cycle. He then went on to apply the chronic single unit recording technique to the motor system with great success, and his seminal contributions include the representation of movement parameters by activity in motor cortex neurones, the changes that occur during the preparation for an instructed movement, and the interaction between central and peripheral inputs within the motor system. It was largely his efforts that brought about the subsequent revolution in our understanding of central integrative neurophysiology. He died quite suddenly in 1985.

providing indicators of the discharges of the receiving cells are simultaneously available, and to examine the particular functional associations with parameters of movement performance which these correlations demonstrate.

5.2 DISCHARGES ASSOCIATED WITH A CONDITIONED MOTOR RESPONSE

Evarts exploited the examination of impulses generated by individual pyramidal tract neurones (PTNs) in conscious free-to-move monkeys. At a surgical operation under aseptic conditions, stimulating electrodes were inserted into the pyramidal tract and a defect in the bony cranium was created, providing for later access to the arm area of the precentral motor cortex through the intact dura mater. On subsequent occasions, and repeatedly, fine metal microelectrodes could then be driven slowly through the dura and into the motor cortex without causing the animal any discomfort and while the monkey was engaged in natural behaviour.

When the tip of the electrode was positioned sufficiently close to a cell in the motor cortex to record its discharges selectively, the responses of the cell to pyramidal tract stimulation could be examined. A neurone projecting its axon into the pyramidal tract (a PTN) could be identified by the antidromic response within it, which occurred with a brief, constant latency and could follow brief trains of stimuli delivered to the pyramidal tract at high frequency. The collision test provided additional proof that the discharges were being produced by a PTN (see Phillips and Porter 1977, pp. 54–56; Fuller and Schlag 1976). Indeed, the collision test still represents one of the best tests available to the neurophysiologist for confirming that recordings are being made from one and the same neurone throughout the experimental procedure and also that the device used to convert the spikes recorded from the neurone into logic pulses (usually some form of window discriminator) is actually recognizing spikes only from one cell (Lemon 1984, p. 102). Any pulses generated by spikes from other neurones in the vicinity will fail to collide with the antidromic impulse. This is an essential point, because it is these logic pulses that will eventually be used to reconstruct the nature of the association of the single cell's discharges with movement performance. Lemon *et al.* (1986) used STA to detect the *orthodromic* impulses of such neurones. Because of considerable uncertainties as to the relative contributions to the antidromic latency of the utilization time (the time taken to electrically excite the axon) and the conduction time, the latency of these orthodromic impulses probably yields a more reliable estimate of axonal conduction velocity than does the antidromic latency (see Lemon 1984, pp. 102–6). From these latency measurements and the estimated conduction distance through the internal capsule, an approximate conduction velocity of PTN axons can be calculated.

Evarts (1966) trained monkeys to perform a conditioned wrist extension movement to release a bell push and to execute this task briskly in response to a light flash. Release of the bell push in a response time of less than 350 ms was rewarded by the delivery of a squirt of juice into the monkey's mouth. Electromyographic activity in wrist flexor and extensor muscles was monitored using surface electrodes, and recordings were made of the discharges of identified PTNs in the motor cortex simultaneously with the performance of repeated conditioned response movements. PTNs which showed changes in their discharge in association with the performance of the conditioned movement task did not respond to the sensory stimulus of the light flash. They only changed their firing when this

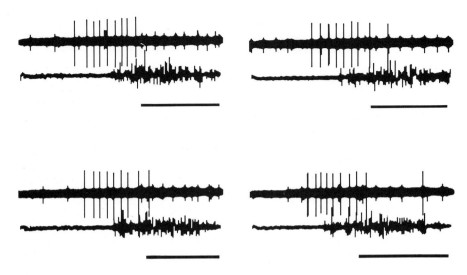

FIG 5.2   Monkey motor cortex PTN activity during performance of a conditioned hand movement. Each set of traces is initiated by the onset of a light flash which signals a monkey to release a bell-push by performing a brisk conditioned wrist extension movement. The release of the bell-push occurs when the lowest trace appears, after about 300 ms. This event is preceded by the onset of muscle activity (EMG recorded from the wrist extensor muscles) in the middle trace. The upper trace in each panel records the discharges of an identified PTN in the motor cortex contralateral to the moving wrist. In every trial, the discharge of the PTN in response to the light flash precedes the onset of muscle activity and the conditioned wrist extension response. The duration of the oscillograph sweep is 500 ms. (Reproduced with permission from Evarts (1966).)

signal resulted in performance of the movement task. A population of PTNs produced a burst of impulses 50 to 80 ms before the onset of EMG activity in the extensor muscles of the wrist and well before the beginning of wrist extension. For individual cortical cells, the latency of onset of neuronal discharge following the conditioning stimulus was positively correlated with the reaction time in response to that stimulus: the longer delayed the onset of PTN discharge, the greater the reaction time. Taken together, all of these observations demonstrate a close temporal association between the discharges of PTNs and a conditioned movement response, and allow of the possibility that the PTNs, leading the onset of muscle contraction by 50 ms or so, could be *causing* motor unit activation. (Fig. 5.2).

5.3 TEMPORAL RELATIONSHIP OF NEURONAL DISCHARGE TO
MOVEMENT PERFORMANCE

Evarts (1972) studied the temporal relationship of the discharges of a large
number of individual cortical neurones to an abruptly executed flexor or
extensor movement of the wrist. These neurones exhibited firing which
covaried with one direction of movement. They were identified according
to their location – in either the precentral or postcentral gyrus. However,
in these experiments, no separate categories, segregated in accordance with
the destination of their projecting axons, were distinguished; rather, all
precentral and all postcentral recordings were aggregated. Moreover,
because different muscles became active at different times before the onset
of the brisk wrist flexion or wrist extension, the timing of the onset of a
given cortical cell's activity was, in these studies, related not to the muscles
with which its discharge was correlated, but to the onset of movement in
that direction. Figure 5.3 plots the onset times of the discharges of the
populations of precentral and postcentral neurones in relation to the
beginning of the movement response. Precentral neurones could begin to
discharge as early as 140 ms before the onset of the movement response
and the greatest number of the neurones sampled changed their activity

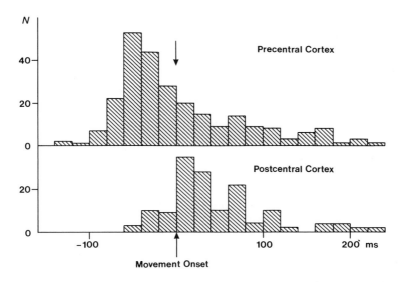

FIG 5.3   The relationship between the onset of neuronal discharge exhibited by a
large number (*N*) of monkey precentral and postcentral cortical neurones and the
beginning of a movement with which each neurone's discharge was associated. In
general, precentral neuronal firing preceded the onset of movement (wrist flexion
or extension). (Redrawn from Evarts (1972).)

60 ms before the movement. Similar temporal relations were found by Lamarre *et al.* (1981) for a reaction time task involving rapid elbow movement. The mean interval between onset of discharge in precentral neurones and movement onset was 122 ms.

In contrast to the precentral activity, Evarts (1972) found that most neurones in the postcentral gyrus changed their firing after the movement, as though they could have been influenced by it. Similar conclusions were reached by Fetz *et al.* (1980) from their sample of unidentified pre- and postcentral neurones recorded during a self-paced elbow flexion and extension task, and by Wannier *et al.* (1991) for a precision grip task. Thus for cells active before elbow flexion, mean peak activity in precentral cells occurred 156 ms before peak activity in biceps. In contrast, most postcentral units became active at the same time as biceps; their mean peak activity differed by only 1 ms from peak biceps activity.

Such clear contrasts in the timing of activity exhibited in different central nervous system structures has not been observed elsewhere. The timing of neuronal activity in motor cortex, in advance of movement, overlaps with the timing of discharges in premotor cortex, SMA, deep cerebellar nuclei and basal ganglia (Thach 1978; Hepp-Reymond 1988; Crutcher and Alexander 1990). There are differences in the timing of activies in these different structures, but the idea that such motor areas of the brain are recruited to activity in a simple serial fashion before a movement is performed is not supported by the data. Much of the activity in these connected parts of the brain appears to occur in parallel (Crutcher and Alexander 1990; Fetz 1992).

The fact that the delay between the onset of neuronal discharge in the precentral motor cortex and the commencement of self-initiated muscle contractions is much longer than the time taken (10 ms or less) to activate a forelimb muscle by means of a synchronous corticospinal volley stirred up by electrical stimulation of the efferent projections from the motor cortex, should not be claimed to undermine the functional significance of this cortical activity in relation to motor performance. Cheney and Fetz (1980) selected for study only those precentral neurones whose probable direct monosynaptic linkage with motoneurones was demonstrated by a short latency (average 6.7 ms) postspike facilitation of the EMG's of particular wrist flexor or extensor muscles. Yet when the overall responses of these cortico-motoneuronal neurones and their target muscles were examined for individual performances of the motor task, in most cases the onset of the EMG in target muscles also followed the beginning of cortico-motoneuronal discharge by 60 to 70 ms. While the first impulse in the cortical cell's train of activity clearly increased the probability of motor unit discharge, it must have required the addition of subsequent synaptic impacts and temporal facilitation from the repetitive discharges of the cell to produce motor unit activation. Figure 5.4 illustrates the temporal

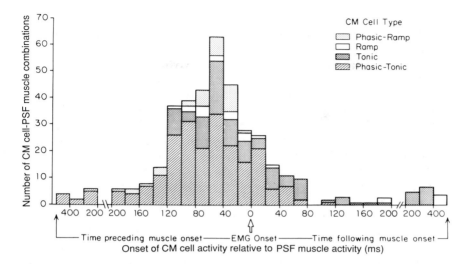

FIG 5.4 The temporal relationship between the onset of discharge of a population of identified cortico-motoneuronal (CM) cells and the onset of EMG activity in the muscle in which the CM cell could be shown to produce postspike facilitation (PSF). The CM cells were classified according to their characteristic firing patterns during a ramp and hold movement task (see text). (Reproduced with permission from Cheney and Fetz (1980).)

relationship of identified cortico-motoneuronal cells to a movement response and is to be compared with the upper half of Figure 5.3.

According to Porter (1987),

The earliest discharges of the cortico-motoneuronal cells obviously influenced the probability of motor unit activation with a tempo consistent with a monosynaptic cortico-motoneuronal excitation of their motoneurones. Yet this influence remained subthreshold for motor unit activation until summed with the effects of succeeding impulses in the CM cell's pattern of firing and until added to the subthreshold influences of other members of the colony of cortico-motoneuronal cells presumed to be converging on the same motoneurones. This temporal and spatial summation could occur in the 50 ms or so before activation of muscle contraction, during which period each of the contributing cortico-motoneuronal cells would be expected to produce a few impulses.

It is possible that the summation which occurs during this period involves the activity of other elements (reticulospinal, propriospinal, or interneuronal) called into action by the important collateral connections that have been described already in Chapters 2 and 4. As we have indicated, however, it is at least possible for the maximal total depolarization of the motoneurone to be brought about by the convergence of the influences of perhaps around 100 or so members of a cortico-motoneuronal colony (Section 4.15). As we have documented, some of the unitary synaptic contributions, to some preferentially innervated motoneurones, may be quite large, and no information exists as to whether or not there is any obvious relation between the time of onset of neuronal discharge before movement and the strength of the PSF exerted by a given CM cell. And it is likely that the inhibitory influences, which are clearly generated by intraspinal cortico-motoneuronal collaterals, are highly organized and focused on antagonistic motoneurones, so that they would not be expected to reduce the incrementing excitatory actions of the cortico-motoneuronal colony.

The internal temporal features of the cortico-motoneuronal cell's burst of firing could have significance for the receiving motoneurones if temporal facilitation of synaptic effectiveness is a general feature of these connections. The high frequencies of cortical spikes at the beginning of the burst of phasic–tonic discharge could be especially effective in determining the precise timing of motoneurone discharge and motor unit activation (Porter 1972; Lemon and Mantel 1989). Such temporal factors may be of particular importance in relation to the fine control of the timing of motor unit activation in precision movements about distal joints of the limb. Some evidence exists which relates the occurrence of the time of the least interval in a burst of cortical cell firing to the time of onset of muscle contraction in successive trials of a movement task (see Phillips and Porter 1977, pp. 273–81).

Although for an individual neurone, the relation between its discharge frequency and the onset of movement may be very precise, all studies to date have reported a wide variation in the time of onset of discharge over the whole population of motor cortex neurones investigated (Evarts 1972; Porter and Lewis 1975; Thach 1975; Fetz *et al.* 1980). As Hepp-Reymond (1988) has pointed out, the large scatter of the latencies raises a significant problem of interpretation. Since even single joint movements require a complex set of muscular actions to be set in progress, it may be that this variation reflects differences among the members of a group of neurones having different projections to heterogenous targets. But against this is the evidence of Cheney and Fetz (1980) who found a similarly large scatter discharge in onset times for a group of CM cells which all facilitated EMG activity in the same group of wrist muscles. A further possibility is that the scatter represents a recruitment process within the motor cortex (Porter and Lewis 1975). The cortico-motoneuronal cells which modulated their activity earliest in relation to movement showed phasic–tonic or phasic patterns of activity, while tonic cells modulated their firing only just before or after movement onset (Fetz and Cheney 1980; Wannier *et al.* 1991; see Fig. 5.4); to some extent these categories correspond to fast and slow PTNs, respectively (Fromm and Evarts 1981), although this dichotomy is by no means absolute (Hepp-Reymond 1988, pp. 550).

It is also important to realise that changes are occurring in all the descending pathways and in the receiving motoneurones throughout this 60 ms interval. Because of these changes, and the bringing of motoneurones into a state of progressively heightened excitability, the reaction time to a change of instruction, occurring during the emergence of a motor response, is much briefer than in the conventional conditioned response situation (Vicario and Ghez 1984; Pettersson 1990; Paulignan *et al.* 1990; Georgopoulos *et al.* 1989). Both reaction time and motor cortex neuronal activity can be influenced by the information available before movement occurs. For instance, Riehle and Requin (1989) showed that when monkeys were informed of both the direction and extent of a required wrist movement, motor cortex neurones became active earlier in relation to movement onset, and the reaction time was shorter than in situations when only information related to the extent of the movement was available.

5.4 THE RELATIONSHIP OF NEURONAL DISCHARGE IN THE MOTOR CORTEX TO FORCE DEVELOPMENT IN CONTRACTING MUSCLES

While studying the discharges of identified PTN, Evarts (1968) examined the effects of dissociating the position achieved by the wrist, in a repetitive flexion–extension task, from the force required to be produced in flexor and extensor muscles in order to achieve and maintain a given position (see Fig. 5.5). For 26/31 PTNs examined, he demonstrated clear changes in firing rate when additional loads were added to oppose either wrist flexion or extension. Since the displacement of the lever was the same in all trials, the changes in PTN firing were clearly related to the force needed to achieve that position rather than to the position itself. The activity of the remaining 5/31 PTNs was better related to displacement.

The relationship between the discharge rate of motor cortex neurones and static force demonstrated by Evarts has since been confirmed many times. These investigations have examined the control of force in a variety of tasks (Smith *et al.* 1975; Hepp-Reymond *et al.* 1978; Cheney and Fetz 1980; Hoffman and Luschei 1980; Evarts *et al.* 1983; Kalaska *et al.* 1989; Werner *et al.* 1991; Wannier *et al.* 1991; see Hepp-Reymond 1988). The conclusions from these different studies may be summarized as follows.

First, a variable proportion of the neurones sampled within the motor cortex showed activity related to static force: sometimes the proportion was found to be as low as 20–25 per cent (Evarts 1969; Hoffman and Luschei 1980), but more usually it was in the 40–50 per cent range (see Hepp-Reymond 1988; Crutcher and Alexander 1990; Werner *et al.* 1991). The studies which yielded the highest proportion of force related neurones were those in which the sample was restricted either to identified PTNs (Evarts

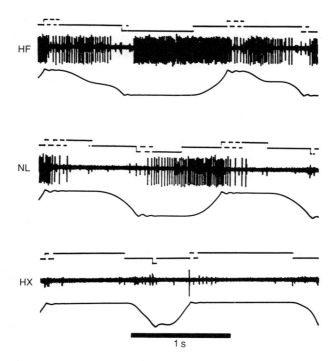

FIG 5.5   Evidence for correlation of the discharges of a PTN with the force needed to move the wrist to a flexed position, rather than with the displacement of the wrist to that position. These results were obtained in the classic study reported by E. V. Evarts (1968). The figure illustrates the discharges of a PTN associated with movements of a lever between an extensor stop and a flexor stop (upwards movement of the third trace indicates displacement to the flexor stop). In the traces labelled HF, a load of 400 g was added to the lever to require increased force development in the flexor muscles during the displacement (to move the lever plus the load) and during 'paying out' of the load at the onset of the extensor displacement. NL reveals the discharges when no load was added to the lever. HX indicates that, with a load so placed as to assist the flexor displacement, movement to this position occurred without significant discharge of the PTN. (Reproduced with permission.)

et al. 1983; 62 per cent) or to identified cortico-motoneuronal cells (Cheney and Fetz 1980; see below). These results indicate that static force is an important but not the sole parameter encoded by neuronal activity in M1, the primary motor cortex (Thach 1978).

Secondly, some M1 neurones modulated their discharge over the entire range of forces tested, while others tended to code for force over a much more limited range (Hepp-Reymond *et al.* 1978; Hoffman and Luschei

1980; Evarts *et al.* 1983). Amongst their large sample of 94 PTNs with significant changes in discharge frequency with static load, Evarts *et al.* (1983) found that slow PTNs (antidromic latency (ADL) >1.5 ms) tended to encode over the entire load range tested, while most fast PTNs (ADL <1.5 ms) exhibited sigmoidal relationships (see Fig. 5.6).

Third, many M1 neurones showed a striking modulation of their activity at low force levels. This important feature of M1 activity was first demonstrated by Hepp-Reymond *et al.* (1978) when they reported M1 neurones which became active during an isometric precision-grip task, which was adjusted for very low forces (<1.0 N total force exerted between the tips of the thumb and index finger: see Fig. 5.9). The fast PTNs illustrated in Fig. 5.6b showed large changes in firing rate at low forces, close to the point of load reversal from supination to pronation or vice-versa. Further evidence suggesting augmented motor cortex activity during production of small force increments was furnished by Evarts *et al.* (1983), who concluded that 'M1 outputs are especially important in controlling the early recruited motoneurones that are involved in precise fine movements'. The rate of change of force (dF/dT) may also be encoded by some neurones (see Smith *et al.* 1975).

While frequency modulation of the discharges of these output elements appears to be the major means of encoding changes at low levels of force, what happens at high force levels? In contrast to the behaviour of the motoneurone pool, where large, late-recruited motoneurones are activated when high forces are needed, relatively few M1 neurones are found to be recruited specifically at high force levels (Cheney and Fetz 1980; Evarts *et al.* 1983). It is difficult to train animals to sustain such strong contractions for long, and relatively little work has been done to explore the contribution, if any, of M1 to the generation of large forces.

A final property of M1 neurones revealed by these studies has been the demonstration that, for the majority of neurones, there is a congruence of their torque and displacement sensitivities. Evarts *et al.* (1983) examined 273 M1 cells, which modulated their activity when the monkey was rewarded for resisting different external torques applied to a handle; 206 of these cells also changed their firing when the monkey controlled the position of the handle. Those cells which increased their discharge with loads which required increased pronator activity, became more active when the forearm was actively moved into a pronated position against a constant load. Kalaska *et al.* (1989) demonstrated that, in the monkey, M1 neurones which showed continuously graded changes in activity related to the direction of a reaching movement, also exhibited similar large graded changes in discharge when inertial loads were applied to the device moved by the monkey. Such load related activity was particularly strong in cells recorded at low threshold ICMS sites, many of which were probably in lamina V.

An important advance was made by Cheney and Fetz (1980) when

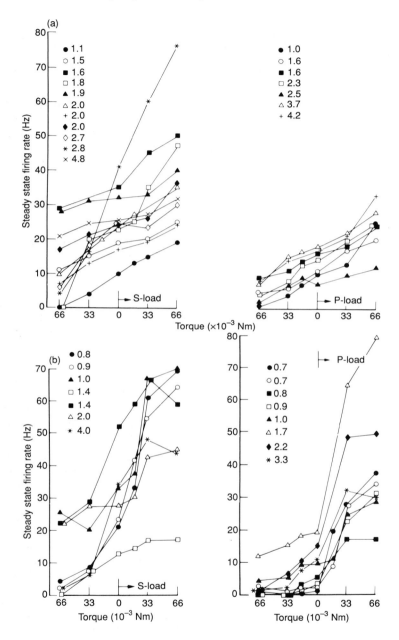

FIG 5.6 Relationship between firing rate of motor cortex PTNs and the static force exerted by a monkey. The monkey grasped a handle and maintained it in a position with the forearm midway between supination and pronation, against steady external torques (33 and 66 $\times$ 10^{-3} N m) applied to the handle in either direction.

they examined the relationship to force generation of identified cortico-motoneuronal cells discharging in association with a repetitive stereotyped wrist flexion–extension task. The monkeys were rewarded for the correct performance, on each occasion, of a ramp-and-hold performance of the movement at the wrist. This could be auxotonic, wherein the wrist moved against an elastic load requiring generation of active torque proportional to wrist displacement, or the animal could be required to generate isometric responses in which a ramp-and-hold torque was generated without wrist displacement. All cortico-motoneuronal cells related to these tasks could be classified into one of four groups on the basis of the profile of their discharge with the ramp and hold performance; these different categories are illustrated in Fig. 5.7. More than half (59 per cent) were phasic–tonic, 28 per cent were tonic, 8 per cent were phasic–ramp and 5 per cent had a ramp profile of firing in relation to the task.

To investigate the relationship between the discharges of these cortico-motoneuronal cells and the development of force in their target muscles, the monkeys were required to exert different levels of torque for the same displacement or, in the isometric condition, without displacement. During the hold periods, tonic activity of the cells was a linearly increasing function of the level of the static torque over the whole range of torque levels tested. The increase in firing rate per increase in static torque was similar for auxotonic and isometric responses. Graphs of the relationships between cell firing and static torque for 14 extension-related cortico-motoneuronal cells are illustrated in Fig. 5.8. These cells were investigated under auxotonic conditions; their PSF effects are also shown. The mean slope of the firing rate–force relationship for all extension-related cells was higher than the mean slope for all flexion-related cells (4.8 and 2.5 Hz/Ncm, respectively). Most cortico-motoneuronal cells in this test situation were inactive when the monkey was at rest and silent during movements in the direction opposite to that associated with contractions of their target muscles. Only one CM cell (SI 64-3 in Fig. 5.8) showed a clear torque threshold for tonic discharge.

The control of force in a precision grip represents a functionally impor-

---

(a): Linear gradation of firing rate over the entire torque range tested was found for 11 PTNs (shown on the left) which increased their activity with the load opposing supination (S-load), and for 7 PTNs increasing activity with the load opposing pronation (P-load). Most of these neurones were slow PTNs with antidromic latencies (ADLs) of 1.5 ms or longer (ADL in ms given beside each cell symbol). (b): Non-linear relation of firing rate to load shown by 7 PTNs with higher discharge rates for S-load (on left) and 8 PTNs with higher rates for P-load (right). Most of these neurones showed a steep increase in firing rate between zero load and the 33×10^{-3} N m load. Many were fast PTNs with short ADLs (<1.5 ms). (Reproduced with permission from Evarts *et al.* (1983).)

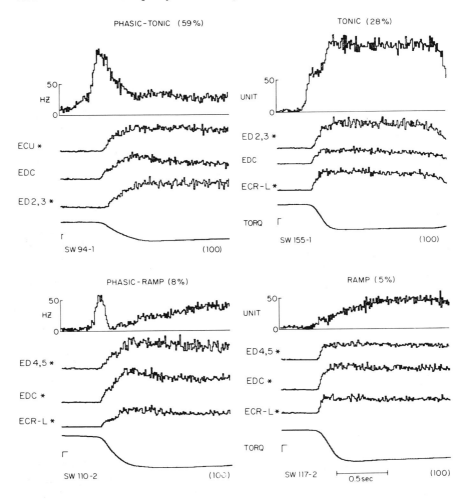

FIG 5.7 The four types of response patterns characteristic of CM cells during ramp-and-hold wrist movements in the monkey. The illustrated responses are isometric torque trajectories; similar patterns occurred when torque was accompanied by wrist displacement. The four categories are distinguished by: (a) the firing rate during the static hold period, which was either constant (tonic types, top) or increasing (ramp cells, bottom); and (b) the presence (left) or absence (right) of an additional dynamic burst response during the initial increase in torque. Percentages in brackets indication proportion of 135 CM cells studied with this pattern of activity. Also averaged were rectified EMG activity of three coactivated forearm muscles; those facilitated by each cell are indicated by an asterisk. Torque calibration bar: 5×10^5 dyn cm. 100 trials were averaged for each cell. (Reproduced with permission from Cheney and Fetz (1980).)

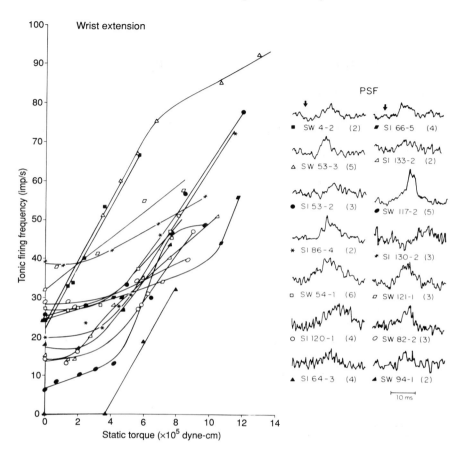

F IG 5.8 Relation between tonic firing rate and static torque for 14 CM cells related to wrist extension. For each cell, an example of PSF of one target muscle is shown at the right; arrows at top indicate time of triggering spike in CM cell. The number of facilitated muscles is indicated in parentheses. Cells were selected solely on the basis of the strength of their PSF and the adequacy of the range of loads studied. The firing rate of all plotted cells was measured from response averages, compiled for at least four load levels. All cells showed activity linearly related to torque over at least part of the tested torque range. (Reproduced with permission from Cheney and Fetz (1980).)

tant aspect of primate hand function. It is a biomechanically complex task, requiring the activity of many different intrinsic and extrinsic hand muscles (Smith 1981; Muir 1985; Maier *et al.* 1990, 1993). Hepp-Reymond and her colleagues have documented in great detail the behaviour of M1 neurones during an isometric precision grip task, which is illustrated in Fig. 5.9. The paradigm employed a two-step force control at low force levels (up to 1.0 N). In a recent study, Wannier *et al.* (1991) described a total of 331 M1 neurones with either phasic, phasic–tonic or tonic patterns of discharge during the task, and 62 per cent of these cells showed significant changes in firing with force. For the cells with a positive correlation (e.g. those shown in Fig. 5.9c), the average force sensitivity was 69 Hz/N. Interestingly, a high proportion of correlated neurones showed negative correlations with force. These 'decreasing' cells showed a clear reduction in firing rate as grip force increased (see Fig. 5.9d). None of the cells was identified, although many may have been corticospinal neurones since they were recorded at loci yielding digit movements with low ICMS currents.

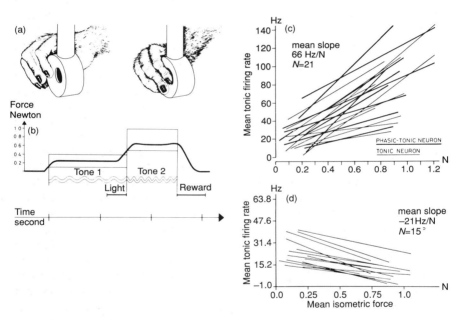

FIG 5.9 Relationship of motor cortex neuronal activity to precision grip force in the monkey. (a) Manipulandum used to measure isometric grip force exerted in the precision grip. The gauge was pressed between thumb and index finger. (From Smith *et al.* (1975).) (b) Experimental paradigm. The force had to be kept constant within narrow limits set at two successive levels; correct force level exerted by the monkey was signalled by tones of different frequencies. A light signal provided the instruction to increase force from the first to the second level. (c) and (d) Regression lines calculated for M1 neurones having a statistically significant monotonic change in their firing rate with force. (c) Regression lines for 33 tonic and phasic-tonic M1 neurones with positive correlations. (d) Negative regression lines for 15 phasic-tonic neurones which decreased their firing rates with increased force. (From Hepp-Reymond (1988). Copyright © 1988. Reprinted by permission of John Wiley and Sons Inc.)

Muir and Lemon (1983) first described a small population of identified cortico-motoneuronal cells which increased their discharge rate with increased auxotonic load. A study of 28 cortico-motoneuronal units was subsequently carried out by Maier *et al.* (1993); these cells all produced medium to strong postspike facilitation (PSF) of intrinsic hand muscles. The relationship of CM cell mean firing rate to static grip force was investigated under either isometric or auxotonic conditions. Although the activity of most of the selected cells showed some relation to force, in only half of them (14/28) was there a statistically significant correlation; the correlation was positive for eleven and negative for three cells. The rate/force slopes were 32.8 Hz/N for positively correlated and -39 Hz/N for negatively correlated cells. The other 14 cells showed either uncorrelated activity, or were completely deactivated during the hold period of the task (three cells). This task, which was somewhat different from that used by Hepp-Reymond *et al.* (1978) and by Wannier *et al.* (1991), required independent control of the force level exerted on two levers by the thumb and index finger. A focused pattern of force control by these CM cells was suggested by the finding that all the correlated neurones exhibited a significant force sensitivity for one digit or the other, but not for both.

Maier *et al.* (1993) examined the 'muscle fields' of their CM cell sample and looked for any relationship between the pattern of target muscle activity and the type and strength of the correlation of their discharge with force. Most of the cells with significant correlations had small muscle fields (one to three muscles showing a PSF) while cells with larger muscle fields had weak or no correlations, again suggesting that the precise level of grip force was better encoded in cells with more focused muscle targets.

The existence of CM cells with a negative covariation of firing rate with force was unexpected, since these cells clearly had an excitatory influence over their target muscles and Maier *et al.* (1993) even showed that the absolute amplitude of the PSF generated increased with increasing force level. But there were no differences in the muscle fields of negatively and positively correlated cells. It is probably significant that neurones with activity negatively correlated to force have not been reported in studies of M1 activity during control of force during other tasks, such as biting, wrist extension/flexion or forearm supination/pronation (Hoffman and Luschei 1980; Cheney and Fetz 1980; Evarts *et al.* 1983, respectively). The biomechanical complexity of the precision grip movement requires accurate adjustment of the level of co-contraction amongst the active muscles, and it can be argued that the decreased level of activity in some CM cells could result in a disfacilitation of Ia inhibitory interneurones, which normally reinforce a reciprocal pattern of muscle activity (Smith 1981; Fetz and Cheney 1987; Maier *et al.* 1993; see Section 5.5 below). Alternatively these 'negative cells' may be important for the controlled release of force: by increasing their activity at a time when most of the positively covarying cells are decreasing theirs, they may provide a more sensitive control mechanism for force control during the release of objects from the grip.

It is perhaps surprising that a relatively small proportion of M1 cortico-motoneuronal cells has been found to show activity correlated with precision-grip force. But cortico-motoneuronal cells which discharge in relation to the use of the small muscles of the hand, in relatively independent movements of the digits, tend to discharge most in association with this essential fractionation of distal muscle activity in the positioning of the fingers, even in the absence of external loads. This intense discharge during the finest movements of the fingers (see Fig. 5.11) was originally reported by Evarts (1967) and has been the subject of extensive discussion in Section 4.12, to which the reader is referred.

5.5 POSSIBLE CORTICOSPINAL INVOLVEMENT IN CONTROL OF JOINT STIFFNESS

Humphrey and Reed (1983) recorded from neurones in the 'wrist' zone of the precentral motor cortex. The animals were required to resist a sinusoidally varying load tending to displace the wrist in a flexion or extension direction at different frequencies. While at low frequencies (< 0.6 Hz) the animals opposed the applied load by exerting appropriate 'reciprocal' extensor or flexor forces by contracting appropriate muscles acting on the wrist, at higher frequencies, co-contraction of the flexor and extensor muscles occurred, increasing the overall stiffness of the joint, and holding the wrist in a steady position in the face of the oscillating imposed loads. These different strategies for resistance of load changes at different frequencies were reflected in the discharges of neurones in the motor cortex, 42 per cent of which were rapidly conducting PTNs and 13 per cent were slowly conducting PTNs.

At low displacement frequencies, neurones in the motor cortex exhibited 'reciprocal' actions and their discharges varied in line with the observations of Evarts (1968) and Cheney and Fetz (1980). At higher frequencies of load change, a class of neurones which fired tonically, and with discharge rates increasing as the frequency of the force perturbation was increased, was identified. This suggested the existence of a population of cells within the precentral cerebral cortex whose discharges were related to the task of co-contraction of antagonistic muscles and to the fixation of the wrist joint by increasing its stiffness in relation to load changes.

5.6 MODIFICATION OF MOTOR CORTEX OUTPUT BY PRIOR INSTRUCTION

Tanji and Evarts (1976) trained monkeys to make one of two responses by either pushing or pulling a vertical handle which was gripped continuously with the fingers wrapped around it. The 'instruction' about the direction of the movement to be made was provided by a coloured light, green to push and red to pull. Having received the instruction about direction, the animals were required to wait until a later signal (a brief perturbation of the lever itself, which might be detected like a tap in the hand) indicated that it was time to push or pull, and then to perform that movement briskly. Records were obtained from identified PTNs in the 'arm area' of the motor cortex and it was found that many of these PTNs changed their firing well in advance of the actual performance of the movement. Many more PTNs (75 per cent of the sample of 122) changed their firing in preparation for future movement than did non-PTNs (23 per cent of 137) and the change in firing rate was greater for the PTNs. These preparatory changes in response to the 'instruction' occurred 200 to 500 ms after the instruction was provided but were not accompanied by any change in EMG activity in the target muscles of the forearm. It was only after the 'move now' trigger had been given that the appropriate muscles for the push or pull action were called into contraction. Additional changes in the discharges of the PTNs preceded and accompanied these voluntary contractions.

The effects of the prior instruction, about the direction of the movement to be executed, seemed to operate differently on different PTNs. A neurone which increased its firing in preparation for the push movement would decrease its firing when the instruction called for a pull movement after the waiting period. In parallel with these changes in preparatory discharge there were modulations of the amplitude of the dynamic stretch reflexes exhibited in the arm muscles in response to the perturbations of the lever which pulled on those muscles. During the period in which the monkey was waiting to produce a pull movement after a perturbation which stretched the biceps muscle, there was an increase in the size of the short latency reflex caused by this sudden stretch. The same reflex response was diminished during periods following an instruction for the animal to prepare to push. It was suggested that the firing of PTNs during the waiting period could be modifying the excitability of subcortical and spinal centres in preparation for the trigger to move. Tanji and Evarts (1976) suggested that this preparatory PTN discharge was resetting subcortical and spinal centres to focus fusimotor drive to appropriate muscles which would become the prime movers in the subsequent task. In this connection it may have been significant that the preparatory effects generated by the instruction were more evident in PTNs than other neurones. As we have seen, the PTNs are connected, through corticospinal systems and extensive collateralization with all the subcortical and spinal neurones which we would expect, from their connectivity, to be involved in the production of a movement response.

Although these overtrained animals made very few errors in their motor responses to the instruction, when a wrong direction of movement did occur in response to the trigger signal, this response was invariably associated with an incorrect 'preparatory' discharge of the PTN. In addition, if the instruction light and the perturbation trigger followed one another after a very short interval, the presentation of the signal to move 'was usually associated with a grossly impaired motor response'. It is implied that a period of preparation of (or by) the motor cortex is required, following an instruction about a direction of movement to be made, so that the motor centres in the brain and spinal cord can be primed for appropriate motor outputs. Preparatory activity in motor cortex can be shown to encode movement direction, but does not appear to reflect either current or anticipated loading conditions or amplitude of movement (Alexander and Crutcher 1990a; Riehle and Requin 1993). It must be presumed that the changes in firing of PTN during preparation for movement are indicators of such priming modulation of widespread neuronal activities which occur in many parts of the central nervous system. These preparatory changes depend on cortico-cortical influences impinging on the motor cortex from premotor and other regions influenced by the instruction and reflect changes in excitability in other cortical zones and in deep brain structures such as the basal ganglia (see Alexander and Crutcher 1990a,b; Crutcher and Alexander 1990). It is probable that similar changes occur during internally generated movements and may contribute substantially to the delay between the initial discharge of M1 neurones and movement onset (Mushiake *et al.* 1991; see Section 5.3).

5.7 CO-OPERATIVE ACTIVITY OF POPULATIONS OF NEURONES IN THE PRECENTRAL MOTOR CORTEX

In addition to the corticospinal neurones, each projection area of the cerebral cortex contains a large number of other neuronal elements. Moreover, the cortical representation of movement at different joints (finger, wrist, elbow, and shoulder) is now known to show extensive regions of overlap (see Chapter 8). The muscles facilitated by a single cortico-motoneuronal cell can be employed in movements at different joints. It has been reasoned that the summed total neuronal activity in the combined projection areas related to movements about all of these joints will be relevant to the voluntary task of reaching to a target in space: Georgopoulos (1988) states,

It is sufficient to realise that the organisation and neural integration of the reaching movement need not be the concern, or the burden, of the motor cortex: instead, we suppose that the motor cortex is concerned with the specification of the direction of reaching in space according to internally generated goals (as, for example, in drawing) or according to information from exteroceptors (for example, in reaching towards a visual or an auditory object). The initiation of reaching in the appropriate direction would then be accomplished by the activation of neuronal populations in the motor cortex, which, in turn, would engage the spinal reaching circuits.

Georgopoulos *et al.* (1982) examined the discharges of individual neurones in the precentral motor cortex in monkeys trained to move their hand to a visual target in two dimensional space. The activities of single neurones were only broadly tuned to a preferred direction of reaching to the target (see Fig. 5.10). Each cell had its own preferred direction; discharge of individual cells was highest for movements in this direction and gradually decreased with movements in directions progressively further away from the preferred one. It was possible to demonstrate that this firing related to the direction of the active movement, rather than to the position of the target in space, by requiring that the monkey, rather than reaching to a series of targets at different locations, commence each movement from one of these widespread locations and always move to a single centrally placed target location. There was little evidence for any significant coding of movement amplitude in this population of motor cortex cells (Georgopoulos 1987, pp. 137).

It was possible to assign the contribution of each cortical cell in a sampled population to the specification of a particular direction of movement by plotting that cell's *predicted* discharge in relation to that direction of movement as a vector of length related to the cell's change in discharge frequency with that particular movement. The separate sums of all these vectors for all the cells from which sequential recordings had been made were calculated for each direction of movement studied. These 'population vectors', assembled by aggregating the responses of many separately recorded units, illustrated the outcome of the 'ensemble operation' of the neurones in that area of cerebral cortex. They produced a result, for reaching in either two-dimensional or three-dimensional space (Georgopoulos *et al.* 1983) that indicated that the actual direction of movement fell within the 95 per cent confidence limits of the population vector's prediction of movement direction from the summed activities of the discharges of a population of broadly tuned neurones (Fig. 5.10). Moreover, this prediction of direction could be detected in the pre-movement discharges of the cells, even during delay periods imposed before the movement could be executed (Georgopoulos 1987; Georgopoulos *et al.* 1989).

Georgopoulos, having set out to examine the aspects of the neuronal responses that could be aligned with the direction of the reaching movement, concluded that the representation of directional information in the

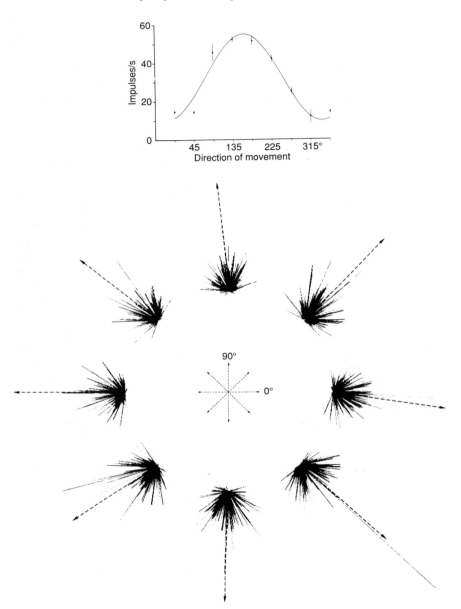

FIG 5.10 Representation of the direction of reaching movements in the monkey motor cortex. Above: directional tuning curve for a single neurone. The data points are the mean (±SEM) frequency of discharge from the target onset until the end of the movement for a neurone recorded in a task in which a monkey had to reach from a central hold zone to one of nine target positions arranged in a circle of 8

motor cortex must be a distributed code, in that each cellular element provides only part of the information and 'the ensemble (i.e. the neuronal population) uniquely determines the direction of the movement in space' (Georgopoulus 1988). He estimated that, in order to specify the direction of the movement within 10 to 15 degrees, the contributions of approximately 150 to 200 cells were required to be included to achieve the population vector. These elements were assumed to have fixed influences on weighted combinations of muscles involved in the reaching task and all were expected to make equally strong contributions, proportional to their directional vector. It may not be appropriate to give equal weighting to the contributions of all these cortical elements because some, those with axons projecting to the spinal cord, must be presumed to have a greater direct contribution to make to the influences exerted on the spinal cord machinery for execution of the reaching movement and hence on the activated muscles.

In these experiments, the population vectors calculated for the discharges of cells in layers II and III (most of whose axons have cortico-cortical destinations) gave predictions of the direction of movements in two-dimensional space, which were as adequate to describe the movement as those calculated for the discharges of lamina V and VI neurones (Georgopoulos 1988). This result suggests that, *if* the receiving areas of the separate projections from the motor cortex that are represented in these complex synthetic populations are able to decode, from the convergent signals they receive, the vectors that are implied in this form of analysis, directional information about the reaching movement is available to all brain structures in receipt of these projections. In the deeper layers, more cells show load related activity. Kalaska *et al.* (1989) defined the 'load axis' of M1 cells as the direction of inertial load opposing the movement direction associated with the cell's highest firing rate. For a majority of cells, the load axis was close to 180° from the preferred direction observed under unloaded conditions, although in some cells a more complex relationship between the two encoded parameters was observed.

Because the majority of the neurones sampled in these studies must be presumed to make connections remote from the motoneurones which

---

cm radius centred on the hold position. The curve is a sinusoid fitted to the means by a least squares method. From this curve the 'preferred direction' of this cell can be calculated to be toward a position at about 160°. Below: population vectors for a sample of 241 motor cortex cells. Each cluster represents the same population; each line represents the contribution of one cell; its angle indicates the preferred direction for that cell, and its length indicates the firing rate in the direction represented by the different clusters. The population vector (thick dashed line with arrow) points in the direction (or near to the direction) of the reaching movement, which is indicated by the thin dashed lines in the centre diagram. (Reproduced with permission from Georgopoulos *et al.* 1982, 1983).)

will activate the co-ordinated muscle contractions involved in the reaching movement, it is not possible to specify the transforms to which these neuronal discharge signals will be subjected in connection with movement execution. In other words it is not possible to identify any causal relationship between the *representation* of the population vector and the *execution* of the movement in the same direction. This is particularly true for the shoulder girdle muscles in the macaque monkey, which appear to lack any strong cortico-motoneuronal projection (Kuypers 1981; Flament *et al.* 1992c). Earlier attempts to give a summary of the quantitative relationship between the aggregate of firing rates of cells in the motor cortex and the output variables of a movement performance which involved the rotation of a joystick were made by Humphrey (1972). The response of a theoretical linear control system, receiving the summed cortical discharge as input, was optimally matched to the real movement performance if, after a delay of 50 to 100 ms, the output had been transformed by a function which had temporal characteristics resembling the twitch tension profile of skeletal muscle. In the experiments of Humphrey *et al.* (1970), and in line with the more recent studies of Georgopoulos and his colleagues, the calculations for groups, including increasing numbers of neurones, gave a smoother output for the proposed control system than did single cells. A larger assembly of neurones provided more accurate predictions of the movement outcome. These were almost equally accurate for displacement achieved, velocity of the movement and rate of change of force with time (Humphrey *et al.* 1970): all of these are, of course, correlated variables and derive from co-ordinated contractions of co-operating muscles.

Fetz and Shupe (1990) have used a neural network model to examine the contribution of a population made up of different types of cortical 'hidden units' to a wrist flexion–extension tracking movement. Dependent on the relative weighting given to these different units (which weightings represented the strengths of their linkages to the flexor or extensor motoneurones) it was possible to transform a simple stimulus (a visible step change in a target position) to the patterns of motoneurone discharge which have been observed to occur during the performance of a movement to the target. It was possible to produce this result by appropriate combinations of units showing tonic, phasic–tonic, ramp, or decrementing activity, similar to those shown in Fig. 5.7, and to include contributions of units whose activity appeared to be uncorrelated with the task. But there was no unique solution to the problem. Fetz (1992) states: 'Relevant to the coding issue, one significant result of these simulations is the demonstration that a large number of network solutions can produce the same transform'. This point is relevant to the general flexibility which is characteristic of the motor system, and the large number of degrees of freedom within which it appears to operate.

5.8 NEURONAL ACTIVITY IN THE MOTOR CORTEX IN ASSOCIATION WITH CONTRALATERAL, IPSILATERAL, AND BILATERAL MOVEMENTS OF THE DIGITS

Even in the conditioned response experiments of Evarts (1966), a small proportion of PTNs in the motor cortex discharged a burst of impulses in association with a brisk wrist extension movement performed by the ipsilateral limb. Lemon *et al.* (1976) reported discharges of the same cell in the motor cortex accompanying either ipsilateral or contralateral hand movements in a small proportion of their PTNs. A similar small proportion of neurones in the precentral gyrus of human subjects was found to discharge with ipsilateral hand movements (Goldring and Ratcheson 1972). Matsunami and Hamada (1978) also reported bilateral associations with movement of PTN discharge in experiments on conscious monkeys. Tanji *et al.* (1987) designed an experiment specifically to examine the involvement of different areas of the cortex in ipsilateral, or bilateral, as well as contralateral movements. They trained monkeys to press a small key with the right or left hand or with both hands, each in response to an appropriate signal. A small proportion (8.2 per cent) of neurones in the precentral motor cortex changed their firing before ipsilateral and bilateral, but not before contralateral, movements. A further 5 per cent of neurones in the precentral motor cortex (similar to the proportion found by Lemon *et al.* 1976) demonstrated bilateral associations, that is, they discharged when both the contralateral and the ipsilateral limb were used. In both cases, the pre-movement lead time was similar to that for cells with exclusively contralateral associations. We have already alluded to the potential role of the small proportion of ipsilateral and bilaterally projecting corticospinal fibres which could produce these effects (see Section 2.7).

5.9 FLEXIBILITY OF THE RELATIONSHIP BETWEEN CORTICOSPINAL DISCHARGE AND MUSCULAR CONTRACTION: TASK-RELATED ACTIVITY

To test the security of the relationship between cortical discharge and force development, Fetz and Finocchio (1971, 1972) trained a monkey to produce isometric contractions of particular forelimb muscles while its arm was immobilized in a cast. Using the EMG activity recorded from arm muscles as reinforcement criteria, they were able to train the monkey to produce contractions in one of these muscles while suppressing, more or less completely, the EMG responses in the other muscles from which simultaneous recordings were being made. With appropriate reinforcement, the monkey could be trained to produce relatively isolated contractions, in turn, in each of four muscles from which EMGs were recorded. Some precentral cortical cells, including PTNs, produced bursts of impulses commencing about 70 ms before the onset of EMG activity in one of the muscles (e.g. biceps brachii) as would have been anticipated from earlier studies. These cells were inactive when relatively isolated contractions of other muscles (e.g. triceps) were produced. The stability of this relationship was tested by rewarding the animal for producing bursts of discharge of the cortical cell while simultaneously suppressing all muscle contraction, including that of the muscle with which the cortical cell's firing had been closely related (e.g. biceps, in this example). After many trials, this dissociation could be achieved. Phillips and Porter (1977, pp. 293) pointed out that this dissociation could have depended on other cortical connections with the spinal cord machinery for movement being so modified in this conditioned situation that motor output was prevented in spite of the influence of the test cells.

The reverse dissociation was attempted, when the monkey was rewarded for producing contractions in the biceps muscle without concomitant cellular discharge in the sample cortical neurone. This dissociation was not achieved completely. Contraction of the muscle could be accompanied by less than the normal cortical cellular discharge. This could have implied that, in order to initiate contraction of the biceps muscle, some cortical discharge of cells related to the innervation of motoneurones of this muscle was essential.

Other dissociations between PTN firing and motor responses are also well documented. Evarts (1964) found that, in sleep, bursts of high-frequency discharge may occur in PTN without any overt motor response. Cheney and Fetz (1984) indicated that many cortico-motoneuronal cells fired impulses in response to passive joint rotation or cutaneous stimulation, yet these neuronal responses were not accompanied by contractions of the target muscles of those cortico-motoneuronal cells. Cheney and Fetz (1980) reported that little discharge in cortico-motoneuronal cells accompanied the 'intense activity' of their target muscles in association with rapid ballistic movements. These authors reported that some monkey cortico-motoneuronal cells which showed reciprocal activity during wrist flexion–extension movements were almost completely deactivated during a power grip (Fetz and Cheney 1987).

A clear dissociation between the amount of cortico-motoneuronal discharge of a particular cell and activity in its target muscle was revealed by changing from a precision grip to a power grip in the experiments of Muir and Lemon (1983) and Buys *et al.* (1986). They examined the task related discharges of monkey cortico-motoneuronal cells which all facilitated muscle activity in at least one intrinsic hand muscle. Each of these cells was discharged at higher frequency during the precision grip task, despite the fact that in most cases the cell's target muscle was more active during the power grip (see Fig. 5.11). According to Muir and Lemon (1983), 'These cortico-motoneuronal PTNs can thus be taken to have a

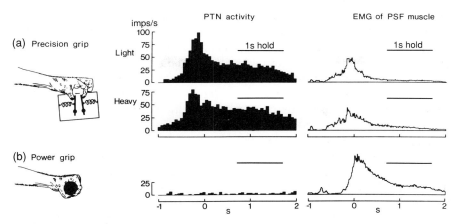

Fɪɢ 5.11   Activity of a monkey PTN during precision and power grip. (a): Response averages for a PTN and for the muscle (1DI) in which it produced a PSF, showing activity before and during a precision grip task. Histograms of PTN discharges for 16 repetitions of the task with either light (above) or heavy force were constructed in relation to the earliest detectable lever movement (time zero). The gross EMG recorded at the same time with percutaneous wire electrodes was recti-fied and averaged (shown at right). (b): Corresponding task-related analysis for the same PTN and muscle during the power grip. Time zero represents the earliest detectable pressure increase in the rubber cylinder. This cell was almost completely deactivated during the power grip, despite the fact that its target muscle showed increased activity during this task. (Reproduced with permission from Muir and Lemon (1983).)

particular role during the fractionation of muscle action required for discrete movements of individual digits'. Differences in firing rate have also been observed for some CM cells when monkeys performed two different 'precision' tasks, both involving independent movements of the index finger and thumb: a pincer grip and a rotation grip (Bennett 1992). So flexibility of functional association, even for monosynaptically connected cortical neurones and motoneurones, may be dependent on the task in which the total muscular apparatus is engaged. One of the operations that this may represent is the change in muscle synergy that is required for different tasks (see Section 4.12).

5.10 CORTICAL DISCHARGE DURING LOCOMOTION: OBSERVATIONS MADE IN CATS

Although it has been clear, since the early experiments of Graham Brown, that cats subjected to decerebration at a high level are capable of co-ordinated walking on a moving belt and that their gait is appropriately adjusted to the rate of movement of the belt, the cerebral cortex must be capable of engaging this locomotor machinery for purposive rather than for externally initiated locomotion. Armstrong and Drew (1984a,b) used a series of implanted microwire electrodes to examine the discharge properties of cells in the motor area of the cat's cerebral cortex while these animals walked at controlled speeds on a moving belt. Records were made from identified PTNs with both fast and slow conduction velocities of their axons (Lance and Manning 1954; Armstrong 1965). The conduction velocities fell into two groups, with most common values at $10–15 \, \text{m.s}^{-1}$ and $40–55 \, \text{m.s}^{-1}$. In line with other conventions, the dividing line between the fast and the slow group of axonal conduction velocities of the PTN was set at $21 \, \text{m.s}^{-1}$ (Takahashi 1965).

During locomotion at $0.5 \, \text{m.s}^{-1}$, just over half the cortical cells discharged more rapidly than they had at rest and the greatest increases occurred in the PTNs with rapidly conducting axons. The actual discharge rates of the PTNs during locomotion ranged from 5 to 60 impulses s^{-1}. Altogether 80 per cent of the neurones studied discharged rhythmically during locomotion, generating a discrete burst of impulses in association with each step. The changes in firing that occurred in these cells with different speeds of walking were insignificant. More important, from the point of view of the above discussion concerning cortical coding of force, however, was the observation that, when the locomotion was changed to an uphill gradient, which required a major increase in muscle activity in the extensor muscles of the hindlimb and in both the flexors and extensors of the forelimb, there was no significant change in the modulation of firing of the PTNs compared with their discharge while walking on the flat. Armstrong and Drew (1984a) suggested that cortical cellular activity was more concerned with the timing of the activation of the spinal and brainstem machinery for locomotion, and that adjustments of muscle force in relation to the mechanical requirements of the task in steady walking may be delegated to these lower centres. Indeed, Graham Brown's decerebrate cats adjusted their gait to uphill walking. As the cats walked at higher rates, some PTN showed progressive changes in the timing of their bursts of activity in the step cycle, in line with the changed timing of EMG activities in some of the muscles.

5.11. CORTICAL ACTIVITY IN ASSOCIATION WITH VOLUNTARY MOVEMENTS IN HUMAN SUBJECTS

Our approach to the study of the output functions of the precentral motor cortex has been weighted heavily towards attempts to understand the behavioural relationships of the discharges of single neurones identified according to the connections made by their axons. Especially in the case of cortico-motoneuronal elements, the fact of their monosynaptic excitatory impact on spinal motoneurones innervating particular muscles provides the opportunity to analyse exactly, and to specify precisely, the functional meaning of the discharges projected along their axons during self-initiated (i.e. voluntary) movements. Yet these cortico-motoneuronal cells comprise only a few per cent of the pyramidal neurones in the precentral motor cortex, and the study of their activities can give little indication of other related functional associations of the majority of intermingled and interconnected neurones in that zone of cortex. Finally, the necessity to examine the discharges of such identified single neurones sequentially, through many different trials and frequently on separate occasions separated by days, precludes the description of functional associations of a whole integrated intra-cortical system of connected neural elements. In spite of such limitations, we advocate a continuation of the quantitative study of associations between the discharges of single, identified neurones and measured aspects of movement performance as the most fruitful approach to the study of function.

The small number of observations of single neurone discharges in precentral motor areas that has been made in human subjects performing voluntary movements indicates that parallel findings to those reported for conscious monkeys may be obtained. Naturally, the neurones in the human cortex cannot be classified according to the destination of their axonal projection. However, the conscious subjects may be asked to perform a range of different movements and the changes in activity of the one cell may be followed through all of these without the need for prolonged periods of training (Goldring and Ratcheson 1972). As a consequence, very great emphasis must be given to the data obtained in human subjects. In particular, these indicate that cortical neurones which discharge impulses in association with consciously initiated voluntary movements of the fingers do so in a manner indistinguishable from the bursts of activity recorded from single cortico-motoneuronal cells in a monkey. Secondly, these studies indicate that a small proportion of cortical neurones discharge such bursts of impulses in association with voluntary movements of the fingers of the ipsilateral as well as the contralateral hand. Finally, as we will discuss in the next chapter, these same cells are in receipt of signals generated by passive manipulation of the fingers.

The overall change in neuronal activity in a region of the human cerebral cortex, such as the 'arm area' of the precentral motor cortex, in relation to voluntary movement of a limb, may be estimated in conscious subjects by studying changes in regional cerebral blood flow (rCBF) or regional cerebral metabolism. Increases in local neuronal and synaptic activity in a region of normal human cerebral cortex will be accompanied by an increase in local metabolism. Because the brain uses glucose almost exclusively as an energy source, measures of local glucose metabolism and local oxygen consumption will be related directly to the total energy cost of neuronal activity (including synaptic actions and neural/glial responses). These changes are said to occur predominantly in the neuropil and in relation to increased activity at synapses (Roland 1987).

Changes in metabolism may be measured directly using positron emission tomography (PET) to study glucose metabolism, using a positron-emitting ^{18}F-labelled or ^{11}C-labelled deoxyglucose injection. Alternatively, oxygen consumption (with a bolus of a short-lived isotope of oxygen available for utilization by brain tissue) may be measured. Since, in the normal brain, rCBF is adjusted to local metabolic demands, changes in regional cerebral glucose metabolism or oxygen consumption should be reflected in proportional changes in rCBF. Regional blood flow, then, may be used as an indicator of overall changes in local neuronal activity. In all of these human studies, changes in cerebral activity with voluntary movement must be assessed against a background resting state, and baseline measurements of rCBF or regional metabolism must be made under conditions 'in which the subject does not move, has no detailed plans for moving, and no intention of moving' (Roland 1987). In the same individual, then, changes from these baseline measurements which accompany the performance of a particular voluntary movement, under particular conditions, may be documented.

The precentral motor cortex, in association with other localised brain regions, demonstrates a consistent increase in rCBF or regional metabolism whenever voluntary movements are performed (Oleson 1971; Roland and Larsen 1976; Mazziotta and Phelps 1984; Deiber *et al.* 1991). While local changes may be dramatic, blood flow through the whole brain remains remarkably constant through changing levels of cerebral activation (Kety and Schmidt 1946; Lassen 1959). Oleson (1971) studied focal changes in the rate of wash out (by local blood flow) of the single photon-emitting radioactive isotope ^{133}Xe which had been injected into the carotid artery as a bolus dissolved in saline to load the brain tissue (Lassen and Ingvar 1961). In the early experiments, a relatively small number of detectors could be arranged over the surface of the skull, and the localization procedures involved X-ray identification of the bony landmarks of the skull with which these detectors were associated. Resting and test states were compared in up to four repeated measurements. During the test state, in these early observations, the subject was asked to open and close his hand as vigorously as possible at a frequency of 1 to 2 movements per second throughout the period of the test measurement. Measurements of both the rest and the 'voluntarily moving' state were carried out over two-minute periods in each case.

During physical work with the contralateral hand, focally increased blood flow, which averaged 54 per cent above resting levels, was measured in all subjects except one. The size of the focus appeared to differ from subject to subject and, whereas most of the central parts of the hemisphere appeared to exhibit an increase in blood flow in one subject, localized increases corresponding to, and approximately limited to, the sensorimotor hand area of the cerebral cortex were seen in five individuals.

The measurement of rCBF by estimating local clearance of ^{133}Xe was improved by the use of narrow collimation, and large numbers of small detectors (254 detectors were assembled over one hemisphere). It was also possible to reduce the sampling period to one minute. The method, which is illustrated in Fig. 5.12, was limited to the estimation of blood flow

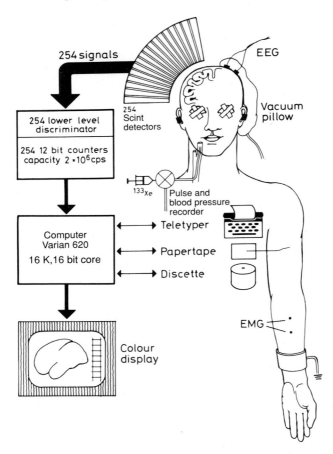

FIG 5.12 A diagram of the method used for estimating changes in regional cerebral blood flow (rCBF) from the clearance rates of the single photon-emitting isotope ^{133}Xe, following its injection into a carotid artery. (Reproduced with permission from Roland *et al.* (1980a).)

through the most superficial structures. Focal regions of increase in rCBF could be identified clearly and the location over which these functional changes were measured varied as the body musculature employed in the voluntary movement was changed. Hence, movements performed with the foot caused focal changes most medially, while those involved in speaking caused these changes most laterally over the sensorimotor region (Lassen 1985).

Roland *et al.* (1980a) required their subjects to perform a series of flex-ions of the index finger to compress a spring-loaded cylinder between index finger and thumb at a rate of once per second. This motor activity caused an increase in rCBF localized to the 'finger area' of the sensory and motor cortex. The region in which increased blood flow occurred in association even with this limited movement 'occupied almost the whole middle third of the primary motor area' (Roland 1985). Precisely this same region of motor cortex exhibited a local increase in rCBF when a much more complex task involved sequential movements of each of the fingers in quick succes-sion to touch the thumb in an organized, stereotyped learned pattern (Fig. 5.13). The area over which the blood flow change could be detected and the magnitude of that change was not dependant on the force developed by the moving fingers (Roland *et al.* 1980a).

The use of PET following administration of ^{15}O-labelled water or car-bon dioxide has allowed measurement of rCBF within short time periods, of the order of a few minutes. It also provides the opportunity for repeated observations to be made in the same subject on the same day (Raichle *et al.* 1985; Maziotta and Phelps 1985). Using approaches of this kind, Roland *et al.* (1982), Roland (1984); Maziotta and Phelps (1984); Fox *et al.* (1985) and others were able to repeat the studies of rCBF which had been measured in association with voluntary movements. Roland (1987) summarized his observations on the 'snapshots' of blood flow changes observed during one-minute measurement periods during which blood flow changes occurred in a number of neocortical areas. Because all the observa-tions available from a complete cylinder of detectors arranged round the subject's head in the PET scanner could be used to construct, by computer manipulations, a series of tomographic 'slices' through the human brain it was possible to illustrate modifications of neuronal function in deep brain structures whose changed metabolic demands were now matched by changes in rCBF to them.

We shall return to the changes in brain regions other than the motor cortex in later chapters of this book. Some, like the supplementary motor area and premotor area, are not always active during all voluntary motor tasks. Here we wish to concentrate on the motor cortex itself where the use of PET confirms in a dramatic manner that the contralateral precen-tral cortex is always activated in topographically identifiable regions when voluntary motor tasks are performed using widely spaced body parts

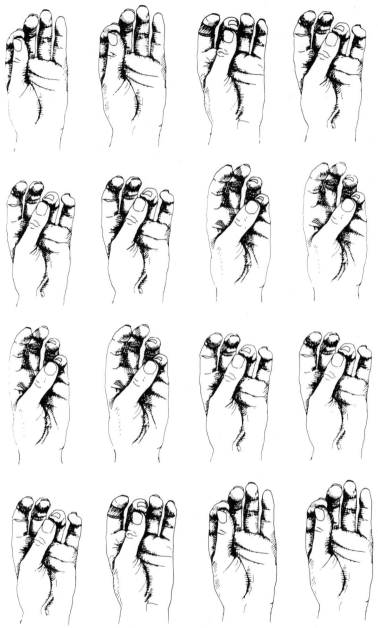

FIG 5.13   The sequence of finger-touching performances which subjects were required to learn and then perform repetitively while regional cerebral blood flow (rCBF) measurements were made is indicated from above downwards. (Reproduced with permission from Roland *et al*. (1980a).)

(Colebatch *et al.* 1991). When no voluntary motor activity is being undertaken, this primary motor area does not exhibit an increase in regional
metabolism or regional blood flow. Figure 5.14(a) illustrates the motor cortical field in the 'finger area' of the motor cortex which increased its rCBF
by 23–26 ml $100\,g^{-1}min^{-1}$ during repetitive flexion of the contralateral
index finger against a spring (Roland *et al.* 1977).

The left hand tomogram (Fig. 5.14(b)) indicates a mean percentage

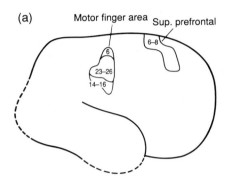

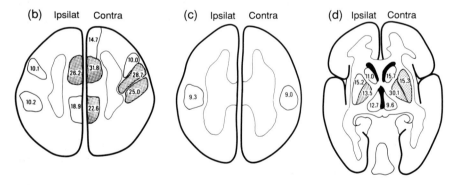

FIG 5.14   (a): Diagram to indicate the regions of the right cerebral hemisphere
in which an increase in regional cerebral blood flow (in ml $100\,g^{-1}\,min^1$) occurred
when a subject was required to repetitively flex the left index finger. (From
Roland *et al.* (1977).) (b), (c), (d): Computer-constructed tomograms illustrating the
percentage changes (averaged over 10 subjects) in regional cerebral blood flow
(rCBF) measured with PET in the human brain and occurring in association with
the performance of repetitions of the complex, learned finger-touching task
illustrated in Fig. 5.13. Three sections of the brain are shown with a separation of
17.5 mm. Cross-hatched areas $P < 0.001$, hatched areas $P < 0.01$, other areas
$P < 0.05$. (Reproduced with permission from Roland *et al.* (1982).)

increase of 28.7 per cent in the rCBF extending into the sulcal depth of the middle region of contralateral precentral cortex, averaged over 10 subjects performing the complex motor sequence task necessitating execution of a learned series of finger movements (Fig. 5.13).

There are still limitations to the detail that can be derived from PET studies in human subjects. Its spatial resolution is not yet sufficient to focus local metabolic activities or rCBF within circumscribed anatomical structures. And the temporal period within which the measurements must be made will require that other electrophysiological or magnetoencephalographic methods will be needed to understand the within-region and the between-region neural changes which are associated with these metabolic consequences. No localized increases in metabolism occur in the motor cortex during the absence of voluntary movement. This suggests a uniform level of synaptic activity through all parts of the precentral gyrus during these periods. During one-minute periods of repetitive movement performance, using the fingers of the contralateral hand, a major increase in synaptic activity is presumed to occur in the 'hand' area of the motor cortex. Some of this may be derived from other regions of the brain and may be excitatory to those output neurones which need to be recruited to the voluntary motor task and from which bursts of neuronal discharge might be detected electrophysiologically. Other synaptic actions will be suppressing, by inhibitory effects, those neurones which do not participate in the execution of these voluntary movements. The parallels of these events have been seen in conscious monkeys from whom single cell cortical recordings have been obtained.

5.12 SUMMARY

Both single-unit and rCBF studies confirm the involvement of the motor cortex in the execution of a voluntary movement. The causal nature of its contribution is confirmed by the observation that many motor cortex cortico-motoneuronal cells, with proven connections to spinal motoneurones, are active in advance of movement. However, the temporal relationship of motor cortex neuronal activity to the onset of movement is by no means unique, and some of its outputs are activated in parallel with neurones in other important motor structures. Even identified cortico-motoneuronal cells exerting strong facilitation at short latency (6–7 ms) on their target muscles are active long in advance of movement (60–70 ms). Although temporal facilitation and summation will account for some of this delay, it is also possible that processing of activity in other structures must occur before the motor cortex output is able to generate a movement. These other structures would include the basal ganglia and cerebellum, which are linked through major, reciprocally-connected loops to the motor cortex.

Motor cortex neurones can be shown to encode a variety of movement parameters, including force, rate of change of force, direction of movement, and muscle stiffness. Several different parameters may be encoded within the discharge properties of a single neurone. We emphasise the difference between neuronal activity that may encode the description of a movement and that which is required for the execution of the movement. The encoding of muscle force appears to be best represented in the output neurones of lamina V, including the cortico-motoneuronal cell population, although the CM population controlling the hand muscles may be more specifically concerned in the precise patterning of these muscles for finger movement rather than in the control of precision grip force. The encoding of movement parameters by a given cell's activity appears to be dependent upon the task performed, and it is possible to demonstrate considerable flexibility in the relationship between the neural discharges of a cortico-motoneuronal cell and the contractions of its target muscle. There may also be differences in the strength of this relationship during different phases of an executed movement. This could, in part, reflect the particular synergy in which that muscle is active for a given task. PET and other imaging techniques illustrate the overall level of activity in motor cortex during movement and have provided important clues about the contribution of different motor structures in the human brain to different voluntary movements.

6

Inputs from peripheral receptors to motor cortex neurones

6.1 THE RELATIONSHIP BETWEEN SENSATION AND MOVEMENT PERFORMANCE

At the outset, we made it clear that one of the major issues which has been addressed since the earliest studies on the neurophysiological basis of voluntary movement has been the relationship between sensation and movement performance. Although their conclusion has been questioned by the findings of later work (Nathan and Sears 1960), Mott and Sherrington (1895) described a greater deficit in motor function in animals following dorsal nerve root section than following ablation of the motor cortex. Moreover, the question of the existence of motor output pathways originating from the 'sensory' receiving areas of the cortex was hotly debated through the whole period of domination of experimental work by the methods of electrical stimulation of the brain and imperfect anatomical methods for tracing connectivity. We have reported, in Chapter 2 (Section 2.7), the evidence which demonstrates that, while the origins of the corticospinal tract may be concentrated within the primary motor cortex, substantial contributions to the tract are made by the somatosensory cortex, and the precise organization and connections of these projections may vary in different species.

Rothwell *et al.* (1982) were able to study motor performance in a man deafferented by a severe peripheral sensory neuropathy of the hand and forearm. This patient was able to perform a remarkable repertoire of movements of the hand. They reported that, 'Individual digits could be activated independently without practice and he could even touch his thumb with each finger in turn using either hand. Repetitive alternating movements of the wrist and hand such as tapping, waving or fast flexion–extension of the fingers were executed easily.' The patient could outline shapes and figures in the air using his wrist and fingers and with his eyes closed. He continued to drive a car with a manual gear change, presumably relying on motor programs already stored within his central nervous system and not requiring sensory 'feedback' for their activation. Yet this patient did demonstrate that, for some tasks involving sensorimotor co-ordination, performance was greatly impaired in the absence of afferent signals from the moving limb. Hence feeding himself, holding a cup and co-ordinating the movements of his fingers in fastening buttons on his clothes were almost impossible. Moreover, this patient found it impossible to learn new motor tasks. A graphic description of the enormous problems facing a deafferented patient, and the long term struggle to regain even simple motor skills is given by Cole (1991).

Recent understanding of the nature of the connections between different brain regions provided by more reliable neuroanatomical methods, and of the functional co-operation between many regions, revealed by studies in human subjects engaged in tasks requiring sensorimotor co-ordination, has allowed many of the issues of concern in the past to be clarified and some of the apparent anomalies to be explained. Sensory signals conveyed from specific peripheral receptors in the limbs of primates have relatively direct access to the motor cortex. Indeed, identified PTNs and cortico-motoneuronal (CM) cells have been shown to be influenced at short latency by peripheral stimuli capable of affecting particular populations of receptors in the limb whose movements may be influenced by those PTNs or CM cells.

The anatomical basis of both this 'external feedback' to the motor cortex, as it was then described, and of the internal projections to motor cortex from other regions of the brain which could be involved in the selection and co-ordination of motor cortex outputs were detailed in Phillips and Porter (1977, Chapter 6). There, the evidence relating to the internal organization of these connections within the motor cortex was explored. It was concluded that, in the motor cortex, in contrast to arrangements in sensory receiving areas, this organization could not be described in terms of separated, functional 'columns' specified by a common thalamic or cortico-cortical input. Moreover, the rigid hard-wired relationship between the influence of a peripheral input on a corticospinal projection and the motor effect of electrical activation of that projection which had been described by Rosén and Asanuma, (1972) for the tranquillized monkey, could not be supported by the extensive studies of input–output relationships of PTNs in conscious monkeys and cats. In these conscious animals, the output associations of the responsive PTNs could be assessed in relation to natural self-initiated movements and the association of PTN discharge with movement performance could be studied (Lemon and Porter 1976a; Lemon *et al.* 1976; Armstrong and Drew 1984c). Such associations have been described in Chapter 5.

Because of the central importance of corticospinal connections for the accomplishment of voluntary movement, we shall concern ourselves, in this chapter, only with the influences detected in the motor cortex and closely associated areas, and caused by the activation of peripheral receptors. We shall examine the evidence for the prevalence of particular receptor populations in these projections to the motor cortex, discuss the pathways by which such access is available, and comment on the possible functional significance of these particular afferent projections for the control of voluntary movement. In concentrating this account on inputs from the moving limb, and especially those from the muscles themselves, we do not imply that the involvement of other sensory systems, such as vision, in guiding voluntary movement should be neglected. However, we wish to focus this discussion on the supraspinal influences of muscle spindles, earlier regarded as being involved in 'unconscious' proprioception.

6.2 INPUTS TO THE MOTOR CORTEX FROM PERIPHERAL RECEPTORS

It was clear, even from the early experiments of Adrian and Moruzzi (1939), that in the chloralose anaesthetized cat, stimulation of a variety of peripheral receptors was capable of evoking a synchronized volley of impulses which descended in the pyramidal tract. Such relayed pyramidal discharges could be produced by a flash of light, a loud sound or a strong stimulus to a limb (Buser 1966). They were associated with an evoked potential over the motor cortex and could have been involved in the 'myoclonic' jerks exhibited in such animals in response to peripheral stimuli. The analysis of the 'receptive fields' from which individual PTNs in the cat could be influenced revealed that, even without the effects of chloralose, which could have operated to extend the field of influence from which excitatory effects could be obtained (Baker *et al.* 1971; Lemon and Porter 1976b), output cells in the motor cortex could be affected by a variety of peripheral stimuli. Some PTNs had localized receptive fields limited to part of a contralateral limb and responded to movement of hairs, light touch, pressure over the limb or movements of joints (Brooks *et al.* 1961a,b; Towe *et al.* 1964). Other PTNs had more widespread receptive fields and labile responses to a range of modalities of stimulation. The variety of the relationships of these influences, generated by activation of peripheral receptors, to the output characteristics of the projection cells in the cat motor cortex, and the presumed significance of these PTN responses (Asanuma *et al.* 1968; Brooks and Stoney 1971) were discussed in detail in Phillips and Porter (1977, pp. 234–64).

6.3 PROJECTIONS FROM MUSCLE AFFERENTS TO AREA 3a

Amassian and Berlin (1958) drew attention to the fact that afferent volleys set up by stimulation of the nerves to forelimb muscles in deeply anaesthetised cats could produce localized, short-latency evoked potentials in the cerebral cortex, even when the strength of these stimuli was graded to activate less than 20 per cent of a maximum Group I volley. Receptors in muscle or tendons, with afferent fibres among the largest in the muscle nerve, must have access to pathways projecting relatively directly to the cerebral cortex. These projections from the forelimb of the cat were studied by Oscarsson and Rosén (1963, 1966). A secure projection from the Group Ia afferents of primary endings of muscle spindles to the contralateral postcruciate dimple (area 3a) of the cat's cortex was established.

Phillips *et al.* (1971) examined responses of neurones in area 3a of the baboon's cerebral cortex, at the nadir of the central sulcus, when afferent volleys were generated in the deep radial and ulnar nerves of the contralateral forelimb. They concluded that area 3a was a specific site to which Group I muscle afferents projected. None of the individual neurones from which they recorded short-latency responses to Group I volleys could be identified as a corticospinal neurone, even though, anatomically, a proportion of corticospinal projections arise from area 3a, as we have documented in an earlier chapter. The afferent projection to the cells of area 3a was conducted to this region of cortex via the dorsal column of the spinal cord and caused discharges of single cells within this region of cortex at latencies of 5 to 10 ms (Fig. 6.1).

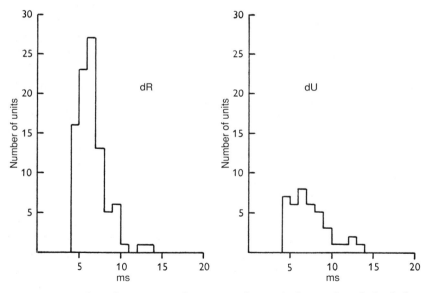

FIG 6.1   Latencies of response of neurones in cortical area 3a of the baboon, excited by single volleys of Group I strength in deep radial nerve (dR, 93 units) and deep palmar branch of ulnar nerve (dU, 40 units), measured from time of arrival of volley at dorsal root entry zone. (Reproduced with permission from Phillips *et al.* (1971).)

Heath *et al.* (1976) examined the behaviour of single neurones throughout the whole depth of the bank of the postcentral gyrus of the baboon. Units that responded only to muscle nerve stimulation were located within area 3a but overlapped into the deepest part of area 3b. Units that responded only to cutaneous nerve stimulation were found mainly in area 3b, but some were located in area 3a. Cells receiving a convergent input and responding to both muscle and cutaneous nerve stimuli were found throughout area 3a and the rostral part of area 3b. The latencies of the responses to muscle nerve stimuli (mean of approx. 8.0 ms, which accorded with the results shown in Fig. 6.1) indicated that those cells responding could be considered as a single population of neurones. Yet their responses were not indicative of the whole response repertoire of area 3a. Hence, according to their observations, area 3a is not uniquely a receiving area for only Group I afferents from muscle nerves. Heath *et al.* (1976) clearly regarded it as a specialized region of the sensory cortex with a special responsiveness, dominated by this submodality of afferent signals from muscle receptors, a view they shared with Jones and Powell (1969). Attempts by Phillips and his colleagues (Andersen and Phillips, quoted in Phillips *et al.* 1971) to demonstrate, in the anaesthetised baboon, that the cells of area 3a, which were in receipt of such short latency projections from muscles, relayed these signals directly to the output neurones of area 4, were unsuccessful.

Jones *et al.* (1978) identified area 3a in the monkey by recording the short-latency Group I afferent evoked potential generated in it by weak muscle nerve stimulation. At this site, they injected tracers that would allow the plotting of both anterograde and retrograde transport through the afferent and projection fibres of the localized region. They found that area 3a was reciprocally connected with area 1. If areas 3a and 3b were considered as parts of sensory receiving cortex, they both projected backwards to areas 1 and 2, which posterior zones were, in turn, reciprocally connected with area 4 (Fig. 6.2). In summarizing his anatomical findings on the connections of area 3a and the cortico-cortical inputs to area 4, Jones (1986) indicated that 'the principal inputs to area 4 are those from areas 1, 2 and the anterior part of area 5, to all three of which it returns cortico-cortical fibres as well as to area 3a. Yet it receives no input from area 3a and appears to stand totally unconnected with area 3b'. Jones clearly stated that, in the light of connectivities revealed in the monkey's cerebral cortex, both cutaneous and muscle afferents could have access to area 4 neurones (from 3b and 3a) only by exercising their influence through areas 1 and 2.

It is pointed out by Jones and Porter (1980) that the descriptions of connectivity that are obtained from experiments of this kind depend on the definition used for the location of area 3a. There may be a more anterior part of the 'transitional' zone, between sensory and motor cortex, in which an attenuated or discontinuous granular layer overlaps the most posterior of the giant pyramidal cells of lamina V. Histologically, this is usually

(a) Inputs to limited zone of area 4

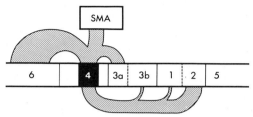

(b) Inputs to whole arm representation of area 4

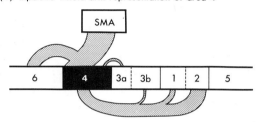

FIG 6.2   A schematic summary of the ipsilateral cortico-cortical projections to the forelimb region of area 4, in the monkey, prepared as a diagram to illustrate the relative densities (by the width of the shaded projections) of afferents from other cytoarchitectonic zones: from the quantitative studies of Ghosh, Brinkman & Porter (1987). (a): A limited small injection of HRP into the 'finger' representation only of area 4 revealed that the majority of cortico-cortical projections to this region were derived from within area 4 itself (these projections are not illustrated). Area 4 contained about half of the retrogradely labelled pyramidal cells. The remainder of the retrogradely labelled cortico-cortical neurones were located within premotor cortex (area 6), SMA, area 2 and area 3a. Note that other authors (e.g. Jones 1986) deny the existence of projections from area 3a to area 4. (b): When the injection of HRP into the arm representation of area 4 is more extensive and includes the total forelimb region, intra-areal connectivity cannot be revealed. The cortico-cortical connectivity which can be quantified by counting retrogradely labelled neurones is now as much as 10 times greater and is dominated by projections from SMA, area 2 (and 5) and premotor area 6. A small contribution from area 3a is again revealed, and it is possible that this is restricted to the connections with the 'finger' region because it has not increased significantly in absolute number of cortico-cortical neurones, above those illustrated in (a). (Reproduced with permission from Porter (1984). Copyright © 1984. Reprinted by permission of John Wiley and Sons Inc.)

included in area 3a, even though the electrophysiological focus of Group I afferent activity frequently seems to be located nearer the 3a/3b border (Phillips *et al.* 1971). At least this anterior part of area 3a in the monkey does appear to provide projections from cortico-cortical neurones in lamina III to area 4 of the precentral motor cortex. The cells of origin of this

3a-to-4 projection may be labelled by the retrograde transport of HRP from small localized injections in the hand area of the motor cortex and constitute a few percent of the cortico-cortical connections to a limited region of area 4 (see Fig. 6.2; Ghosh *et al.* 1987). As yet, it is not possible to ascertain whether such cells receive short-latency projections from muscle afferents and we are not aware of any studies in the monkey which have first located those cortico-cortical neurones which project from area 3a to the motor cortex and then examined the responsiveness of such cells to muscle nerve stimuli. Alternatively, the complete intracellular staining of individual cells in receipt of projections from muscle afferents could reveal whether or not projections or collaterals of their axons crossed into area 4.

DeFelipe *et al.* (1986) made small injections of HRP into the white matter immediately beneath the sensory cortex of monkeys and studied the individual pyramidal neurones whose somata and axons had been labelled by uptake of the HRP. They illustrate cells with long-range axon collaterals taking influences, through several separate sprays of terminals, into a number of cortical zones. Neurones in area 3a could project such collaterals into area 4.

In the cat, Zarzecki *et al.* (1978) and Zarzecki and Wiggin (1982) have described projections from area 3a cells which were activated by muscle afferents and which could transmit this influence to motor cortex neurones. Zarzecki's studies have emphasized the degree of convergence of different thalamic, callosal, and cortico-cortical inputs upon individual neurones in the cat's sensorimotor cortex (Zarzecki 1991). Most of these inputs were revealed by intracellular recording; they may go undetected in the extracellular record. However the convergence was by no means complete, and few neurones received inputs from all three sources tested. The specific combinations of different inputs may be important in the selective activation of different classes of projection neurones, including corticospinal cells.

Iwamura *et al.* (1983a) studied the receptive field properties of single neurones recorded from areas 3a and 3b in the conscious monkey. They found that receptive fields were almost invariably confined to a single finger and that the cells of area 3a responded to movement of the joints of one finger only. Recordings made from neurones in area 3a of conscious monkeys during the performance of movement tasks (Yumiya *et al.* 1974; Tanji 1975) have not clarified their role in signalling aspects of muscle state or in transmitting to other regions (such as the motor cortex or parietal sensory regions) signals relevant to muscle length or rate of change of length during active movements. Tanji's results indicate that many of the cells in area 3a which receive projections from Group I muscle afferents discharge impulses in a manner that suggests a role for area 3a in tasks which require tonic activity in the muscle from which the afferent projections derive.

6.4 PROJECTIONS FROM MUSCLE AFFERENTS TO NEURONES IN THE PRECENTRAL MOTOR CORTEX

Albe-Fessard and Liebeskind (1966) demonstrated topographically organized projections to individual neurones in the motor cortex of chloralose anaesthetized monkeys. Convergence of influences from a variety of peripheral sources was revealed. Characteristically, however, the cells in the motor cortex were caused to discharge by movements of joints. They responded to traction on the tendons of muscles and to light pressure over the surface of denuded muscles. In a clear demonstration that the origin of part of this influence must derive from muscle spindles, Albe-Fessard *et al.* (1966) stimulated fusimotor fibres to muscle spindles, after critical curarisation had abolished the contraction of extrafusal muscle fibres, and showed that this stimulus caused activation of precentral cortical neurones. Wiesendanger (1973) confirmed in baboons and monkeys, the convergence of afferent inputs from both superficial and deep territories on to individual PTNs in the motor cortex. Lucier *et al.* (1975) and Hore *et al.* (1976) studied the responses of individual neurones in area 4 to controlled ramp stretches and to sinusoidal stretches of forelimb and hindlimb muscles of the anaesthetised baboon and monkey. In these experiments, the cells in area 4 seemed to show greater sensitivity to the static changes in length of test muscles and to have less responsiveness to the dynamic changes in velocity of muscle stretch, suggesting that the projections were preferentially from the secondary endings of muscle spindles.

A large number of investigations has addressed the characteristics of the 'afferent input zones' (Lemon and Porter 1976a) of individual PTNs whose natural discharge is associated with a defined component of active movement performance. These studies have examined the nature of the peripheral stimulus which is most effective in causing the PTNs to fire when the conscious animal is relaxed and not moving (Fetz and Baker 1969; Rosén and Asanuma 1972; Lemon and Porter 1976a; Wong *et al.* 1978; Fetz *et al.* 1980; Lemon 1981a,b; Strick and Preston 1978a). The findings all agree that the afferent input zones may be strictly localized, for example, to a single direction of movement about a single joint (Fig. 6.3). Table 6.1 shows that, while convergence from cutaneous and deep receptors may occur, the influences exerted on single PTNs are dominated by receptors which signal joint movement, except for those PTNs which are associated in their natural discharge with finger movement, when localized cutaneous receptive fields may have a major projection to the PTNs (see Section 6.5).

It must now be regarded as without doubt that it is, indeed, discharges of muscle spindle receptors which are projected to PTNs in the motor cortex of conscious monkeys during natural behaviour. Such projections would account for the results of experiments conducted in many laboratories in which animals were required to hold a particular position of their wrist,

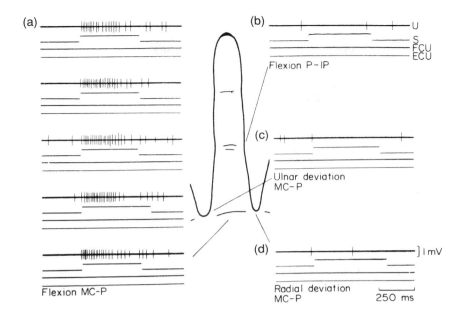

(a)

(b) U
S
FCU
ECU

Flexion P–IP

(c)

Ulnar deviation
MC–P

(d)] 1 mV

Flexion MC–P

Radial deviation
MC–P   250 ms

FIG 6.3   Response of a monkey precentral neurone to movement at a single joint. This neurone responded only to flexion of the metacarpo–phalangeal joint (MC–P) of the middle finger. For each set of recordings the signal marker (S) gives an approximate indication of the onset and duration of the imposed movement. Records from this cell (U) show a reproducible discharge pattern for each of the five successive flexions shown in (a). Absence of any EMG activity (bottom two records in each set) indicates the relaxed state of the animal during natural stimulation. Movements at other joints (b),(c),(d) did not excite this neurone. (Reproduced with permission from Lemon and Porter (1976a).)

within flexion or extension targets, while records were made from PTNs in the contralateral motor cortex (Evarts 1973; Evarts and Tanji 1976; Tatton *et al.* 1978; Cheney and Fetz 1984). Sudden, unexpected disturbances were then imposed on the manipulandum to stretch or unload the muscles contracting in order to maintain this position. Wolpaw (1979, 1980) provided the disturbance in a different manner, calculated to activate only receptors in the muscle and tendon of a single muscle. He implanted a magnetic pellet within the tendon of flexor carpi ulnaris (FCU) at the wrist of a monkey. The monkey performed a task in which it had to generate a steady level of force in its wrist extensors or flexors to maintain a handle within a target zone. The arm was extended through a coil which allowed electromagnetic force to be applied to the pellet, when current was passed through the coil, thereby stretching the FCU. Activation of the sensitive

TABLE 6.1   Afferent input to MI neurones (adapted from Hepp-Reymond 1988).

	Species	Joint muscle (%)	Skin, hair (%)	Both submodalities (%)	Neurone type	N
(Rosén and Asanuma 1972)						
Hand	Cebus	57	35	8	not identified	87
(Lemon and Porter 1976a)						
Forelimb	Macaque	87	7	6	PTNs + not identified	214
(Wong *et al.* 1978)						
Forelimb	Macaque	73	18	9	not identified	728
(Fetz *et al.* 1980)						
Arm, leg	Macaque	90	5	5	PTNs + not identified	388
(Lemon 1981a)						
Hand, finger	Macaque	38	46	12	PTNs + not identified	216
Forelimb	Macaque	75	20	4	PTNs + not identified	536
(Strick and Preston 1978b) Hand						
rostral	Squirrel	96	3		not	33
caudal	monkey	12	88		identified	59
(Wannier *et al.* 1986) Hand						
rostral	Macaque	74	13	13	not	39
caudal		70	25	5	identified	20
(Picard and Smith 1992a) Hand						
rostral	Macaque	67	33		not	44
caudal		39	61		identified	164
(Tanji and Wise 1981) Leg						
rostral	Macaque	91	9		not	188
caudal		12	88		identified	229

muscle spindle receptors in this single muscle clearly had a powerful influence on PTNs in the motor cortex. Wolpaw's results demonstrated that most of the PTNs that were selectively excited by muscle stretch were also the more active when that same muscle was contracted to maintain handle position: units excited by FCU stretch were more active when the monkey was producing flexor forces than extensor. However, other input-output relationships have been found also (cf. Porter and Rack 1976; Lemon *et al.* 1976; Cheney and Fetz 1984). Perhaps surprisingly, the influence of activation of receptors in only a single muscle was detected in a large number of PTNs widely spread throughout the cortex and associated in their natural discharge with a wide spectrum of motor performances. This suggests that the projection path from a given population of muscle spindles, while oligosynaptic and relatively secure in its transmission capacity, is nevertheless distributed to a wide precentral territory and not focused on the corticospinal population which projects to the motor centres for the one muscle (see Section 8.5). It has been pointed out that this widespread distribution of the effect to large zones of the motor cortex could have resulted, in part, from the unphysiological isolation of the local muscle spindle responses to the tendon vibration. In such circumstances, activity in FCU muscle spindles was dissociated from the peripheral activation of other receptors in muscles, joints, tendon, fascia and skin which would accompany natural stimulation, for example, by joint movement (Porter 1990).

Colebatch *et al.* (1990c) studied the responses of individual precentral neurones, whose association with movement performance was categorised on the basis of their discharges during self-paced natural movements, when muscles were passively stretched by movement of joints and when the tendons of these muscles were percussed (to produce a phasic disturbance) or vibrated transcutaneously. Figure 6.4 compares, for the one precentral neurone, the discharges of the neurone accompanying repeated brisk flexion movements of the wrist imposed by the experimenter while the monkey remained relaxed, with the effects produced by gated periods of vibration applied over the extensor tendons of the wrist or over the flexor tendons of the wrist. In this case, the response to extensor tendon vibration, which had an onset latency of 16 ms, was plainly revealed only when the vibration was applied over the tendons whose muscles would have been stretched by passive wrist flexion. Such responses could underlie stretch or vibration induced 'transcortical reflexes' (see Section 6.7).

6.5 INFLUENCE OF CUTANEOUS AFFERENT INPUTS UPON MOTOR CORTEX NEURONES

Early studies showed that most motor cortex neurones were responsive to natural stimuli, such as joint rotation and muscle palpation, that were likely to excite deep receptors. However, a proportion of neurones did respond to cutaneous stimulation (see Table 6.1). As might be expected, most of these neurones were those concerned with movements of the hand and

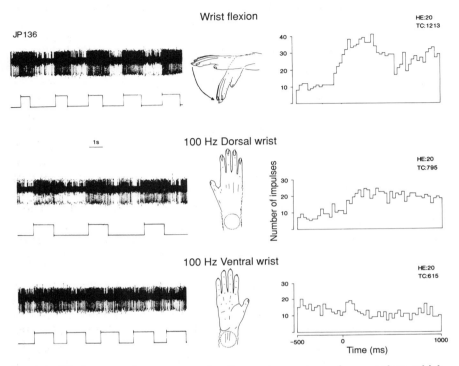

FIG 6.4 Discharges of a neurone in the motor cortex of a monkey which responded with a sustained burst of impulses to passively imposed flexion of the wrist (upper section). When vibration at 100 Hz was applied to a pad situated over the extensor tendons on the dorsum of the wrist (upward displacement of the signal trace), the neurone exhibited an increase in firing (middle section). The latency to onset of the vibration induced discharge was 16 ms. Vibration applied to same pad when it was placed over the flexor tendons on the ventral surface of the wrist, produced only a small transient change in background firing of the unit, and no sustained response. This pattern of response was consistent with an input from vibration-sensitive afferents within the muscle passively stretched by the imposed movement of wrist flexion. (Reproduced with permission from Colebatch *et al.* (1990c).)

fingers (Rosén and Asanuma 1972; Lemon and Porter 1976a; Strick and Preston 1978b; Lemon 1981a; Hepp-Reymond 1988; Picard and Smith 1992a) or of foot and toes (Tanji and Wise 1981). Table 6.1 presents the evidence that cutaneous and proprioceptive information may be projected, respectively, to caudal and rostral regions of M1 (Strick and Preston 1978b; Tanji and Wise 1981). However, this separation is by no means complete, and in the anterior bank of the central sulcus, neurones with proprioceptive and cutaneous inputs are intermingled (see Table 6.1; Lemon 1981a; Wannier *et al.* 1986; Picard and Smith 1992a).

Lemon (1981a) found that 46 per cent of 216 neurones in area 4, including 38 PTNs, which responded to natural stimulation of the hand, were responsive only to cutaneous stimulation. Very similar proportions were recently reported by Picard and Smith (1992a) for 208 neurones active during a task which involved lifting an object between the thumb and index finger (Johansson and Westling 1984; Espinoza and Smith 1990). Most of these cells were excited by light brushing of the glabrous skin (39 per cent, Lemon 1981a; 42 per cent, Picard and Smith 1992a), and responses to hair movement were rare. Responses to hair movement are more common amongst cat motor cortex neurones (Welt *et al.* 1967; Armstrong and Drew 1984c). In the monkey, afferent input zones are small (typically about $2\,cm^2$) and restricted to the glabrous skin of a single digit. Neurones responsive to both cutaneous and proprioceptive stimulation make up a small proportion of the whole responsive population (12 per cent, Lemon 1981a; 2 per cent, Picard and Smith 1992a). Motor cortex responses to tactile stimuli can occur at short latencies (8–15 ms), with the shortest latency responses being recorded from neurones lying in laminae III and V (Lemon 1981a).

Lemon (1981a) demonstrated a clear relationship between the cutaneous afferent input to a motor cortex neurone and the activity of the neurone during prehension movements. In his sample, most of the 80 neurones with cutaneous inputs were much more active during a task which required the monkey to remove small food rewards from a rosette than during the grasping and pulling of a lever. Most of them exhibited an increase in discharge frequency before hand contact was made, and many showed strikingly high firing frequencies during exploratory behaviour (e.g. searching the experimenter's hand for a sunflower seed). Picard and Smith (1992a) have shown that the majority (63 per cent) of neurones with cutaneous input are responsive to the texture of the lifted object; a smaller proportion (45 per cent) of neurones with proprioceptive input were texture sensitive. Interestingly, when the motor performance required an object to be lifted between thumb and forefinger, a greater proportion of task-related neurones had activity related to the texture than to the weight of the object (52 per cent and 29 per cent of tested cells, respectively). About half the texture sensitive neurones increased their discharge with smooth textures, such as smooth metal. A higher grip force is required to prevent an object with this texture from slipping through the fingers. The other half showed the reverse behaviour, and discharged more frequently when the object carried a rough-textured surface (e.g. sandpaper). Many of these texture-sensitive neurones responded to object slip with a short-latency burst of impulses. This activity seems to be important for the muscular response to slip, which typically takes place around 50 to 100 ms after slip (Picard and Smith 1992b). In man, it is known that the integrity of signals from cutaneous mechanoreceptors is essential for the scaling of grip forces to object texture, and for these 'automatic' reflex responses to slip (Johansson and Westling 1987b; Westling and Johansson 1987; Johansson *et al.* 1992). Since motor cortex neuronal activity can be shown to be modulated by the passage of textured objects across the skin (Darian-Smith *et al.* 1985; Picard and Smith 1992b), it is possible that this cutaneous input is also important for tactile exploratory behaviour.

6.6 PATHWAYS BY WHICH PERIPHERAL AFFERENTS PROJECT TO THE MOTOR CORTEX

The pathway from receptors to the PTNs in the motor cortex must be relatively direct and involve few synapses because, in the monkey, the shortest latencies for responses to natural stimulation of either the skin or muscle were sometimes less than 10 ms, and frequently had values between 10 and 30 ms (Lemon and Porter 1976a; Lemon 1979). These latencies accord precisely with those measured by Evarts (1973), Evarts and Tanji (1976), Porter and Rack (1976), Tatton *et al.* (1978), and Wolpaw (1980) when sudden perturbations were used to disturb movement performance, by briefly displacing a joint and stretching muscles acting round that joint. Mean latencies for changes in PTN firing in response to these perturbations were of the order of 16 to 24 ms. Even the shortest latency responses of PTNs to muscle stretch, however, seem to occur some milliseconds after cells in area 3a will have responded to the peripheral stimulus, perhaps because the effects are relayed to area 4 only after being received in area 3a, or perhaps because the pathway to area 4 is separate to that for area 3a and contains, as seems possible from the results of Hore *et al.* (1976), a greater component of the more slowly conducted static length signals. In the cat, Herman *et al.* (1985) have shown that some motor cortex neurones that can be activated from area 3a also receive a more direct input from the forelimb, possibly mediated by direct thalamic projections.

Brinkman *et al.* (1978) studied the responses of precentral cortical neurones to natural activation of peripheral receptors in trained, conscious monkeys which had been subjected to bilateral surgical interruption of the cuneate fasciculi of the dorsal columns at the C1–C2 level some weeks before testing. In line with expectations from the observations of Phillips *et al.* (1971), section of the cuneate fasciculi either removed or greatly diminished the short-latency responses of precentral neurones to activation of peripheral receptors and to passive movement of joints. Although the animals with these lesions exhibited disturbances of discriminative ability, especially when using the fingers, movement performances to which they had been trained continued to be quite skilfully executed (see Section 3.5). Moreover, the natural discharges of the cortical neurones, including those of PTNs, associated with these movements, were not modified in any obvious way by the absence of 'feedback' from the peripheral receptors. Asanuma *et al.* (1980) also demonstrated that the pathway for short-latency projections from the periphery to the motor cortex in the monkey must include the dorsal columns, and Asanuma and Arissian (1984) have shown that combined lesions of both the dorsal columns and somatosensory cortex in monkeys are far more devastating in their effect on motor performance than are lesions to either structure alone. They concluded that, under normal circumstances, sensory input to the motor cortex arrives both directly over the thalamic route, and indirectly via the somatosensory cortex, and, in relation to motor performance, either projection can compensate rapidly for the absence of the other.

As we have indicated earlier, because of the anatomical cortico-cortical connectivities established in the monkey, Jones (1986) considered that the route taken by these afferent signals must involve cuneo-thalamic projections via the sensory cortex (areas 3a and 3b), with a subsequent relay to the motor cortex through areas 1 and 2. Although nucleus ventralis posterolateralis, pars oralis (VPLo of Olszewski 1952) of the thalamus was known to project to area 4 and to receive inputs at an appropriately short-latency from muscle nerves in the contralateral limb (Horne and Tracey 1979; Lemon and van der Burg, 1979; Jones *et al.* 1979; Horne and Porter 1980), Jones and his associates were unable to demonstrate projections from the cuneate nucleus to VPLo (Tracey *et al.* 1980a). However, projections from the dorsal column nuclei and from the external cuneate nucleus to the VPLo have been demonstrated by Berkley (1983) and by Boivie *et al.* (1975), respectively. The dispute concerning the existence of this projection is in large measure due to difficulties in defining thalamic border zones (Berkley 1983). If there is no lemniscal input to VPLo, it seems most likely that the dorsal column afferents are relayed in the cuneate nucleus and projected to the somatosensory cortex via nucleus VPLc. Alternatively they may become a part of the 'cerebellar' projection to the motor cortex, the relay of which is regarded as the dominant function of VPLo. A modern summary of the pathways through the thalamus to the somatic sensory-cortex, motor cortex and the supplementary motor area is provided by Jones (1986) (Fig. 6.5). Recent work by Holsapple *et al.* (1990) has shown that the hand representation in the bank of the central sulcus receives an important input from the VLo nucleus. However, since neurones in this nucleus are not generally responsive to peripheral sensory stimulation, this seems an unlikely source of the short-latency responses of neurones in this hand area of the primary motor cortex.

A further alternative or rather, parallel, pathway is that provided by collaterals of afferents travelling in the dorsal columns which themselves ascend in the ventral white matter as part of the spinothalamic projection. Relova and Padel (1989) have demonstrated that, in the cat, motor cortex PTNs can be excited at short latency (mean 7.2 ms) by stimulation of the

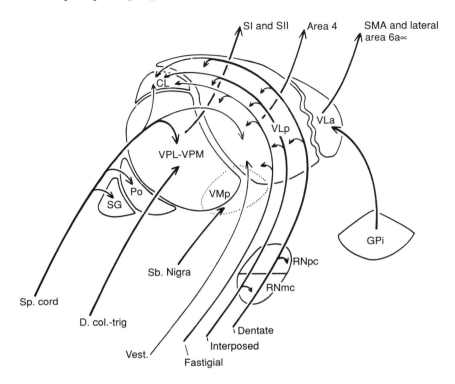

FIG 6.5   A summary of the relays through the thalamus of afferents from the spinal cord, cerebellum, and basal ganglia and their projections from several thalamic nuclei to the sensory and motor areas of the macaque cerebral cortex. This scheme emphasizes the segregation of lemniscal, cerebellar, and pallidal routes through to the cortex. (Reproduced with permission from Jones (1986).)

dorsal columns *caudal* to a complete transection of these columns at the level of C2. They showed that lesions of the ventral half of the spinal cord abolished these effects. Relova and Padel (1989) have proposed that this pathway is part of an ascending somaesthetic system providing both the red nucleus and the motor cortex with rapid feedback from the moving limb (Padel *et al.* 1988).

In the monkey, receptors activated by joint movement produce discharge not only of cells in area 3a, but also of those in area 2 (Powell and Mountcastle 1959; Wolpaw 1980). Iwamura *et al.* (1980) and Iwamura *et al.* (1983b) found that the neurones in areas 1 and 2, in contrast to those in areas 3a and 3b, had large and complex receptive fields suggestive of a high degree of convergence of inputs from different populations of area 3 neurones representing different submodalities and from different small peripheral receptive zones. Since area 2 clearly projects to area 4 (Jones *et al.* 1978), it was reasonable for Friedman and Jones (1981), Wolpaw (1980), and Asanuma *et al.* (1983) to suggest that it might mediate the short-latency effects transmitted via the dorsal columns to the motor cortex. But, in the conscious monkey, the organization of afferent input zones is simpler and restricted to smaller peripheral territories for cells in area 4 than it is for cells in area 2. Nevertheless, re-sorting and recombination of these convergent complex signals could conceivably occur between area 2 and the motor cortex.

Brinkman *et al.* (1985) examined the responses of neurones in the precentral motor cortex of conscious monkeys before and after producing reversible suppression of neuronal activity in area 2 with a surface cooling probe. Effective cooling of area 2, so that synaptic transmission was blocked within it, and behavioural changes were observed in the monkey, did not alter the return of signals to neurones in area 4, generated by passive movements of the limb. Some parts of area 2, deep in the intraparietal sulcus, and parts of area 5 adjacent to this, should have been less affected by the cooling and could have been responsible for the preservation of the responses in the motor cortex to peripheral stimuli, even when the animal's sensation of its limb had been severely impaired so that it neglected to use the limb. Moreover, if direct projections from area 3a to area 4 exist in the monkey, these would have remained relatively intact in this experiment and been unaffected by the cooling. It is challenging to consider that the preservation of responses in the motor cortex under the conditions of this experiment argues for a projection of these influences from area 3a directly to area 4. The details of the precise pathways by which peripheral receptors in a moving limb gain access to neurones in the motor cortex still await further experiment. The potential inclusion of second-order spinothalamic fibres, which could travel within the dorsal columns and have access to VPLo, deserves further exploration because these could provide an alternative to the '3a to 4' route. A separate spinothalamo-cortical system for bringing peripheral afferent influences directly to the motor cortex has not been excluded.

6.7 THE SIGNIFICANCE OF PROJECTIONS FROM MUSCLE SPINDLES TO THE MOTOR CORTEX: TRANSCORTICAL REFLEXES

In his Ferrier Lecture, Phillips (1969) reiterated that the cortico-moto-neuronal projection from the precentral gyrus to motoneurones provided the most direct access for the brain's voluntary commands to exert influences on the motor machinery of the hand. In commenting on the experimental observations made by Evarts (1968) that PTNs associated in their discharge with a movement such as wrist flexion showed increased firing when this movement had to be performed against a load (Section 5.4), he suggested the possibility that the increased discharge could be 'in response to a signal of mismatch between "intended" and actual displacement. Whether this signal is a crude one from the muscle spindles, or whether the mismatch has been computed by the cerebellum is still unknown; nor, in this experiment, can the contributions of joints, skin and vision be assessed.' He went on to consider that, if the cortico-motoneuronal system were part of a control loop, the most important function of fusimotor coactivation during voluntary movement might be 'to maintain the inflow of muscle length to the cortex and cerebellum'.

Load compensation adjustments occur in the movements of the human digits. Marsden *et al.* (1972, 1973) and Day and Marsden (1982) examined the performance of human subjects in producing linear ramp movements by flexing the distal phalanx of the thumb against a constant force, while they measured both angular displacement and the integrated EMG of the flexor muscle. The linear movement could be suddenly disturbed by introducing a forcible extension of the thumb, by halting the movement or by suddenly reducing the force against which the movement was required to be made. The changes in the EMG records which accompanied these disturbances had a latency of 50 to 60 ms, a similar latency to that of the long-latency stretch reflex described in human subjects by Hammond (1956, 1960). Marsden *et al.* considered that the responses observed in the flexor of the thumb was also a stretch reflex and that its timing was such that it could be mediated transcortically. The automatic compensations for suddenly imposed disturbances of voluntary muscle contraction which are revealed in these studies of normal human subjects were abolished by dorsal column lesions and modified by focal cortical lesions affecting the sensorimotor cortex or its outflow through the internal capsule (Marsden *et al.* 1977a, b).

The deafferented patient referred to in Section 6.1 (Rothwell *et al.* 1982) showed no responses whatsoever to unexpected stretch of his thumb during linear movements. When, rather than moving the thumb, he was expected to exert, over several seconds, a constant level of force by flexion of the thumb, he was quite unable to achieve this. Apparently random, large fluctuations in force characterized his attempts to maintain a constant level. So afferent feedback clearly had a major role in controlling the maintenance of steady force levels and the patient's inability to perform simple everyday tasks like holding a cup could have been compromised by his lack of ability to control the force exerted in his grip on the cup. If Marsden is correct in ascribing to the muscle spindle projection to the cortex a major role in this function of sustained force control, it may be that the recordings made in area 3a of the monkey by Tanji (see Section 6.3 above) illustrate an involvement of this projection in steady force maintenance.

The projections from muscle spindle receptors in a limb to engage neurones of the motor cortex of the monkey could provide an anatomical and functional basis for long-loop transcortical reflexes operating in the manner proposed by Phillips (1969) to allow servo-assistance to the control of voluntary movements. Cheney and Fetz (1984) produced evidence to demonstrate that cortico-motoneuronal cells do contribute to long-latency stretch reflexes in the Rhesus monkey. They recorded the responses of both CM cells and their target muscles to imposed perturbations of active wrist movements. For each CM cell–target muscle pair, the timing of the responses to sudden lengthening perturbations of the target muscle was measured in a number of trials. The latency for the CM cell to respond after the peripheral disturbance gave a measure of the time occupied in traversing the afferent limb of a transcortical reflex loop. It was consistent with the times measured by these and other authors (e.g. Evarts and Tanji 1976) for PTN responses to a peripheral disturbance (see above). The latency to the onset of the postspike facilitation of the EMG which followed the discharges of the CM cell gave a measure of the time occupied in the efferent limb from cortex to the muscle. The mean value of the sum of these afferent and efferent times (30.5 ± 10.2 ms) for a large number of CM cell–target muscle pairs was comparable to the mean onset time of the second EMG peak (M2 or the 'functional stretch reflex') in the recordings made from the muscles which were stretched (27.9 ± 5.1 ms). Moreover, the duration of the CM cell's response to the disturbance was closely matched to the duration of the M2 peak in the EMG of the muscle.

The proof of the effectiveness of the burst of impulses produced in CM cells by stretching of a target muscle was provided by spike-triggered averages of the muscle EMG using only the spikes contained within the burst of responses to the peripheral disturbance. These cortico-motoneuronal impulses effectively facilitated the muscle response.

The question of whether or not all the influences operating in servo-assistance of voluntary movement use this transcortical route to allow muscle spindle detectors of mismatch between intended and actual performance to modify functional stretch reflexes has been raised by many. Under some conditions, in spinal or decerebrate monkeys, stretch of a muscle can produce long-latency EMG changes with an M2 latency and form (Ghez and Shinoda 1978; Tracey *et al.* 1980b), and patients with Huntingdon's disease, who typically lack the long-latency M2 response in hand muscles, show clear long-latency responses in more proximal arm muscles (Thilmann *et al.* 1991). These long-latency effects are most likely produced within the spinal cord and, if they operate in the normal state when voluntary movements are being performed, they would be working in parallel with the transcortical effects. Matthews (1991) had sought an explanation of the later muscle responses to stretch in the spinal actions of slower group II muscle spindle receptors, which could thereby account for the long-latency

(a)

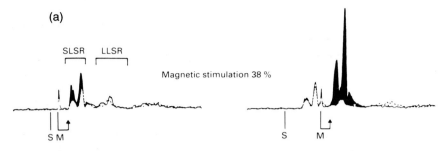

Magnetic stimulation 38 %

(b)

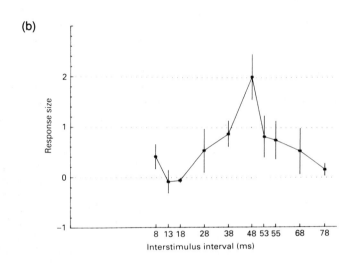

(c)

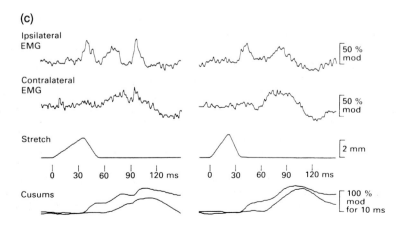

reflexes with a purely spinal mechanism (Matthews, 1984). He has now acknowledged that it is essential to recognize that a long-loop reflex through the cerebral cortex must have a role in the generation of these functional stretch reflexes.

Vibration, which should be a powerful stimulus for the primary endings of the muscle spindles and for any long-latency reflexes which depends on their firing, is, however, unable to elicit such a response with the magnitude that attends stretch of the muscle. Matthews (1989) argued that the slower afferents from secondary endings, which are activated by stretch, could therefore be responsible for the long latency reflex. By cooling the human arm, he set out to delay the time taken for afferent volleys to travel from the hand to the spinal cord, the degree of which delay depends on the size of the fibres involved and on their conduction velocity. The result of this experiment demonstrated that cooling of the limb slowed the long-latency reflex by the amount appropriate for fast conducting afferents. The excess delay in the long-latency reflex must therefore arise centrally and the reflex could not be caused by afferents from secondary receptors. It remains a problem as to why the long-loop reflex actions which are initiated by

---

Fig 6.6 Interaction of muscle stretch and magnetic brain stimulation to provide evidence for the existence of a transcortical stretch reflex in man. (a): Responses from one subject contrasting the effect of muscle stretch (S) on the response to magnetic (M) cortical stimulation. Superimposed are the average ($n = 32$) surface-rectified EMG response from finger flexor muscles in the forearm to stretch alone (dotted lines), together with the response to stretch plus a magnetic stimulus to the contralateral cortex (continuous line). The increase in motor torque displaced the fingertip about 17 mm with a peak velocity of around 0.5 m.s^{-1}. The shaded areas indicate the extra EMG response produced by the cortical stimulus. The EMG response to the cortical stimulus was timed to appear either on the short-latency stretch reflex (left) or the long-latency reflex (right). (b): Pooled data from four subjects showing the mean ($\pm$ S.E.M.) EMG response size to the magnetic cortical stimulus at one intensity when combined with a stretch stimulus using ten interstimulus intervals. The response size is expressed as a fraction of background EMG activity. The peak effect, at 48 ms, can be interpreted as resulting from the synchronous arrival at the cortex of excitatory afferent volleys evoked by muscle stretch together with the excitatory effect of the magnetic stimuli. (Reproduced with permission from Day *et al.* (1991).) (c): EMG responses of the short thumb flexor (FPB) to stretch at constant velocity of the thumb in a patient with Klippel–Feil syndrome and mirror movements affecting the hands. Left, stretch velocity 755 mm.s^{-1} (255 trials). Right, stretch velocity 150 mm.s^{-1} (510 trials). The stretched (ipsilateral) muscle (upper averages) showed both early and late responses, while the contralateral muscle (lower averages) gave just the late response. EMG rectified and averaged; calibration bar represents 50 per cent of pre-existing EMG level before stretch. Bottom traces are CUSUMs of the EMG averages. Stimulation of left hand. (Reproduced with permission from Matthews *et al.* (1990).)

Group Ia afferents are larger when the Group Ia input is generated by stretch than when it is generated by vibration.

Further evidence for a transcortical pathway mediating the long-latency reflex response to muscle stretch has been provided by the observation that it can be strongly facilitated by magnetic stimulation of the cortex contralateral to the stretched muscle; the time course of this facilitation indicates the interaction of the magnetic stimulus and an afferent volley from the stretched muscle at the cortical level (Day *et al.* 1991). This is illustrated in Fig. 6.6(a); magnetic stimulation which was timed to produce an EMG response in the long finger flexors at the same time as the long-latency stretch reflex (LLSR), produced a much larger effect than stimuli delivered to evoke responses during the short-latency, presumed spinal, reflex (SLSR). The peak effect was observed for an interval of around 50 ms between the stretch and the magnetic stimulus (Fig. 6.6(b)), and this would mean that the magnetic stimulus was influencing the cortex at the moment at which corticospinal neurones were being maximally excited by the stretch stimulus. The action of the magnetic stimulus on corticospinal neurones, be it direct or indirect (see Edgley *et al.* 1990), would be to enhance the number of them that respond to the stretch and thereby to increase the size of the descending volley and the pool of responsive motoneurones. The results shown in Fig. 6.6(a,b) are therefore consistent with, but do not prove, that the LLSR is indeed transcortical. Further evidence has come from patients with mirror movements. These patients exhibit normal, crossed somatosensory evoked potentials, but magnetic stimulation of one hemisphere produces bilateral EMG responses in the hand muscles, suggesting a branched corticospinal projection to these muscles (Section 4.6). In such patients, stretch of a muscle on one side evokes both short- and long-latency reflexes on the same side, and a long-latency reflex on the opposite side (see Fig. 6.6(c)), a finding that is never observed in normal subjects (Matthews *et al.* 1990; Capaday *et al.* 1991).

6.8 DESCENDING CONTROL OF TRANSMISSION OF SENSORY INPUT TO THE SENSORIMOTOR CORTEX

As Hammond (1956) clearly showed in human subjects, the amplitude of the late functional stretch reflex depended on the instructions given to a subject about his reaction to the muscle stretch. If subjects were asked to resist the disturbance, the late reflex response was large. If the subjects were instructed to 'let go', the late response did not occur or was greatly diminished. So the functional stretch reflex could be 'gated' depending on the instruction provided to the subject. We have already described the experiment in which Evarts and Tanji (1974) trained a monkey to make a push or pull movement of a lever depending upon the instruction to move in this direction. The trigger to move, however, was a brief perturbation of the lever itself which could be in either the push or pull direction and so stretch the muscles involved in one of these tasks. Recordings made from PTNs in the monkey's motor cortex revealed that the response of the cortical cell to these sudden brief muscle stretches also depended on the instruction which had been given to the animal. Hence a PTN could be shown to produce a burst of impulses 20 to 40 ms after a brief perturbation in the push direction (stretching the 'pull' muscles) providing that the instruction had been for the animal to pull when the trigger signal arrived. With the alternative instruction to push, the same disturbance failed to produce a burst of impulses in the PTN or else the response was very much smaller. So the afferent limb of the transcortical reflex loop could be made operative (closed) or inoperative (open), depending on other influences relating to the preparation for movement.

These other influences could exert their effects directly on the excitability of the PTN and so modify the response to the same incoming signal from peripheral receptors. Clearly, in the Evarts and Tanji experiment, the excitability, and indeed the firing rate, of the PTN was modified during the phase of preparation to move. However, because the pathway from the peripheral receptors to the PTN involves a number of synaptic relays, cortico-cortical or corticofugal activity consequent upon changes in the brain generated by the instruction to move, could also affect transmission along the afferent limb of the loop. There is a great deal of evidence suggesting that sensory transmission can be modified at many different levels of the neuraxis (for a review, see Prochazka 1989), and, as has been discussed previously, descending corticofugal projections to the trigeminal nuclei, dorsal column nuclei, and spinal dorsal horn may play an important part in such sensory modulation (Section 2.5). Animal and human studies have demonstrated a depression of sensory transmission immediately before and during movement (e.g. Ghez and Pisa 1972; Coulter 1974; Chapman *et al.* 1988). In most of these studies, transmission has been tested with a sensory input that is not relevant to the movement performed, such as electrical stimulation of a peripheral nerve, and this may account for the rather non specific pattern of sensory modulation that is observed. For example, Jiang *et al.* (1990, 1991) recorded both the cortical evoked potentials and single-unit responses recorded in the arm region of macaque somatosensory cortex (areas 3b and 1) to an air-puff stimulus directed at the skin of the forearm. These responses were depressed during rapid elbow movements, but the degree of modulation was not affected by either the type of movement (isometric or isotonic) or its direction (elbow flexion or extension).

In reviewing the evidence, Lemon (1981a) stated: 'It therefore remains possible that afferent input directly related to the task may still exert a powerful influence on the motor cortex and other structures', a view echoed by Jiang *et al.* (1991): '. . . controls over sensory transmission may vary as a function of the behavioral significance of the input'. Indeed, there is growing evidence that inputs 'relevant' to the performance of a given movement produce enhanced responses during movement. Nelson (1984) had shown that somatosensory cortex responses to vibration of the hand were greater when monkeys had to move in response to the vibratory cue, compared to when no movement occurred, and Ageranioti and Chapman (1989) found neurones with enhanced responses to textured stimuli when monkeys had to discriminate different textures. Although the discharge of some motor cortex neurones, which were excited by tactile stimuli in the passive animal, was suppressed when their receptive field came into contact with an object, this type of response was in the minority. Most cells showed enhanced activity once contact was established (Lemon 1981a; Picard and Smith 1992b). In the cat, Tsumoto *et al.* (1975) have described corticofugal influences that can differentially modify transmission of cutaneous and kinaesthetic information through the thalamus.

6.9 SENSATIONS PRODUCED BY ACTIVATION OF MUSCLE SPINDLES

It is well known that vibration applied transcutaneously over muscle tendons in conscious human subjects activates muscle spindle receptors and causes tonic reflex activation of the muscle (Hagbarth and Eklund 1966; Lance and DeGail 1965; DeGail *et al.* 1966). It is probable that this transverse vibratory stimulus activates the dynamically sensitive primary endings of the muscle spindles, even though secondary endings may also be affected (Matthews 1984). Percutaneous vibration of tendons at a frequency of 100 Hz produces illusions of movement (Goodwin *et al.* 1972). Vibration over the biceps tendon in a subject with the arm comfortably positioned, caused an illusion of extension of the elbow. The vibration-induced discharges of muscle spindle receptors mimicked the firing that would be transmitted along their afferents if the biceps muscle were being lengthened.

McCloskey and Torda (1975) and McCloskey (1978) conducted a large number of experiments to demonstrate the involvement of muscle spindle responses in the production of sensations of movement. If movement is paralysed, for example by local curarization of the forearm and hand (McCloskey and Torda 1975), subjects know that they cannot move and have no illusions of movement generated by making a conscious effort to move. Internal 'feedback' within the brain, presumably impinging on neurones in the motor cortex, is not capable of producing a sensation of movement. On the other hand, passively imposed movements of paralysed joints were accurately perceived. Other experiments excluded the role of receptors other than those in the muscles themselves in signalling this perception of movement. McCloskey (1985) has described the effects of local anaesthesia of skin receptors and has also documented the experiences of those with total joint replacement and the absence of joint receptors capable of contributing to sensations about movement. McCloskey was able to experience a sensation of movement when the extensor tendon of his own great toe was exposed at a surgical operation, divided, and pulled upon in a controlled experiment aimed at determining the accuracy with which a human subject could estimate imposed joint movements on the basis of muscle spindle derived information alone (McCloskey *et al.* 1983).

Whatever the pathway employed to deliver muscle spindle projections to the motor cortex, and whether this depends on a relay through area 3a or upon a separate pathway through the thalamus to area 4, these projections must also exist in man. While the projections to the precentral motor cortex may not themselves subserve sensory experience and the perception of movement, conscious sensation and perception will be expected to depend on the parallel activation of the sensory cortex by activity in these afferent pathways. The influence of the afferent projections to precentral regions in producing, in association with vibration of muscle tendons, increased excitability of the corticofugal projections from the motor cortex, however, has been demonstrated. Increased excitability could exist at a cortical or a spinal level or both. Changes at a cortical level may be judged from the facilitation of the muscle responses of conscious human subjects to transcranial stimulation of the motor cortex (Berardelli *et al.* 1983; Rossini *et al.* 1987).

6.10 SUMMARY

We have concentrated in this chapter on the obvious fact that the vast majority of the muscles that will operate in the performance of voluntary movement are endowed with specialized muscle spindle receptors for the detection of the length of the extrafusal contractile elements of those muscles and for rate of change of this length. In addition to their involvement in monosynaptic excitation and other reflex actions upon spinal motoneurones, the afferents from the muscle spindles, along with the projections from a large number of other peripheral receptors, gain access to contralateral somatosensory receiving areas of the cerebral cortex, and to the motor cortex itself. A major projection of muscle spindle afferents is found within area 3a, between the predominantly cutaneous sensory receiving zone of the cortex (area 3b), and the motor cortex itself (area 4). Whether the projections of influences from muscle spindles to the motor cortex are relayed in area 3a or whether a separate pathway exists for projections to area 4 is still uncertain. Kinaesthetic sensations are, however, produced by the afferent projections from muscle spindles, presumably by means of influences exerted on area 3a and the projections from it to areas 1 and 2. The projections to the motor cortex are involved in the production of long-loop transcortical effects which are manifest as long latency functional stretch reflexes and may be implicated in the production of muscle tone and in load compensation.

7

Motor functions of non-primary cortical motor areas

7.1 REGIONS OF CEREBRAL CORTEX CLOSELY CONNECTED WITH THE PRIMARY MOTOR CORTEX

Early maps of the motor areas which relied on histological methods or on the delineation of regions from which movements were obtained in response to electrical stimulation, identified a number of zones (e.g. premotor or intermediate precentral cortex, and supplementary motor area) which appeared to have a close association in structure and function with the primary motor cortex (M1). We provided some of the historical basis for the identification of these zones as non-primary motor areas in Chapter 1. Examination of the connectivity of these associated cortical areas, using a variety of methods of tracing projection fibres, demonstrated that both the postarcuate premotor area and the supplementary motor area (SMA) project directly to the primary motor cortex. Both are parts of Brodmann's area 6. Mettler (1935a, b) had studied cortico-cortical connections in the monkey using the Marchi method to trace degenerating fibres. He found diffuse inputs to area 6 from the frontal lobe (prefrontal cortex) and also from parietal cortex (areas 5 and 7). Ward *et al.* (1946) used the strychnine neuronographic method of Dusser de Barenne and McCulloch to seek electrophysiological evidence of regional connectivity. Again the most consistent finding was the projection from parietal cortex to area 6, although the approach adopted in their work was considerably influenced by contemporary interest in suppressor strips between premotor and motor cortex and the study attempted to distinguish a separate connectivity for these strips.

Matsumura and Kubota (1979) used the retrograde transport of HRP from an injection in the physiologically defined hand area of the primary motor cortex (identified by electrical stimulation of the cortical surface) to map the projections into this motor zone from area 6. Labelled neurones were found on the ipsilateral side in the lower and upper limbs of the posterior bank of the arcuate sulcus, including the medial and lateral areas of the arcuate spur, in the dorsomedial part of area 6 and in the middle portion of the supramarginal gyrus (SMA). In addition, cells in similar regions of the cortex of the contralateral hemisphere were labelled, indicating a bilateral projection from area 6 into area 4. Muakkassa and Strick (1979) identified the arm area of the cortex in some of their studies by intracortical microstimulation (in others they relied on Woolsey's motor map). They then made multiple small injections of HRP into the motor cortex. Essentially their results confirmed those of Matsumura and Kubota (1979). However, they distinguished a number of separate projection areas within area 6, each of which contributed to fibre connections with the face, arm, and leg zones of M1. The main two of their four projection areas were again the postarcuate premotor cortex (lateral area 6) and the SMA (medial area 6). Godschalk *et al.* (1984) also used different retrograde tracers to produce a delineation of the anatomically separate projections in which neurones below the inferior bank of the arcuate sulcus projected to the face area, while neurones in the posterior bank of the inferior limb and in the region of the arcuate spur projected to the arm area of motor cortex. The upper (medial) limb of the arcuate sulcus was not retrogradely labelled by M1 injections.

Wiesendanger (1981b) defined secondary motor areas of the cerebral cortex as those capable of producing motor effects when stimulated electrically, but usually requiring longer periods of stimulation and higher current intensities to elicit these movements. Moreover, the responses obtained were frequently of a complex nature (see Chapter 1). Although we now know that there are multiple motor areas within the frontal lobe (Matelli *et al.* 1985; Rizzolatti 1987; Dum and Strick 1991), it is the premotor cortex and SMA that especially command our attention. The major input and output connections of these cortical regions are schematically illustrated in Fig. 7.1 (adapted from Humphrey 1979). Ghosh *et al.* (1987) counted retrogradely labelled neurones and found that, in terms of the relative numbers of neurones projecting axons into the hand area of the primary motor cortex, these two zones were clearly preponderant. For the three monkeys investigated, 11–31 per cent of all retrogradely labelled cortical neurones were found in lateral area 6, and 6–26 per cent in the SMA. The great majority of these neurones were in lamina III. The potential importance of these cortico-cortical projections is underlined by the fact that the number of cortical neurones retrogradely labelled outside area 4 was between two and eight times as many as all the thalamocortical neurones labelled after the same M1 injections.

Wiesendanger (1981b) emphasized the point that has already been made in Chapter 2: both the premotor cortex and the SMA contribute significantly to the corticospinal projection in monkeys. Both zones also contribute major corticostriate and corticopontine contributions to the re-entrant circuits which will return to modulate motor cortex activity. So multiple pathways for interaction exist through which the 'secondary' motor areas may influence spinal cord function and movement outcomes.

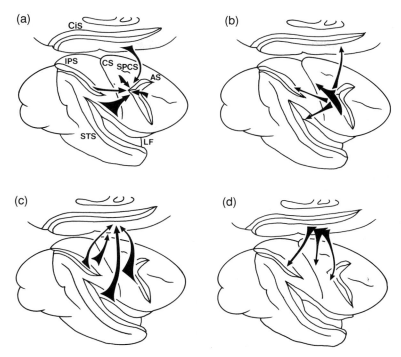

FIG 7.1 Schematic diagrams to summarize the ipsilateral input regions from which cortico-cortical afferent projections are provided to the postarcuate premotor cortex (a) and the supplementary motor area (c). In turn, the cortico-cortical efferent projections from the premotor cortex (b) and the supplementary motor area (d) include projections to the precentral motor area (M1). (Redrawn to illustrate the data included in Humphrey (1979) and Wiesendanger (1981b).)

In what follows, we shall deal with each of these prominent secondary motor areas separately.

7.2 CONNECTIVITY OF THE SUPPLEMENTARY MOTOR AREA

Wiesendanger and Wiesendanger (1984) provided a schematic summary of the ipsilateral cortico-cortical connections with the SMA (Fig. 7.2) revealed by the use of both anterograde and retrograde tracing methods. In addition to the ipsilateral connections, we should emphasize the bilateral nature of the efferent projections from the SMA. These project to the corresponding regions of SMA, premotor, and motor cortices of the other hemisphere. The proportion of corticospinal neurones arising from the SMA has been

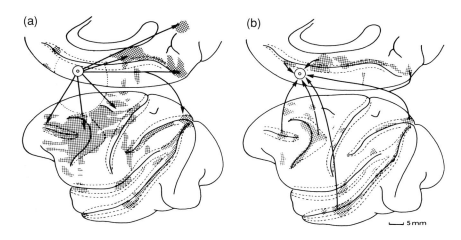

FIG 7.2 Schematic representation of afferent and efferent ipsilateral cortico-cortical connections of the SMA in *Macaca fascicularis*. (a): Outputs from the SMA. Arrows point to areas in which substantial labelling was found (hatched areas without arrows were weakly labelled). (b): Inputs to the SMA. The regions marked by arrows contained a substantial number of retrogradely labelled cells. The hatched area without arrows contained some scattered cells only. (Reproduced with permission from Wiesendanger and Wiesendanger (1984).)

illustrated in Fig. 2.15 (p. 72) and Table 2.4 (p. 70) (Künzle 1978; Macpherson *et al.* 1982b; Dum and Strick 1991). The SMA also sends fibres to the red nucleus and, as we have indicated above, it projects to the basal ganglia and to the pons. Ipsilateral cortical inputs to the SMA arise in the parietal lobe (areas 5 and 7), the second somatic sensory area, SII, the motor cortex itself and the postarcuate premotor area. In addition, the SMA is reported by Schell and Strick (1984) to receive its input from that part of the thalamus (nucleus VLo) receiving the major output from the basal ganglia (Fig. 7.3). Strick (1987) has emphasized that each of the cerebral cortical motor areas had reciprocal connections with the others (illustrated in the upper part of Fig. 7.3) but received their afferents from distinct cortical and subcortical territories.

A comprehensive account of the movement responses revealed by electrical stimulation of the SMA in man has been provided in Chapter 1. Woolsey *et al.* (1952) mapped both primary motor area responses and those obtained following stimulation of the SMA in barbiturate anaesthetised monkeys. They did not detect the bilateral responses which Penfield and Welch (1949, 1951) had described in both monkeys and man and they considered that the deep anaesthesia used in their study may have suppressed ipsilateral occurrences. They did identify a topographically organized repre-

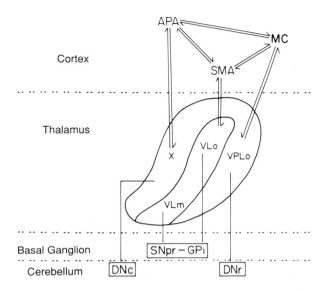

FIG 7.3 Summary of anatomical relationships between cerebellar and basal ganglia efferents and motor and premotor cortical areas in the monkey. This diagram illustrates: (1) the pathway from caudal portions of the deep cerebellar nuclei (DNc) to area X and the arcuate premotor area (APA), (2) the pathways from the pars reticulata of the substantia nigra (SNpr) and the internal segment of the globus pallidus (GPi) to VLm and VLo and the supplementary motor area (SMA), (3) the pathway from rostral portions of the deep cerebellar nuclei (DNr) to VPLo and the primary motor cortex (MC), and (4) the reciprocal connections between the MC, APA, and SMA. (Reproduced with permission from Schell and Strick (1984).)

sentation in the SMA with movements of the face located most anteriorly, followed by movements of the forelimb and then the hindlimb as the stimulating electrode was moved progressively more caudally. The location of the monkey's SMA is indicated in Fig. 7.4.

7.3 RECORDINGS FROM NEURONES IN THE SMA

Brinkman and Porter (1979) recorded the discharges of individual neurones in the SMA of conscious monkeys trained to carry out self paced movements. A high proportion (almost 80 per cent) of the cells recorded within the 'arm area' of the SMA exhibited modulation of their discharge in association with some aspect of movement performance. The firing of these cells was associated with either proximal movements (about the shoulder and the elbow) or distal movements of the wrist, hand, and fingers (see also

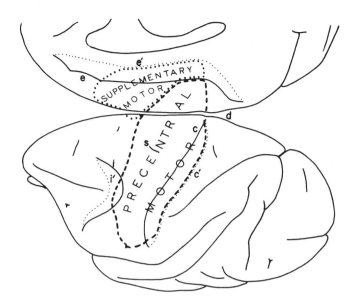

FIG 7.4   Medial and dorsolateral views of the left hemisphere of *Macaca mulatta* showing the extent of the precentral and supplementary motor areas. The posterior bank of the central sulcus, the anterior bank of the arcuate sulcus, and the lower bank of the cingulate sulcus have been cut away. c, central sulcus; c′, bottom of central sulcus; i, arcuate sulcus; i′, bottom of arcuate sulcus; d, medial edge of hemisphere; e, cingulate sulcus; e′, bottom of cingulate sulcus. (Reproduced with permission from Woolsey *et al.* (1952).)

Tanji and Kurata 1979). Around 5 per cent of these cells could be identified as PTNs by the antidromic responses generated in them by pyramidal tract stimulation. Figure 7.5 illustrates the discharges of a neurone in the SMA of the left hemisphere occurring in advance of flexion of the elbow during a lever pulling task. The neurone produced a burst of impulses about 300 to 400 ms before the movement commenced whether the right hand (a) or the left (c) was used to move the lever. Panel (b) of Fig. 7.5 illustrates the periresponse time histogram of the EMG activity of the brachioradialis muscle of the right arm during the same 20 performances of the task as those used for constructing histogram A. The onset of EMG activity in this muscle preceded movement by about 100 ms.

The vast majority of the neurones in the arm area of the SMA from which recordings were made in these experiments (94 per cent) discharged in association with the same aspect of movement performance whether this movement was performed by the ipsilateral or the contralateral limb. The majority of the quite small sample of PTNs located within the SMA also exhibited a bilateral association of their discharge with movement.

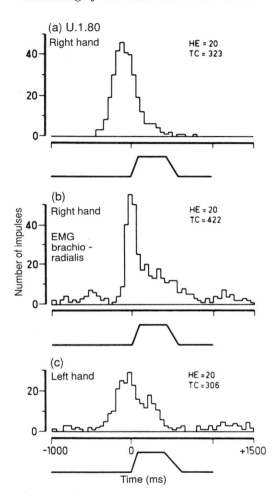

Fig 7.5 The discharges of a neurone in the left supplementary motor area which fired in advance of elbow flexion during each performance of a lever pulling task by a macaque monkey. (a): Discharges of the neurone accompanying twenty repetitions of the task using the right hand. (c): Discharges of the same neurone in association with twenty repetitions of a similar task the left hand. (b): A histogram of the EMG activity recorded in the right brachioradialis muscle during the movements during which the discharges in (a) were recorded. The neurone increased its discharge well before EMG activity increased. This was the case for the majority of SMA neurones of which the discharge pattern could be compared with EMG changes. (Reproduced with permission from Brinkman and Porter (1979).)

The firing with ipsilateral movements was often less intense than with contralateral movements and this applied especially to those cells whose discharge was associated with movements about the distal joints of the limb. This pattern of behaviour, in which the one cell's discharges occurred in association with both ipsilateral and contralateral actions, illustrates a major difference between the SMA and the primary motor cortex, a difference confirmed in recent experiments which set out specifically to examine relationships of cortical activities in different areas to ipsilateral, contralateral, and bilateral movements of the digits in monkeys (Tanji *et al.* 1988).

These changes in firing occurred in advance of the movements. In such cells, many of which may not be closely coupled to motoneurones (Kuypers and Brinkman 1970; Dum and Strick 1991), it is not realistic to attempt to assess the significance of changed firing which begins several hundred ms or up to one second before the commencement of movement. Yet it is clearly not a reaction to the occurrence of the movement; rather, the change in firing signals that the cell anticipates the performance of a movement. The association of discharges of cells in the SMA with movements of the forelimb when either the ipsilateral or the contralateral limb was employed and, for some cells, when the movement was occurring about a proximal joint, while other cells discharged in relation to movements of a distal joint of the limb, deserves special comment in relation to the known regional connectivities of the SMA. Some of the associations could depend on bilateral influences exerted by PTNs arising from the SMA. Some corticospinal neurones, even in the precentral motor area, exert bilateral influences on the spinal cord (Kuypers and Brinkman 1970). The regional connections of the SMA are themselves indicative of a major potential for bilateral influences, because each SMA projects to the motor cortex on both sides, and also receives inputs from the homologous SMA and from premotor cortex on the other side. Brinkman, in unpublished results referred to in Brinkman and Porter (1979), studied the behaviour of cells in the SMA after section of the corpus callosum. Although she now found a higher proportion of neurones with only contralateral associations, the majority of cells continued to be associated in their discharge with movements of either the ipsilateral or the contralateral limb. If these observations could be confirmed they would seem to indicate that a major drive for the behaviour of these cells must come from subcortical structures such as the basal ganglia and cerebellum and that integrated inputs must reach the SMA via the thalamus.

From the responses recorded while individual cells were discharging in association with self paced arm and hand movements, Brinkman and Porter also reported a general somatotopy in the organization of the SMA. In a single animal, responses associated with movements about the distal joints of the limb tended to be located more anteriorly than those associated with movements about proximal joints although there was a high degree of overlap (Fig. 7.6). Neurones related to movement of the upper extremity tended to be found in the first 2 mm of each penetration and could be shown, on histological reconstruction of the electrode tracks, to be located at the medial edge of the hemisphere on the crown of the superior frontal gyrus. A 'clustering' of neurones which exhibited similar responses was evident in that neurones located close together and sampled in the same electrode penetration discharged similarly in association with proximal or distal movement performances.

While natural stimulation of peripheral receptors in the relaxed animal (stroking of hairs, touching the skin, passive movement of joints, etc.) provided an effective input which caused discharges of a high proportion (of the order of 75–80 per cent) of the neurones in the primary motor cortex (see Chapter 6), such natural activation of peripheral receptors was much less effective in causing discharge of cells in the SMA. Only 14 per cent of the sample of cells recorded by Brinkman and Porter could be shown to respond to natural stimulation of peripheral receptors. This must suggest that the 'sensory' input which is anatomically linked into the SMA by means of connections from parietal cortex and from the second somatic sensory area (SII) must already be so highly processed that projections from particular afferent input zones are often no longer separately identifiable. When responses to natural stimulation of peripheral receptors were obtained, the individual neurone could frequently be driven by passive movements of more than one joint. Sometimes the responses could be driven by passive movement of more than one limb, and some inputs derived from both sides of the body. It may be significant that complex responses from wide territories including more than one limb have been reported in area 5 (Duffy and Burchfiel 1971; Sakata *et al.* 1973; Sakata and Iwamura 1978), and that bilateral receptive fields are common in SII (Whitsel *et al.* 1969). Both of these regions project influences to the SMA. In contrast to these results, Smith (1979) reported that 61 per cent of a small sample of 24 SMA neurones recorded in their experiments responded to stimulation of the contralateral arm. But the sampling of neurones in these two studies was likely to be very different given the differences in the task being performed.

In line with the paucity of influences detected in the SMA when natural stimulation of peripheral receptors was employed in the experiments on relaxed animals we have here documented, only a small proportion (5–8 per cent) of neurones in the hindlimb or forelimb area of the SMA were found to be influenced by an imposed perturbation of movement performance (Wise and Tanji, 1980, 1981; Tanji *et al.* 1980). So, whether the animals were passive or actively moving, little evidence of peripheral 'feedback' to the majority of these neurones exists.

Tanji *et al.* (1980) examined the behaviour of neurones in the SMA

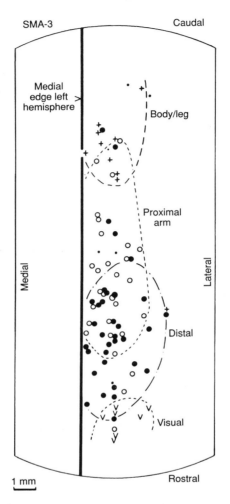

FIG 7.6   A rostrocaudal somatotopic organization of the responses of neurones in the SMA places the forelimb representation in front of the hindlimb representation. In addition, neuronal responses associated with movement about the more distal joints of the forelimb tended to be found more anteriorly than the responses of neurones associated with movements about proximal joints. (Reproduced with permission from Brinkman and Porter (1979).)

during periods following a visually presented instruction to move, but while the animals awaited disturbance of the hand as a trigger to move. In about half of a large number of neurones from which recordings were maintained during the 'prepare to pull' or 'prepare to push' instructed state, which lasted for 2.5 to 5 seconds, changes in discharge of the neurone

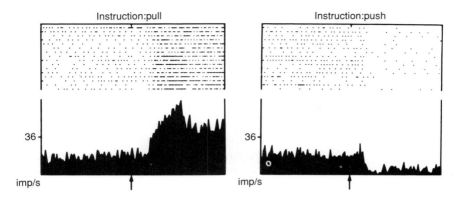

FIG 7.7   Differential responses in the one 'preparatory' cell, recorded within the monkey SMA, occurred after an 'instruction to pull' (left) or an 'instruction to push' (right) signal. Activity of the cell is shown for for 1024 ms before and 1024 ms after the appearance of a red or green light instructing the monkey to pull or push, respectively. Cell activity is shown both in raster form and as a peri-event histogram for 16 trials. Bin width is 16 ms. The time of occurrence of the instruction signal is indicated by an arrow. The motor response to the instruction did not occur until at least 2.5 s afterwards. (Reproduced with permission from Tanji *et al.* (1980).)

were differential. In these cells, if the instruction to pull caused a maintained increase in firing of the cell, the instruction to push caused a decrease (Fig. 7.7). In the other half of the cells, responses to the instruction occurred; however, they were similar irrespective of which instruction about direction of movement was provided. The latencies of onset of these preparatory responses to the instruction could be as short as 140 ms. It is important to note that, of the 201 neurones described by Tanji *et al.* (1980), only four altered their firing in association with the motor task when it was performed and none exhibited a short-latency response to the perturbation of the lever which served as a signal to move. This population of cells, active during preparation to move, therefore represents a different functional group to the neurones which Brinkman and Porter (1979) and Tanji and Kurata (1979) had described as discharging in association with the actual performance of movement. Tanji suggested that the 'preparatory' cells may be cortico-cortical neurones in lamina III of the SMA. Accordingly, Tanji *et al.* (1980) considered that they had observed the development, within a population of neurones in the SMA, of the neural correlates of a preparatory state ('motor set') that would allow the animal to respond adequately to a trigger to move when it was presented. The magnitude of the instruction effects varied in parallel with the development of enhanced motor skill as the monkeys responded more efficiently to the triggering stimulus.

A higher proportion of the differential responses of cells in the SMA

(26 per cent) than of PTN in the motor cortex (8 per cent) had response latencies to the instruction about direction of movement to be performed that were shorter than 200 ms. Tanji *et al.* therefore argued that these preparatory SMA cells could have been involved, through their projections to the motor cortex, in producing the preparatory changes in PTN discharge which were specific to the direction of forthcoming movements which the animal had been instructed to make (see Section 5.6). The possibility is raised that this influence on the motor cortex, exerted by the SMA, may be involved in setting the gain of transcortical reflexes (Section 6.7). In the absence of this form of gain control, for example after ablation of the SMA in man and monkeys, some observers have reported that forced grasping may occur (Travis 1955; Smith 1979; Smith *et al.* 1981).

Tanji and Kurata (1982) examined neurones both in the SMA and in the motor cortex of the same animal on alternate days while that animal performed repetitions of movement response commanded by an external coloured light or auditory cue. Only a small proportion of their SMA neurones could be identified as PTNs (11 of 399). SMA neurones, in contrast to those in the primary motor cortex tended to exhibit 'temporally coupled' responses to visual and auditory as well as tactile stimuli, when these stimuli were used as a signal to move. Movement related activity in the SMA was less intense and less 'closely coupled' to the actual movement performance than was observed for cells in the primary motor cortex. It was concluded therefore that the neurones in the SMA could not be directly involved in initiating the simple brisk movements which these monkeys had been trained to perform. The more remote location of the SMA from the spinal cord machinery for movement which is indicated by its connectivities, would clearly explain some of the differences observed by Tanji and Kurata.

Hummelsheim *et al.* (1986) re-examined the responses obtained by stimulation of the SMA, this time using single-pulse intracortical micro-stimulation (s-ICMS). While they considered the possibility that the motor responses they obtained could be explained by influences projected to the motor cortex by neurones in the SMA, they proposed that the presence of corticospinal neurones with their somata in the SMA provided the opportunity for SMA to 'exert a control on the motor apparatus *in parallel* with the motor cortex' (see also Wiesendanger *et al.* 1987; Dum and Strick 1991). Hummelsheim *et al.* (1986) were able to demonstrate short-latency facilitation of EMG comparable in latency with those observed with s-ICMS applied to the primary motor cortex, although thresholds were higher and the effects weaker. The most clear-cut effects were in the more proximal arm muscles. Single pulse microstimulation avoids the temporal summation of activity that is caused by repetitive ICMS, and is more likely to exert its effects directly upon motoneuronal activity through corticospinal projections than indirectly through the motor cortex, although this has yet to be proven. Wiesendanger *et al.* (1973) reported that the movements caused by repetitive ICMS in the SMA were abolished by primary motor cortex lesions.

Another nearby zone of cortex which is potentially implicated in motor aspects of emotional or motivational behaviour is the cingulate cortex, adjacent to the SMA and possessing both its own corticospinal projections and connections with precentral motor areas. Shima *et al.* (1991) found that a high proportion of task-related neurones, recorded within the cingulate cortex of monkeys, exhibited discharges which preceded activity in distal flexor muscles. Both an anterior and a posterior cingulate region were found to contain such task related neurones. The neurones in the posterior region were located within cingulate zones which projected cortico-cortical afferents to the forelimb region of the primary motor cortex. In neither region were the discharges of these cells time-locked to the onset of sensory signals used to trigger the movement responses.

7.4 ACTIVITY IN THE HUMAN SMA ASSOCIATED WITH VOLUNTARY MOVEMENTS

Roland *et al.* (1980a) used intracarotid injections of radioactive ^{133}Xe to study regional cerebral blood flow (rCBF) in 28 human subjects who were required to perform repeatedly the learned sequence of finger/thumb touching movements already described in Chapter 5 (Figs. 5.12, 5.13). The rCBF was estimated for each zone underlying one of the sensors and was calculated for a period of 45 seconds during which the finger touching task, according to a prelearned sequence, was repeated continuously with the contralateral hand. These measures of blood flow were then compared with those obtained from the same detectors while the subjects remained at rest and also during periods when similar tasks, such as rapidly repeated flexion of one finger or isometric finger flexions, were performed. These alternative tasks did not require a learned sequence of movements to be followed.

When voluntary movements of the contralateral hand, to execute any one of the finger movement tasks, were performed, an increase in rCBF always occurred in the region identified as the hand area of the sensorimotor cortex. This has been described in Chapter 5 (Section 5.11). In addition, whenever the voluntary movement task involved the programmed execution of fast sequential unilateral finger movements, in a learned order, there was a significant increase in rCBF in the vicinity of the SMA in *both* hemispheres: Fig. 7.8(a,b). The mere repetition of isolated movements of the fingers, such as repeated flexions of one finger, or a maintained isometric contraction of finger and thumb to compress a spring throughout the recording period, did not cause a significant change in rCBF in the

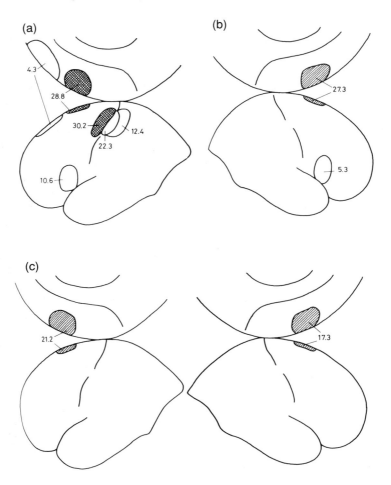

FIG 7.8   (a) Contralateral and (b) ipsilateral changes in regional cerebral blood flow (rCBF) accompanying repeated performances of the learned finger touching movement sequence illustrated in Fig. 5.13. Increases in rCBF occur over the contralateral motor (hand) area and over SMA on both sides. When the subjects were required to think through the learned sequence, but not produce any movement, only the SMA showed an increase in rCBF and this change was evident in both hemispheres (c). (a), from 5 subjects; (b), from 4 subjects; and (c), from 3 subjects (left hemisphere) and 5 subjects (right hemisphere). Numbers indicate mean percentage increase in rCBF. Significance levels for rCBF increases: cross-hatched areas, 0.0005; hatched areas, 0.005; and open areas, 0.05. (Redrawn from Roland *et al.* (1980a).)

SMA, although the focus of increased activity was still clearly recognized over the contralateral sensorimotor hand area, whatever the movement task that was being performed.

During one set of recordings of rCBF, these subjects were required to think through (rehearse) the motor sequence 'in their head' at the same rate and in the same order as they had been trained to perform the movements, but without actually executing the task. This internal simulation of the sequential motor task was referred to by Roland *et al.* (1980a) as 'internal programming' of the movement sequence. In some subjects, EMG recordings confirmed that no movements were made during this internal programming. The important finding from these studies was that, while no increase in rCBF occurred over the contralateral motor cortex, there was a significant increase in rCBF over the SMA of both hemispheres when the subjects rehearsed the task mentally, and this region was the only one from which consistent changes in blood flow could be recorded during 'internal programming' (Fig. 7.8(c)). The temporal limitations of the method determine that regions of cerebral cortex which could have been briefly and transiently involved in aspects of the task would not be detected, and make it impossible to comment on the relative timing of the increases in activity in the SMA compared with that in motor cortex or other regions. Yet the obvious conclusion of these experiments was that the SMA of both hemispheres must participate in generating the pattern of the time-ordered sequence of commands which would be needed for the execution of a complex learned motor task with the fingers of one hand.

Reference to Fig. 5.14(b) (p. 244) reveals a mean percentage increase in rCBF of about 30 per cent in the midline cortex of the SMA of both hemispheres in association with the voluntary performance of the learned finger touching sequence by 10 subjects (Roland 1987). The right hand tomogram (Fig. 5.14(c)) clearly indicates that increased metabolic activity occurs concurrently in the globus pallidus from which the SMA receives input.

The same general zones of cerebral cortex also exhibit bilateral increases in rCBF with other voluntary movement tasks (Orgogozo and Larsen 1979). Hence the SMA is activated along with the sequential movements required to be performed by the mouth or the foot. Larsen *et al.* (1978) described the involvement of the SMA in voluntary articulate speech, in counting aloud or in rehearsing the months of the year. Roland *et al.* (1980b) determined that changes in blood flow in the SMA occurred not only in response to a learned repetitive sequence of ballistic finger movements (internally driven) but also to smooth movements such as drawing in the air with the arm, pointing with the finger, and tracking movements made to follow a target or execute a path through a maze. Fox *et al.* (1985) concluded from their studies of a series of different movements of the hand and of the eyes, including voluntary internally driven or tracking saccades, that the SMA's activity was increased in association with all voluntary movements, whether or not the tasks were complex 'stochastic, non deterministic' (Roland 1987) events. They found that the SMA was active, and exhibited an increase in rCBF, even when the voluntary tasks being performed were simple movement repetitions. Moreover, they found significant differences in the location of the area of peak change in their measures of rCBF depending on the muscle fields involved in the task. The area of peak activation during saccadic eye movements was consistently found to lie anterior to the area of peak activation during hand movements (Fig. 7.9), consistent with the general somatotopy revealed in other experiments (Fig. 7.6).

Deiber *et al.* (1991) have recently used PET to re-examine the question of which cortical areas are active during selection of movement. They were careful to control the rate of voluntary movement in a task which involved moving a joystick in response to a tone. They compared rCBF in conditions in which an external cue was given to the subject to move the joystick in

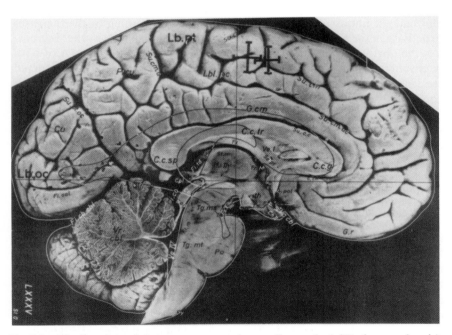

Fig 7.9   The location of the mean stereotaxic coordinates (± 1 SD along each axis) of the area of maximum change in rCBF over the SMA during saccadic eye movements and during the performance of repetitive finger flexion-extension movements. The area for the saccades was, on average, 0.8 cm further anterior than that for the fingers (7 subjects). (Reproduced with permission from Fox *et al.* (1985).)

a particular direction and in which the subject selected the movement direction without an external cue. There was greater activation of SMA for the tasks performed with internal cues, and this was particularly true for the more rostral region of the SMA. However, when they compared rCBF for a 'fixed' condition (moving the joystick forwards) with that for selection of movement direction based on external cues, or for a learned sequence of movements, they could find no significant differences in flow.

7.5 READINESS POTENTIALS ASSOCIATED WITH VOLUNTARY MOVEMENTS

When electrical recordings made from the scalp are averaged in relation to the onset time of a simple voluntary movement (e.g. finger flexion), a slow negative potential which precedes the onset of movement by a period of the order of one second, may be detected with its maximum recorded at the vertex (Fig. 7.10). This is the readiness potential (Bereitschaftspotential) of Deecke *et al.* (1969). The timing of the potential development in advance of movement onset is similar to the timing of the changes in firing of SMA

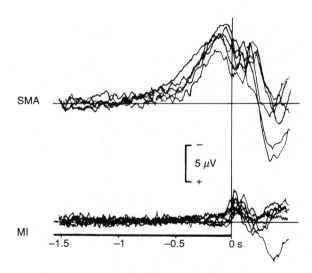

FIG 7.10 Averaged electrical (EEG) recordings made in the same subject on different days in relation to repetitions of fast flexion movements of the right index finger. Time zero coincides with the onset of EMG activity in the finger flexor muscles. The upper trace indicates the readiness potential recorded over the supplementary motor area (SMA), while the lower trace (MI) records the motor potential over the hand area of left motor cortex, detected during the same repetitions of the finger movements. (Reproduced with permission from Kornhuber and Deecke (1985).)

neurones in monkeys engaged in the performance of self-paced movements (Brinkman and Porter 1979). There is evidence that the readiness potential appears first in electrodes positioned over the SMA (Kristeva *et al.* 1979; Schreiber *et al.* 1983) and that it exhibits its maximum amplitude over the SMA in relation to the onset of all voluntary movements whether they are performed by the hand, toe, mouth, tongue, or eye and whether they are complex and programmed (as in speech) or simple, as in flexion of a single joint. Kornhuber (1984) argued that a real-time indicator of SMA neuronal activity may be found in the recordings of the Bereitschaftspotential and that this provided an electrophysiological correlate of the preparation for the onset of a voluntary movement. He suggested that the SMA specifies 'when' a movement is to be made (see also Goldberg 1985 and the commentary on Goldberg's review which follows his article).

The further analysis of the functional associations of the SMA with voluntary movement performance may be expected to depend on techniques which will allow real-time measurement of electrical activities which can be located confidently within the SMA and which may be used during single performances of a motor task, without the need for averaging over many repetitions. Magneto-encephalography has the theoretical capacity reliably to detect signals which arise from electrical events generated in such hidden regions as midline cerebral cortex and the SMA. Deecke (1987) drew the distinction between purely volitional actions initiated from within the brain and movements made in response to stimuli from the environment which he styled 'reactions'. His recordings from the human brain and his study of the readiness magnetic field (Bereitschaftsmagnetfeld) indicated that preparatory activity in the brain preceding volitional movement occurred in widespread regions. However the two principal generators of preparatory activity were the SMA and the primary motor cortex. Activity in the SMA could precede the onset of volitional movement by one second or more and seemed, in these recordings to precede any changes in activity in the motor cortex. In line with Kornhuber's views on the function of the SMA, Deecke therefore concluded that SMA must have a role in the initiation of voluntary movement. This view would be consistent with the greater proportion of 'long lead' preparatory discharges of cells in the SMA of monkeys (Okano and Tanji 1987; Alexander and Crutcher 1990a).

7.6 EVIDENCE RELATING TO THE FUNCTION OF THE SMA
OBTAINED FROM BEHAVIOURAL STUDIES FOLLOWING LESIONS
IN MONKEYS AND IN MAN

Passingham *et al.* (1989) took up the investigation of the involvement of the brain in motor performances in which an animal either reacts to an external event or performs a self-initiated action. Following the line of argument developed by Kornhuber (above) and espoused by Eccles (1982), it might be expected that monkeys with SMA lesions would exhibit disturbances of their performance of self-initiated movements, and they do. Passingham and his colleagues removed the SMA bilaterally in monkeys that had been trained to perform simple arm-raising actions to obtain food rewards, either self-initiated, in their own time ('when they felt like it') or in response to an auditory signal advising them 'when' to move. In addition, animals were tested on their ability to handle a choice between two movements, that is, to decide correctly 'which movement to make' to obtain a food reward. Passingham's results led him to the conclusion that the poor level of performance of monkeys on self-initiated arm raising tasks, immediately following bilateral SMA lesions, was explained by the fact that the monkeys failed to make attempts to raise their arm because they were unable to 'retrieve' the engram of the appropriate movement without an external cue. Even though self-initiated actions were greatly impaired by SMA lesions, the monkeys could react to an external cue and perform the simple motor task well (Fig. 7.11). Passingham (1987) suggested that the SMA was specialized for directing movements on the basis of internal and learned proprioceptive cues about the animal's own actions. The problem which the lesioned monkeys experienced was in

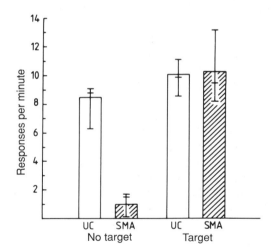

FIG 7.11   Performance of unoperated controls (UC) and monkeys with bilateral SMA lesions (SMA) on a simple arm-raising task. The histograms illustrate the means and the bars provide the scores for individual animals (three in each group). In the 'no target' condition, the animals were required to raise their arm in the dark using internal proprioceptive cues. The 'target' condition required the animal to reach for a peanut in the light. (From Passingham (1987). Copyright © 1987. Reprinted with permission of John Wiley and Sons Ltd.)

retrieving these internal proprioceptive cues and finding the mechanism to allow them to act appropriately (i.e. discovering 'what to do'). Providing that an external cue was available to instruct the animals about the movement to be performed, those with bilateral SMA lesions could learn either to pull or to turn a handle (Fig. 7.13). Hence, the retrieval of the appropriate internal 'proprioceptive' information about the movement to be made could be initiated by an external trigger which signalled what to do and when to do it.

Brinkman (1981, 1984) has conducted a detailed re-evaluation of the influence of unilateral SMA lesions on movement performance in monkeys, paying particular attention to the use of the hand in the production of delicate and precisely controlled use of the fingers. For a few days after excision of the arm region of the SMA on one side, monkeys exhibited a clumsiness of finger movements which was revealed by the fact that they took longer to collect a number of food rewards by manipulating them out of multiple small slots in a wooden board, and they made many more errors in finger movements than pre-operatively. The precise adjustments in finger position and the smooth execution of each food retrieval movement, usually accomplished by extension of the index finger into the slot and then execution of a pincer grip between thumb and index on the food morsel, were disorganized. More importantly, following a unilateral SMA lesion, this disintegration of the precise ordering of a whole range of postural adjustments and finger movements, was exhibited whether the hand ipsilateral to the lesion or the contralateral hand was used in the food collection task. After a few days, this motor problem (clumsiness or a form of apraxia) resolved and could be detected no longer.

Brinkman also examined the monkeys with SMA lesions in a bimanual co-ordination task, similar to that which had been used earlier by Mark and Sperry (1968). A large number of holes in a thick perspex plate were baited with individual food morsels — currants or raisins. Under full visual control, the monkey retrieved the food plugs by pushing with the finger of one hand and catching the food in the other hand cupped beneath the hole. This task required the two hands to adopt different postures and movements simultaneously and to co-operate in sharing aspects of the bimanual task of food collection. Needless to say, even young animals performed the task without the need for elaborate training.

Following unilateral SMA lesions, and even with visual monitoring of the whole performance, the same animals frequently had difficulty in performing this bimanual task. The clumsiness they now exhibited was often caused by the fact that, instead of sharing different aspects of the required performance, both hands were seen to assume the same posture or to be engaged in the same movement at the same time. Figure 7.12 illustrates a monkey attempting to push the food pellet out of the hole

SMX-1

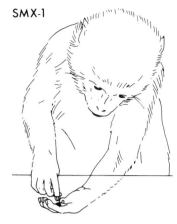 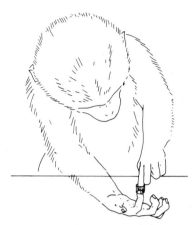

Normal animal   5 months after right SMA lesion

FIG 7.12   Left: normal monkey, pushing from above to collect a bait lodged in a hole in a perspex sheet, uses the index finger of the preferred hand, while the non-preferred hand is cupped underneath, anticipating catch of the falling bait. Right: reversal of hand position and identical behaviour of both hands, 5 months after ablation of the right supplementary motor area. The non-preferred hand is now above the plate, and both hands are used in pushing with the index finger. Even with full visual control the movements are not corrected. (Drawn from individual frames of a movie film. Reproduced with permission from Brinkman (1981).)

with the index finger of each hand, one pushing from above against the other pushing from below. These drawings were made by Dr Brinkman from single frames of high speed movie films of the behaviour of the animals. In the right-hand illustration, this characteristic, but inappropriate, performance using the fingers of both hands, was still obvious five months after a unilateral SMA lesion. The inability to produce the correct shared actions in performing the bimanual task persisted and was still exhibited a year after the surgical lesion had been performed.

This disorganization of bimanual co-operation in a task which should, for its appropriate execution, require different actions by the two hands, is a permanent deficit following unilateral SMA lesions and suggests that an imbalance has been produced by the unilateral lesion, leaving one SMA to deal with the preparation for action by the motor executive apparatus of both sides of the body. It is as if the intact instruction about the movement that is retrieved and available in the remaining SMA results, on occasion, in the same selection of outputs from the motor cortex of each hemisphere. Brinkman (1984) has reported a return to normal in this bimanual co-ordination task if a unilateral SMA lesion is followed by callosal section, suggesting that the intact SMA is now unable to exert a controlling influence on the motor cortex of the opposite hemisphere via callosal connections. She also reported that deficits in bimanual co-ordination do not persist and are revealed only transiently in animals subjected to bilateral lesions of the SMA.

In spite of the fact that early reports by Penfield and others stated that unilateral ablation of the SMA in man was accompanied by 'few permanent symptoms and no permanent deficit in maintenance of posture or capacity for movement' (Penfield and Welch 1951), transient motor defects have been reported in human patients (Laplane *et al.* 1977; Damasio and van Hoesen 1980). Transient impairment of contralateral conjugate gaze, slowness of movement, hypokinesia and paucity of speech have also been observed in man. In response to test situations, patients may exhibit a slowing of alternating finger movements in the hand contralateral to the lesion and awkwardness in the execution of movements involving alternating actions of the two hands. We have referred already to Travis' observation (1955) of contralateral forced grasping in monkeys, although Coxe and Landau (1965) could detect no permanent abnormalities of posture or movement after complete bilateral resection of the SMA in monkeys.

It is tempting to draw parallels between the clumsiness in bimanual co-ordination exhibited in Brinkman's experiments on monkeys and a modern account of the dysfunction experienced by a patient with a unilateral lesion of midline cortex involving the superior frontal gyrus and presumably damaging the SMA. Schell *et al.* (1986) described a patient, a young right-handed woman, who required intra-operative embolization of a left parasagittal arteriovenous malformation and, as a consequence, lost the function of her left SMA. She suffered akinetic mutism and generated no spontaneous speech or movements for a period of four days postoperatively. After recovery from this, 'although the patient could function well when the right or the left hand was used independently, she was not able to co-ordinate motor functions when using both hands simultaneously. Simple tasks, such as buttoning her skirt or transferring a cup from one hand to the other, were performed poorly. Simultaneous pronation and supination of her forearms was very difficult, whereas this alternating movement pattern was executed normally when each arm was tested independently. This bimanual disturbance of alternating movements did not improve during subsequent examinations.'

7.7 TRANSIENT, REVERSIBLE SUPPRESSION OF FUNCTION IN THE SMA

It has been pointed out repeatedly that the interpretation of the deficits in movement performance which accompany lesions in the brain, whether these are created by the experimental surgeon or whether they result from clinical damage or disease in patients, is fraught with difficulties. Because of the transient nature of some of the disturbances, and in the knowledge that all primates exhibit a great capacity for compensation for a demonstrable neurological defect, some of which may be a consequence of functional plasticity in the brain itself, it is very difficult to deduce from the changed behaviour of the animal, the exact functions which were subserved, or the 'information processing' operations which were performed, by the tissue which has been damaged or removed. The experimental physiologist has available the opportunity to interrupt transiently and reversibly the neuronal activities in a given region of the brain by cooling it to suppress synaptic actions within it and so to interrupt its normal operations.

Schmidt *et al.* (1992) examined the effects of cooling of the SMA on one or both sides on the behaviour of neurones recorded in the primary motor cortex in association with the performance of repetitive wrist flexion/extension movements using the contralateral forelimb. Cooling of either the ipsilateral SMA, or both sides, did not prevent the animal from performing this simple repetitive task. The animals were, of course, overtrained and the wrist was moved to track a visual target — a performance which would not have been impaired even in Passingham's monkeys with bilateral surgical lesions of the SMA (see above). Nor did the cooling of the SMA interfere with the responses of the neurones in area 4 to imposed disturbances introduced unexpectedly while the wrist was held in the flexed or extended position. The short latency responses of the motor cortex neurones to peripheral perturbations were not influenced by the suppression of SMA function. The loop through the motor cortex continued to be operative and no evidence was produced in these experiments for a measurable change in the gain of the loop.

7.8 LESIONS OF PREMOTOR CORTEX

Passingham (1985b) studied monkeys which were trained to pull a handle in response to one coloured visual cue, or to turn it in response to another. When the postarcuate premotor cortex on both sides was removed at a surgical operation, it was difficult to retrain the monkeys to perform this task with accuracy. The animals were quite able to perform both of the movements but they had difficulty relearning which response was required to each of the coloured cues (Fig. 7.13). Passingham (1987) concluded that premotor cortex must be involved in instructing the motor cortex about the required output and in selecting the appropriate efferent projections from the motor cortex to be activated in response to visual cues (Halsband and Passingham 1982). Moll and Kuypers (1977) had also reported that lesions in the premotor cortex of macaque monkeys caused these animals

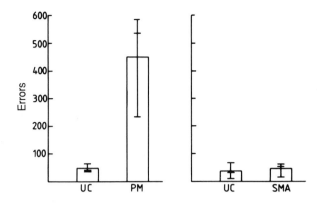

FIG 7.13   Errors in learning a visual conditional motor task after premotor cortex lesions. The task required the monkey to either pull or turn a handle, depending on the colour of the instruction cue. The histograms give the means and the bars the scores for individual monkeys (3 in each group). UC, unoperated control animals; PM, animals with premotor lesions; SMA, animals with supplementary motor lesions. (From Halsband and Passingham (1982) and Passingham (1987). Copyright © 1987. Reprinted with permission of John Wiley and Sons Ltd.)

to have difficulty in using sensory cues to direct movements (see also Rizzolatti *et al.* 1983).

Passingham (1988) has taken the analysis of the movement deficit caused by premotor lesions even further by introducing a requirement for the performance to be delayed following the delivery of the visual cue specifying which movement to make. It had previously been demonstrated that lesions of prefrontal cortex (along the principal sulcus), which region provides input projections to the inferior postarcuate premotor cortex, disturbed delayed reaction tasks (see Goldman-Rakic 1987). Whether the task required motor performance by the hand or by the eyes, these monkeys with prefrontal lesions exhibited difficulty in making appropriate delayed responses on the basis of stored information. Passingham (1988) reported that monkeys with premotor lesions performed badly both when they were required to respond immediately to a visual signal to move and when the appropriate response was required after a delay. He concluded that premotor cortex was not 'primarily concerned with preparation to act in the sense of making the necessary general adjustments before action. Its role is taken to be the specific one of retrieving the correct action.' He considered that premotor cortex must be involved in retrieving this action from memory on the basis of stored information about associations between environmental stimuli and those actions.

7.9 DIRECT PROJECTIONS OF NEURONES IN POSTARCUATE PREMOTOR CORTEX TO THE PRIMARY MOTOR CORTEX

Godschalk *et al.* (1984) confirmed the details of the organization of the regional connectivity to which reference has been made already (Matsumura and Kubota 1979; Muakkassa and Strick 1979) by using several different fluorescent tracers and HRP. Their results confirmed that the major inputs to the postarcuate cortex came from posterior parietal cortex, from SII, and from the superior frontal gyrus and cingulate cortex. Organized, topographically arranged projections from the postarcuate region and its dorsal extension corresponded with the face, arm, and leg regions of the primary motor cortex with little or no overlap between them. These authors mapped the projections of individual neurones from the postarcuate cortex to the precentral gyrus by using weak single stimuli delivered to intracortical electrodes within the motor cortex and searching for antidromic responses in the postarcuate premotor cortex. Records of antidromic responses were obtained from 52 superficially located neurones responding at short latencies ranging from 0.6 to 2.1 ms (mean 1.2 ms), indicating direct projections from these cells to area 4 (Fig. 7.14). All the projections to the arm area of the motor cortex came from the inferior limb of the arcuate sulcus, and, although the superior limb was explored, no antidromically activated neurones were found in this region. These studies provided electrophysiological confirmation of the direct projections of postarcuate neurones into the primary motor cortex (Pandya and Kuypers 1969; Pandya and Vignolo 1971; Künzle 1978).

Godschalk *et al.* also examined the inputs to the postarcuate premotor cortex from parietal areas, using the same electrophysiological methods and guided by their anatomical results (see Fig. 7.1). These inputs originated from the convexity of the postcentral gyrus immediately above the intraparietal sulcus, the banks of the intraparietal sulcus (area 7), the convexity of the rostral part of the inferior parietal lobule (area 7b), and from the dorsal operculum of the lateral fissure (SII, Jones and Burton 1976). The largest projections were from areas 7b and SII, and it appeared from the electrophysiological results that these projections, which could be demonstrated to be reciprocal, were also topographically organized (Stanton *et al.* 1977; Seltzer and Pandya 1980).

7.10 RECORDINGS FROM NEURONES IN THE POSTARCUATE PREMOTOR CORTEX

Wise (1985) summarized the results obtained in a number of laboratories, including his own, and relating to the natural discharges of neurones in

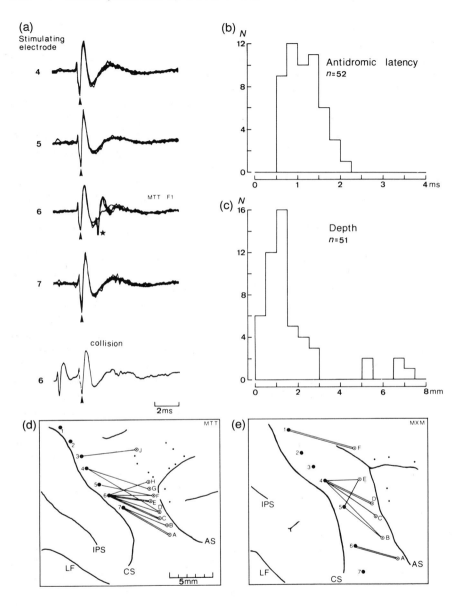

FIG 7.14 Topographic distribution of projections from postarcuate cortex to area 4 in the macaque monkey. (a): Recording from single neurone in postarcuate cortex (penetration labelled F in panel (d)) activated antidromically by intracortical stimulation within area 4 (electrode 6); antidromic spike indicated by asterisk. Four sweeps at threshold stimulus strength (150 µA) have been superimposed together with one at subthreshold strength. Stimulation at three adjacent sites (electrodes 4,

the postarcuate premotor cortex in association with voluntary movement performance. Fuster (1973) examined the behaviour of premotor cortex neurones during periods when animals had been instructed about a movement to be made but required to delay making the movement for a period of time. Neurones in premotor cortex changed their firing in this delay period, and this characteristic discharge during the period of preparation to move (the 'motor set') has been intensively studied by Godschalk *et al.* (1981, 1985); Weinrich and Wise (1982); Wise *et al.* (1983); Weinrich *et al.* (1984); and Wise and Mauritz (1985). Discharges during the delay period may be different, depending on the direction of the movement required to be made after the delay. Premotor neurones responded to 'visuo-spatial' instructions about the movement to be made and commenced firing as early as 120–240 ms after the instruction was provided. In Godschalk *et al.*'s experiments, 75 per cent of cells changed their firing during the waiting period while the food target remained visible. This activity was contingent upon there being a movement: when the monkey was presented with a dummy reward that the monkey did not reach for, no activity was observed in the waiting period (Godschalk *et al.* 1985).

For many neurones, this neuronal activity changed again about 130 ms before the onset of the movement performance itself. Now, for about half the neurones recorded from the premotor cortex, this movement-related discharge occurred differentially in association with the direction of the movement being made (see also Brinkman and Porter 1983). The movement-associated discharge of those neurones in the premotor cortex which behaved in this way could be seen to occur when the same movement was made using the ipsilateral or the contralateral limb, although, in the part of the premotor cortex lateral to the arcuate spur, a higher proportion of the neurones exhibited only associations with contralateral movements. Movement associated discharge was found in premotor neurones associated with movements about distal as well as proximal joints.

There has been much debate about the nature of the external stimuli

---

5, 7) with 500 μA did not excite this neurone. Arrows indicate stimulus artefacts. Antidromic nature of response evoked from electrode 6 is confirmed by collision with orthodromic spike. (b) and (c): distribution of antidromically activated postarcuate neurons according to antidromic latency (b) and depth (c). (d) and (e) show postarcuate penetrations (indicated by ⊙) made in two monkeys (MTT and MXM) in which neurones activated by area 4 stimulation were recorded. Straight lines link these penetrations with stimulus site giving antidromic responses at lowest threshold (D: $<100\,\mu$A; E: $<200\,\mu$A). Results indicate a posteromedial direction of the postarcuate projection to M1. Dots indicate penetrations in which neurones with antidromic responses were not found. (Reproduced with permission from Godschalk *et al.* (1984).)

which are capable of influencing the discharges of neurones in the premotor cortex. Neurones have been shown to respond to visual stimuli (Kubota and Hamada 1978; Sakai 1978; Rizzolatti *et al.* 1981c; Godschalk *et al.* 1981), and to peripheral somatosensory stimuli (Rizzolatti *et al.* 1981a,b). Brinkman and Porter (1979) were unable to detect significant short-latency responses of neurones in the premotor cortex following natural activation of peripheral receptors in the limbs, and they concluded that the convergence of inputs to parietal cortex and the processing of afferent signals which must have occurred before these were projected to premotor cortex must have made it difficult to recognize 'sensory' inputs to these cells.

7.11 SEVERAL FUNCTIONAL AREAS WITHIN THE PREMOTOR CORTEX

Matelli *et al.* (1985) and Rizzolatti (1987) have made use of cytochrome oxidase histochemistry to reveal that the agranular cortex of area 6 is composed of a number of identifiable subareas (Fig. 7.15). It is suggested that some of the confusion that has been generated concerning such issues as the responses of premotor neurones to somatosensory and visual stimuli

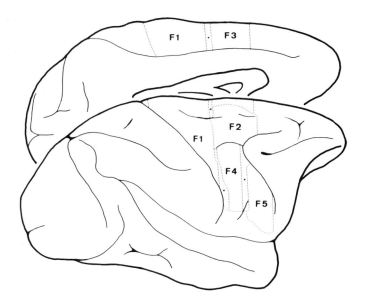

FIG 7.15   The separate subareas within the agranular cortex of area 6 that may be recognized using cytochrome oxidase histochemistry to reveal differences between them. Asterisks indicate transition zones and zones that were impossible to define because of the sulcul pattern. (From Rizolatti (1987). Copyright © 1987. Reprinted with permission of John Wiley and Sons Ltd.)

derives from the fact that the functional associations of neurones in the different subareas of area 6 may be different and that the biochemical substrate of those different functional associations can be detected by such methods as cytochrome oxidase histochemistry.

Rizzolatti and his colleagues have found that neurones in the inferior precentral area demonstrated a gradation of functional properties. Those neurones located in F4, the inferior postarcuate premotor region immediately adjacent to the motor cortex, responded well to tactile stimuli within large receptive fields which were mostly contralateral. They could also be activated by visual stimuli when these stimuli were moving three-dimensional objects within the animal's reach (peripersonal space) and especially when the visual stimulus was being moved towards the cutaneous receptive field, say that on the mouth and face. Fifty per cent of these neurones were reported to discharge with active movements of the contra-lateral limb in reaching or bringing the hand to the mouth. Neurones within F5, further forwards and more inferiorly in the postarcuate region, discharged with active movements and in relation to movements about distal as well as proximal joints. In particular, the discharges of these cells appeared to be related to special purposive movements (e.g. grasping an object with the hand). Less than half of the F5 neurones responded to somatosensory stimuli and very few were affected by visual inputs.

On the basis of these studies, Rizzolatti suggested, along with Haaxma and Kuypers' (1975) ideas, and in agreement with the findings of Godschalk *et al.* (1981), that premotor cortex plays a role in movements which are guided by sensory stimuli and especially by visual inputs. Rizzolatti went further and proposed that the premotor cortex itself stores a vocabulary of movement responses which can be addressed by sensory stimuli. This concept, of the location of this storage of information about purposive movements being within premotor cortex itself, is not consistent with Passingham's evidence that removal of premotor cortex was not accompanied by any defect in the ability to perform motor acts. The deficit revealed in monkeys with lesions of premotor cortex was that they found it difficult to direct actions based on information provided by environmental stimuli and especially by vision, but also using other cues such as sound. According to Passingham (1988). 'The task of the premotor cortex is that of recalling the action that is appropriate for the current situation. The action must be retrieved from memory on the basis of stored information about associations between situations and actions'.

7.12 STUDIES IN HUMAN SUBJECTS: ACTIVATION OF PREMOTOR CORTEX DURING VOLUNTARY MOVEMENTS

When human subjects voluntarily explored the surfaces of solid objects manually in stereognostic discrimination tasks, an increase in rCBF was detected over the contralateral premotor area, along with the changes in the sensory and motor cortex. Similarly, when movements were performed in response to verbal commands (Roland 1984), increases in blood flow occurred over the premotor area in addition to the changes in other zones (Ingvar and Philipson 1977). When the finger was used to track through a maze, by moving from square to square in response to verbal directions, increases in rCBF occurred in the contralateral and in the ipsilateral premotor area and the changes were greater contralaterally. Premotor area changes in rCBF were much greater (27–30 per cent) in these externally directed and guided movement tasks than in the internally driven, finger-touching sequence which we have described already (7 per cent increase in premotor rCBF). 'Pure motor' routines, such as reading aloud and speaking never increased rCBF in the premotor area (Roland 1987). These findings are consistent with a role of premotor cortex in the performance of voluntary movements executed under the guidance of sensory inputs from the environment. Deiber *et al.* (1991) found bilateral activation of the premotor area for a learned sequence of joystick movements, and for movements selected at random by the subject.

7.13 SUMMARY

Voluntary movements of the fingers can be performed with great precision and exquisite accuracy. For example, without the aid of a mechanical stage, and using the visual, cutaneous, and proprioceptive information available to the brain, even untrained students can move a microscope slide to bring to the middle of the visible field first the centre and then the peripheral edge of a single human erythrocyte. The diameter of the red blood cell is of the order of 7 micrometers. So the selection of outputs from the motor areas of the cerebral cortex to the spinal machinery for control of movement has allowed co-ordinated action of motor units in a very large number of muscles to be so organized that their co-operative contractions produced an accurate, controlled movement of the fingers through 3 to 4 micrometers. Since it is through corticospinal (and, we suspect, cortico-motoneuronal) connections that the specific motor units in many muscles are recruited to the task, and that fractionated use of the contractions of distally acting muscles is achieved, we must conclude that it is the function of inputs to the corticospinal system, at the level of the cortical origins of these projections, to engage, in a selective manner, those output projections which will be called into action.

We have considered the potential roles of the SMA and premotor projections in contributing to the selection of output elements to be engaged in a motor task. The connectivities of both of these regions are consistent with the roles that have been deduced for them, both as interpreted from the results of studies of deficits produced by localized damage in these regions in monkeys and human patients, and also from the observations of changes in rCBF during the performance of voluntary movement tasks by conscious human subjects. Yet we are still ignorant about the precise cell-to-cell connectivities and about the information processing that relates these cortical areas one to another. The conclusions which flow from the overall analysis suggest that different regions within cortical area 6 are associated with different aspects of the total management of voluntary movement performance. It is unlikely that the storage of the internal programmes for the whole repertoire of learned movements resides within the SMA, because patients (and monkeys) with SMA lesions can still perform learned, voluntary movements. The SMA is itself the source of some corticospinal projections; however, the specific contributions which these can make to motor outputs, and the capacity they have to produce actions on motoneurones, have not yet been fully evaluated. The bilateral influence of the SMA and its demonstrated involvement in the accessing of the internal programmes for complex, sequential movements and for bimanual co-ordination in co-operative tasks deserve further experimental evaluation and will certainly require detailed electrophysiological analysis of the kind that has been used to study the functional involvement of cortico-motoneuronal projections from the motor cortex. Such experiments are clearly feasible; however, they have not yet been undertaken.

Although a few observations exist concerning the connections made by individual cells in postarcuate premotor cortex, the role of these connections in conveying to the primary motor cortex signals which are relevant to the selection of motor outputs appropriate for the external (environmental) situations which require voluntary actions, deserve further evaluation. The hints that have been obtained from observations in man and monkeys suggest that the analysis of relationships between the projections of individual cortico-cortical neurones in premotor cortex and functionally identified output elements from the motor cortex, using dual electrophysiological recordings in monkeys and cross-correlation analysis, could be a fruitful approach to the understanding of the special significance of this cortico-cortical connectivity in the selection of motor output signals.

8

Dynamic nature of cortical organization

8.1 THE NATURE OF MOTOR CORTEX MAPS: MAPS OF OUTPUTS, INPUTS, AND FUNCTIONS

Modern ideas about cortical localization of function really began with the experiments of Fritsch and Hitzig (1870). Their observations that galvanic stimulation of different regions of the dog's cerebral cortex produced movement of different parts of the contralateral musculature was the first real investigation of a cortical representation. Ferrier (1875) greatly extended these observations in his classic experiments on the monkey cortex using faradic stimulation from an induction coil. But because of the artificial nature of electrical stimulation, the maps he produced, and all of those that have been produced since, were really *maps of outputs.* 'Thus faradic stimulation is disqualified, equally with "galvanic", as a tool for evoking natural function in the projection area. This leaves us free to concentrate on its merits as a tool for mapping the outputs that are available for selection by the intracortical activities that it cannot itself evoke' (Phillips and Porter 1977, p. 37).

The maps of outputs would consist, ideally, of delineations of activities in the separate corticofugal projections from lamina V. This chapter will examine the principal techniques used to detect the effects of these outputs on motoneuronal excitability, muscle contraction and movement. The precise pattern of response detected in this way will be determined both by the structure of the cortical output itself, and by the interaction of this output with the spinal motor apparatus, which has already been discussed in Chapter 4. The early cartographers of the cortical motor representation were not really concerned with how this representation found expression through activation of the corticofugal system. The motor representation was considered to be a cerebral process without reference to the physical machinery needed to reveal it. As Phillips and Porter (1977, p. 36) state: 'matters became confused by failure to disentangle experiments on localisation from experiments on function, and *facts* of localisation from *concepts* of function'.

As well as an *output map*, there is also a map of inputs. Peripheral inputs reaching the precentral motor cortex do so in an organized fashion

(Chapter 6), and this *input map* is generally in register with the output map. We are only just beginning to understand the mapping of other, central inputs to the motor cortex derived from other brain structures. These multiple inputs ultimately select the cortical outputs needed to influence the complex patterns of muscular activity underlying voluntary movement. This operation could be represented as a *functional* map if a complete description of it could be provided. The identity and the topography of these maps is not clear, and indeed will not become clear until further studies of cortical connectivity and neuronal activity give us better insights into the defined operations carried out by the intracortical circuits of the motor cortex. In this light, it is not really surprising that the search for a simple, somatotopic map within the motor cortex, with an orderly representation of the body musculature, an undertaking which occupied the time and energy of so many experimental neuroscientists in the middle of this century, should have failed to come up with any very sophisticated ideas about the functional operations carried out within the motor cortex. There still remains a huge gap between the mapping of connections and the elucidation of functions.

8.2 METHODS FOR INVESTIGATING OUTPUT MAPS

Electrical stimulation of the motor cortex remains the most commonly used tool for investigating the output map. Providing that the effects of electrical stimuli upon the complex neuropil of the cortex are fully understood, this method can be useful. The importance of understanding the effects of the stimulus on the responses of the different elements which make up the cortical structure has been underscored recently by the introduction of non-invasive methods of stimulating the human cortex. However, it is not our purpose to review in detail the action of electrical stimuli upon the neuronal elements of the cortex, because this has been done elsewhere (Asanuma and Arnold 1975; Asanuma *et al.* 1976; Phillips and Porter 1977, pp. 77–90; Amassian *et al.* 1987; Lemon 1990).

For the cortical cartographer, an ideal electrical stimulus should directly excite a spatially circumscribed and identifiable population of output neurones in lamina V. Phillips and his colleagues have shown that the output cells of layer V are directly excited by anodal stimulation of the cortical surface with brief pulses (Hern *et al.* 1962; Phillips and Porter 1977). But this is only strictly true for PTNs whose long axis is orthogonal to the cortical surface, and stronger shocks are necessary to excite the many PTNs located in the cortex buried in the anterior bank of the central sulcus and possibly aligned tangentially to the convexity of the hemisphere. In the macaque, surface anodal stimulation is particularly well-suited for exciting the PTNs of the hindlimb representation, because these neurones lie mainly on the convexity of the gyrus rather than in the bank of the sulcus (Jankowska *et al.* 1975a).

Intracortical microstimulation (ICMS), introduced by Asanuma and Sakata in 1967, allows the output to be studied by delivering small stimulating cathodal currents through the tip of a metal microelectrode, the position of which within the motor cortex can be precisely controlled. Effective stimulating currents are typically 5–30 μA, an order of magnitude smaller than with surface anodal stimulation. ICMS can readily be employed in conscious animals, allowing the depressive effects of anaesthesia on motor responses to be avoided.

Although ICMS pulses delivered within lamina V may act directly on PTNs (Stoney *et al.* 1968), there is much evidence to suggest that the principal action of ICMS upon PTNs is indirect or trans-synaptic and this represents a major drawback of ICMS for mapping outputs (Jankowska *et al.* 1975a; Cheney and Fetz 1985; Lemon *et al.* 1987). Repetitive or tetanic ICMS (typically 10–15 pulses at 300 Hz) produces a marked recruitment of additional PTNs with each successive shock, in a manner similar to that originally described for trans-synaptic activation of PTNs by surface cathodal stimulation (Hern *et al.* 1962). Figure 8.1, from Jankowska *et al.* (1975a), illustrates records from the descending corticospinal tract of an anaesthetised monkey, showing that repetitive stimuli produce a continuous growth in the amplitude and duration of the output volleys (Jankowska *et al.* 1975a; Asanuma *et al.* 1976). In the former study, even single ICMS pulses discharged more than two-thirds of the sampled PTNs at latencies significantly longer than were compatible with direct activation. When applied to the superficial cortical layers, ICMS is capable only of eliciting indirect effects upon PTNs.

In conscious monkeys, it has been found that delivery of single ICMS pulses in the immediate vicinity of CM cells produces effects in the EMG that are 1 to 2 ms *longer* than the postspike facilitation (PSF) produced in the same muscles by the discharges of those cortico-motoneuronal cells (Cheney and Fetz 1985; Lemon *et al.* 1987; Bennett *et al.* 1989). This is illustrated in Fig. 8.2(a, b). It can be seen from Fig. 8.2(d) that for a sample of 34 PTNs, most ICMS evoked responses had longer latencies than PSF, and this was true for ICMS of 10 μA (34/43 averages) or for stronger 20 μA pulses (47/61 averages). It has been argued that this occurs because the PSF underestimates the conduction time from PTN to motor unit (Cheney and Fetz 1985), but this is unlikely since, for most clear PSF effects, this conduction time fits precisely with that predicted by direct stimulation of the pyramidal tract (Bennett *et al.* 1989; see Section 4.11 and Fig. 4.18).

An example of this phenomenon of indirect activation of CM neurones by ICMS is shown in Fig. 8.3, which shows the poststimulus time histogram for a single motor unit recorded from an intrinsic hand muscle of a con-

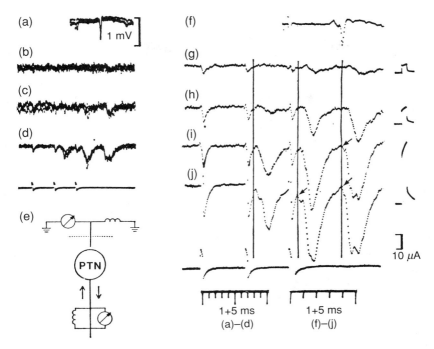

(a) 1 mV

(b)

(c)

(d)

(e) PTN

(f)

(g)

(h)

(i)

(j)

10 μA

1+5 ms
(a)–(d)

1+5 ms
(f)–(j)

FIG 8.1 Indirect activation of PTNs by repetitive intracortical stimulation of the motor cortex in the monkey. The latency of antidromic and orthodromic volleys from PTNs was compared as illustrated in (e). Superimposed traces to the left and the corresponding averaged records to the right. (a) and (f), antidromic potential from a PTN. (b)–(d) and (g)–(j), descending volleys evoked by increasing strengths of ICMS at the same microelectrode position as in (a) and (f), and recorded from a fascicle of the lateral funiculus dissected at the L1–2 spinal level. (j), intracortical stimulation with the same strength as for (d) and (i) but 300 μm deeper. The amplitudes of the stimuli are shown to the right and their timing on the lower traces in (d) and (j). Arrows in (i) and (j) indicate descending volleys with the same latencies as the latencies of the antidromic potentials; these descending volleys were very small, but were followed by much larger volleys at longer latency. These later volleys increased in amplitude with each successive stimulus in the train. Negativity downwards in all the records. (Reproduced with permission from Jankowska *et al.* (1975a).)

scious monkey. This unit responded with a narrow, brief peak at 10.9 ms to shocks applied to the medullary pyramid (Fig. 8.3(a)). When activity in the same motor unit was cross-correlated with spontaneously occurring spikes from an identified cortico-motoneuronal cell, a correlation peak, also with a short half-width, was observed (Fig. 8.3(b)). The latency of this peak was 11.9 ms, i.e. 1.0 ms longer than from the pyramid. This difference

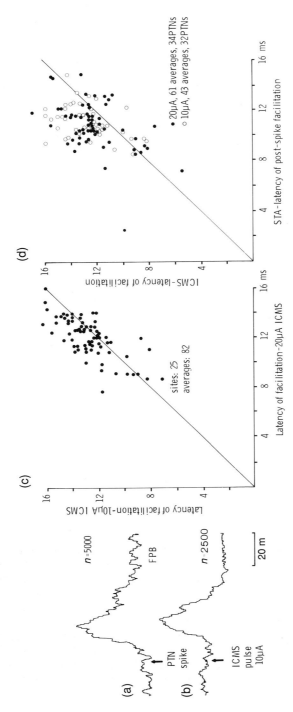

FIG 8.2 Differences in latency between postspike and poststimulus facilitation of monkey hand and forearm EMGs. The sample averages on the left show that the postspike facilitation of EMG from FPB by a PTN (a) had a shorter onset latency than the facilitation evoked by single ICMS pulses (b) delivered at the site of the PTN. (c): Onset latency of responses evoked by single-pulse ICMS. The latency obtained in a given muscle at 20 μA strength has been plotted against the latency of the response to 10 μA from the same site. Most responses showed a shorter latency with the stronger shock. (d): Onset latency of PSF produced by PTNs in a given muscle plotted against the latency of facilitation in the same muscle produced by ICMS at the site of the PTN. PSF latency was usually shorter. (Reproduced with permission from Lemon *et al.* (1987).)

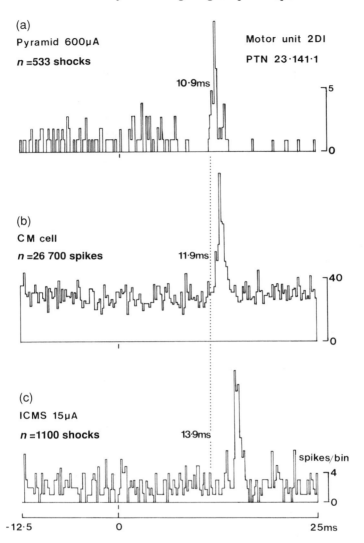

Fig 8.3 Responses of the same hand muscle motor unit to (a): stimulation of the pyramidal tract; (c): single ICMS pulses; and (b) to discharges of a single CM cell. Time zero indicates delivery of the stimulus pulses (a),(c) or discharge of the cell (b). The motor unit responded at 10.9 ms to pyramid stimulation, and at 11.9 ms in the cross-correlation with spikes from the CM cell. The difference between these latencies (1 ms) is attributable to the extra conduction delay from the CM cell to the pyramid (antidromic latency of this cell from the pyramid was 1.1 ms). Single ICMS pulses activated the motor unit at 13.9 ms, at 2 ms longer than expected if ICMS activated the CM cell directly. Motor unit from 2DI muscle; all data recorded during precision grip. Bin width 0.5 ms. (From Lemon and Werner, unpublished observations.)

is attributable to the extra conduction time from cortex to pyramid, and fits almost exactly with the latency of this cell when antidromically activated from the same pyramidal electrodes (1.1 ms). But when single ICMS was delivered through the tip of the cortical recording microelectrode, at the same location at which the cortico-motoneuronal cell was recorded (the discharges of the cell were still in the record at the end of the stimulation period), the motor unit responded at a latency of 13.9 ms (Fig. 8.3(c)), i.e. some 2.0 ms longer than that determined for the cortico-motoneuronal cell-motor unit conduction time. For 27 hand and forearm motor units tested in this manner, ICMS evoked responses which were, on average, 2.8 ms longer than those evoked from the pyramidal tract and 1.4 ms longer than those detected by cross-correlation with the CM cell recorded at the ICMS site (Werner and Lemon, unpublished). The best explanation of this result is that the cortico-motoneuronal cell was not excited directly but indirectly by the intracortical stimulus.

That the delay is cortical, rather than spinal, is further suggested by the observation that the EPSPs produced in spinal motoneurones by single ICMS pulses have significantly longer latencies than those produced by direct stimulation of the pyramidal tract (see Fig. 8.4(a)). The differences (1.5–3.0 ms) are once again longer than can be accounted for by the conduction delay from cortex to medullary pyramid. However, the *segmental* delays of the EPSPs were identical (Fig. 8.4(b)) (see also Jankowska *et al.* 1975b).

We must conclude that, on the basis of the evidence presented above, ICMS exerts its principal action through indirect, trans-synaptic excitation of corticospinal outputs. The cortical elements that are most readily excited by ICMS are probably the bundles of intracortical fibres afferent to the corticofugal neurones. Repetitive ICMS pulses will produce spatial and temporal facilitation in these presynaptic pathways to the PTNs. With repetitive ICMS shocks, the numbers of output elements recruited becomes much greater than with single shocks, and there can be no assurance that all of the neurones activated are located at the point stimulated; they may be found over wide areas of the cortex to which the afferent fibres are distributed. As has been alluded to earlier (Chapter 2), once activated to discharge an impulse, these output neurones are also able to project their influence to other neurones dispersed through the cortex and accessed via long intracortical axon collaterals (Jones 1984; Asanuma *et al.* 1974; Shinoda *et al.* 1985a, b; DeFelipe *et al.* 1986; Huntley and Jones 1991; see Fig. 8.6).

Thus the spatial characteristics of the map determined with repetitive ICMS will depend in part on the tangential spread of the trans-synaptic effects through the cortex. Because the majority of synaptic inputs to a given PTN are derived locally (see Section 2.1), it is unlikely that the physiological spread of stimulating current is extreme (Phillips 1981;

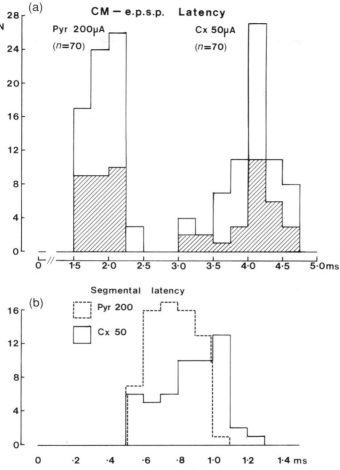

FIG 8.4 (a): Responses of 70 low cervical motoneurones in the monkey spinal cord to stimulation of the pyramidal tract (Pyr 200 μA) at a strength which was supramaximal for fast descending corticospinal volley. This stimulus evoked EPSPs in all motoneurones with latencies varying from 1.5 to 2.3 ms. These were judged to be monosynaptic EPSPs because of their short segmental latencies (shown in (b)), i.e. the delay between arrival of the descending volley and the EPSP onset. Single ICMS pulses (Cx 50 μA) also evoked monosynaptic EPSPs, but at longer latencies (3.0–4.7 ms). The difference in latency (1.5–2.4 ms) is significantly longer than can be explained by the extra conduction delay from cortex to pyramid (0.5–1.0 ms). Since the segmental delays of both ICMS and pyramid evoked EPSPs were the same (see (b)), the additional delay for ICMS-evoked EPSPs must have occurred at the cortical level. Data from 3 *m. fascicularis* monkeys under chloralose and barbiturate anaesthesia. Hatched columns, intrinsic hand muscle motoneurones; open columns, forearm muscle motoneurones. (From Fritz, Illert, Lemon, Muir, and Yamaguchi (unpublished observations).)

Asanuma 1981). The major point is that outputs elicited by ICMS may well reflect the excitation an *organized group of inputs* to PTNs, producing inhibition of some cortical elements and excitation of others so that a particular population of PTNs is recruited. Trans-synaptic activation of PTNs by such a mechanism may be expected to produce a highly organized motor response; and small movements of the electrode, by engaging a new set of inputs, may well produce entirely different movements and EMG responses (McGuinness *et al.* 1980; Sanes *et al.* 1990). The activation of organized input pathways to a specific group of PTNs with appropriately related connections may also explain why ICMS thresholds for movement are generally higher in the white matter than in the overlying grey.

In mapping experiments it is important to realize that trains of intra-cortical stimuli are essential to produce overt movements, and this is particularly true of sub-primates where no direct cortico-motoneuronal connections exist (Asanuma and Sakata 1967; Hore and Porter 1972; Donoghue and Wise 1982). While it is true that the production of movements in such species requires temporal facilitation of the oligosynaptic pathways linking the cortex to target motoneurones (Illert *et al.* 1976a,b; Armstrong and Drew 1985a), the accompanying effects of temporal facilitation at the cortical level should not be ignored.

In some of the chronic studies of macaque motor cortex, the intracortical mapping of the entire motor cortex has taken long periods of up to 18 months. Experiments made over such long periods have inherent problems, such as the thickening of the dura making estimation of precise electrode depth uncertain, and the final recognition and reconstruction of electrode tracks made over such a long period (Kwan *et al.* 1978). This is further complicated by the folding of the cortex, and unfolding procedures are required to produce a two-dimensional map. Such procedures must be extremely accurate, especially for penetrations traversing the radial architecture of the cortex within the anterior bank of the central sulcus. The problem of folding has been overcome by the use of squirrel *(Saimiri sciureus)* or owl *(Aotus trivirgatus)* monkeys, in which there is no central sulcus and where area 4 is found entirely on the cortical surface (Strick and Preston 1982a,b; Gould *et al.* 1986; Donoghue *et al.* 1992). These investigations were undertaken as acute studies in animals under ketamine sedation; ketamine elevates the response threshold to ICMS compared with that found in conscious animals.

8.3 DETECTING THE SIGNS OF CORTICAL OUTPUT

Much of the debate concerning the mapping of motor outputs has arisen because different investigators have chosen to study the output at different levels (Humphrey 1986; Lemon 1990). The means of detecting the output ranges in sensitivity from the production of postsynaptic potentials in single target motorneurones to overt movement. The interpretation of the map depends critically on understanding the essential differences in the chosen index of motor output. The 'false antithesis' of 'muscles versus movements' resulted largely from a failure to grasp the artificial nature of the cortical stimulus and the extent of its motor effects (Phillips 1975).

8.3.1 Movement

The truly 'motor' function of area 4 is reflected in those studies which have chosen the production of an overt movement as the index of cortical output (Leyton and Sherrington 1917; Chang *et al.* 1947; Woolsey *et al.* 1952). Such studies are particularly meaningful in conscious animals and humans where the level of excitability at both spinal and cortical levels is unaltered by the action of anaesthetic agents (Penfield and Rasmussen 1952; Kwan *et al.* 1978; Sessle and Wiesendanger 1982; Huang *et al.* 1989; Sato and Tanji 1989). In such preparations the evoked rather than the spontaneous origin of the responses must be firmly established, and labile, variable responses are difficult to interpret. Independent evidence for activation can be sought by EMG recording (see below). These studies emphasize what Hines (1944) called the 'predominant' pattern of representation, but clearly ignore any effects which are subliminal for detectable movement, including inhibitory influences.

8.3.2 Reflex modulation

A second, more sensitive approach is to study the effects of cortical stimulation on reflexes evoked by stimulation of peripheral nerves (Lloyd 1941; Preston *et al.* 1967; Asanuma and Sakata 1967; Hore and Porter 1972). This allows very precise mapping of both inhibitory and excitatory effects on the motoneurones of the muscles selected for study. But the outputs to other, untested muscles will go undetected. Unfortunately, this method cannot be used to map the disproportionately large representation of the small muscles of the hand, because monosynaptic reflexes are difficult to elicit in these muscles.

8.3.3 EMG activation

This represents another sensitive means of detecting cortical output, and has been used by many investigators (Asanuma and Rosén, 1972; Andersen *et al.* 1975; Cheney and Fetz 1985; Lemon *et al.* 1986, 1987). Spike-triggered averaging from cortico-motoneuronal cells avoids the problems of current spread referred to above, but large numbers of cells must be sampled before any map can be revealed. Monitoring the EMG emphasizes the 'muscle' rather than the 'motor' aspects of cortical output, and it is not always possible to infer the movements that would result from activation of such a 'muscle field'. This is particularly problematical for the complex movements of the hand and digits, and of the tongue, jaw, and lips (Abbs and Cole 1987).

8.3.4 Postsynaptic potentials

This is the most sensitive method of assaying the output, but has not yet been applied to conscious animals. It has been used to detect the synaptic potentials produced by the descending corticospinal pathways in their target motoneurones (Landgren *et al.* 1962a; Jankowska *et al.* 1975b; see Phillips and Porter 1977, pp. 144–51).

All of the above indices are subject to criticism, and strongly depend on whether one is seeking to demonstrate the predominant output of a cortical region (Hines 1944; Chang *et al.* 1947; Asanuma *et al.* 1976) or to investigate the full multiplicity of the region's output connectivities. All of the approaches requiring overt discharge of motoneurones are strongly influenced by the level of motoneuronal excitability (Liddell and Phillips 1950; Kwan *et al.* 1978), as has been demonstrated dramatically in human studies (Hess *et al.* 1987). The production of isolated movements, involving contraction of one or a few muscles, is undoubtedly associated with a subliminal fringe of activity, the extent of which remains unknown. The importance of inhibitory influences must not be overlooked; these effects are widespread in both anaesthetised and conscious animals (Lemon *et al.* 1987); in the latter they will go undetected if movements alone are monitored, or if there is no pre-existing EMG activity which will reveal motoneuronal suppression.

8.4 FEATURES OF THE MOTOR CORTEX OUTPUT MAP

In mapping studies of the primary motor cortex, it has been helpful to distinguish between the *areal* representation, by which is meant the regions whose outputs pass to the main subdivisions of the musculature: orofacial, head, eyes, arm, leg, and trunk; and the organization of outputs within each of these major areas: the *intra-areal representation* (Phillips and Porter 1977, p. 32). The general sequence of body parts represented in the areal map has been confirmed many times since the original study of Leyton and Sherrington (see Fig. 1.2, p. 8), and has become most familiar in the form of the homunculus and simusculus of Penfield and Rasmussen (1952) and of Woolsey *et al.* (1952), respectively. The areal map corresponds approximately with the somatotopic organization of the corticospinal projection to different segments of the spinal cord (Kuypers and

Brinkman 1970; Groos *et al.* 1978; Murray and Coulter 1981; Armand 1982; Sessle and Wiesendanger 1982; Huang *et al.* 1988). There is also a general correspondence between the regions of the primary motor cortex lesioned and the location of deficits in the various body parts (Denny-Brown 1966, pp. 131–35).

It is the fine detail of the *intra-areal maps* that has been the subject of the more recent studies, all of which have revealed that the representation of outputs has four related key features: *multiple representation, convergence, differential accessibility*, and *overlap*. We shall discuss these features in turn.

8.4.1 Multiple representation within the intra-areal map

The existence of multiple yet discrete efferent microzones is now accepted to represent an essential organizational principle of the motor cortex. It has been confirmed for all of the output indicators referred to above. Thus for *movements*, many different investigators have reported that a particular movement can be elicited from different and often discontinuous regions within a particular area (arm, leg, etc.) of the cortex, and this is particularly striking for movements of the digits (Penfield and Boldrey 1937; Craggs and Rushton, 1976; Kwan *et al.* 1978; Sessle and Wiesendanger 1982; Strick and Preston 1982a; Humphrey 1986; Sato and Tanji 1989; Donoghue *et al.* 1992; Huntley and Jones 1991). In the macaque, one of the most complete ICMS studies is that of Kwan *et al.* (1978; see Fig. 8.5). After plotting the location of 585 effective ICMS loci on an unfolded map, these authors described 'a nested organisation with the finger zone in the centre, successive enclosures by wrist and elbow zones and a shoulder zone at the perimeter'. It can be seen clearly from Fig. 8.5 that movements at each of these joints could be elicited from widely separated and often discontinuous zones. Tanji and Wise (1981) found multiple representation of hindlimb movements in the macaque, while McGuiness *et al.* (1980) and Huang *et al.* (1988) described similar results for orofacial movements; they noted many sites from which both contra- and ipsilateral face movements could be evoked. Gould *et al.* (1986) mapped the entire electrically excitable cortex of the sedated owl monkey, including primary motor cortex, SMA, and frontal eye fields. They found that the motor representation 'could not be regarded as strictly somatotopic, yet a somatotopic tendency was apparent in the mosaic of movement-related regions, since in some penetrations, movements of adjoining body parts were elicited from adjoining regions of cortex'. In one monkey, they found five separate representations of the digits and 11 of the wrist.

Huntley and Jones (1991) examined the movements produced by ICMS in the motor cortex of lightly-anaesthetised macaque monkeys and found that 'identical movements could be elicited from multiple, noncontiguous

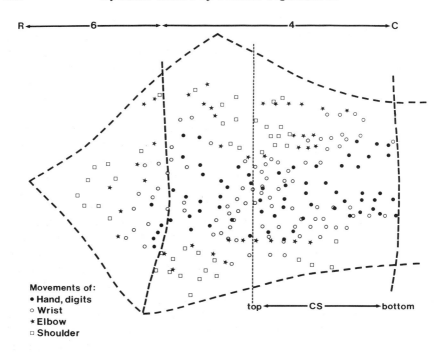

FIG 8.5 Multiple representation and overlap in the map for movements evoked by ICMS from the precentral gyrus of a conscious macaque monkey *(m. arctoides)*. The central sulcus has been unfolded in the rostrocaudal (R-C) direction. The bottom of the sulcus is shown at the far right and its top is indicated by the thin dotted line running mediolaterally. The part of area 4 lying on the convexity of the gyrus, and area 6, are shown to the left of this line. Forelimb movements evoked by repetitive ICMS ($>30 \mu$A) within microelectrode penetrations are plotted on the unfolded map. A region devoted to movement of the fingers is located in the anterior bank of the central sulcus. This region is surrounded by nested rings of tissue from which wrist, elbow, and shoulder movements could be elicited. Note the extensive overlap of regions influencing different segments of the arm and hand. (Redrawn from Fig. 2 of Kwan *et al.* (1978).)

sites'. They made iontophoretic injections of very small quantities of HRP or HRP–WGA at sites at which thumb movement was evoked. An example of their findings is illustrated in Fig. 8.6; the anterior bank of the central sulcus is shown as if projected onto the cortical surface. The injection revealed a profuse set of intrinsic, bidirectional projections that inter-connected digit (D) representations and also those of the wrist, elbow, and shoulder. The cell bodies of retrogradely-labelled neurones were found in patches remote from the injection site and in some cases cells up to 8 mm away were labelled. Anterogradely-labelled axons, 2–5 μm thick, were observed in large numbers streaming in radial fasciculi away from the injection. These axons were again found to terminate in a patchy manner over an extensive region. Multiple representation of movement has been reported also in the motor cortex of the cat (Pappas and Strick 1981a, b; Armstrong and Drew 1984c, 1985a) and of the rat (Donoghue and Wise 1982).

Multiple representation of *muscles* has been reported in both stimulation and STA studies. Thus Lemon (1990) reported that cortico-motoneuronal cells facilitating the same target muscle were distributed over a wide region of the macaque motor cortex. Figure 8.7 shows an 'unfolded' map of the central sulcus in the hand area of a *m. nemestrina* monkey in which a large number of penetrations were made over a four-month period. It plots the relative locations of penetrations (Fig. 8.7(a)) which produced clear postspike facilitation in three different intrinsic hand muscles. Figure 8.7(b) demonstrates the dorsoventral orientation within the bank of the central sulcus of the cortical territory (or 'aggregation of colonies') projecting to these muscles (cf. Andersen *et al.* 1975). The observed distributions occupy as much as 6.5 mm in the dorsoventral and 2 mm in the mediolateral direction. These estimates are probably conservative because of the sampling errors inherent in the STA technique and therefore probably represent only a fraction of the total cortical territory with cortico-motoneuronal projections to these muscles. Large cortical areas devoted to single intrinsic hand muscles were also reported by Sato and Tanji (1989) using ICMS and EMG recording in macaques.

Extensive cortical territories projecting to one muscle (the extensor carpi radialis, ECR) were found by Humphrey (1986) in an ICMS study in conscious monkeys. The area from which clear EMG responses could be evoked by repetitive ICMS in lamina V depended on the current strength (Fig. 8.8(a)). Even at 5 μA, two clear, discontinuous representations were distinguishable. When movements were examined in the same animals, wrist extension only occurred on stimulation within or immediately adjacent to these two low-threshold sites. The movements evoked from the much larger representation of ECR revealed by higher stimulus strengths were at other joints, in which the ECR played a stabilizing role (see Section 8.9 below). The ECR representation is very large; with a stimulus of 25 μA it encompasses an area 5 × 8 mm, which is 70 per cent of the precentral arm area (Humphrey 1986). In the sedated squirrel monkey, Donoghue *et al.* (1992) reported that individual forelimb muscles could be activated from areas varying in size from 2.5 to 20 mm^2, with a mean of 7.6 mm^2.

Multiple representation is even more striking when the extent of cortical tissue projecting to a single *motoneurone* is examined. Using weak surface anodal stimulation in deeply anaesthetised baboons, Landgren *et al.* (1962b) were able to show that the cortical colony projecting to a single cervical motoneurone could be as large as to cover 3-7 mm^2 of the

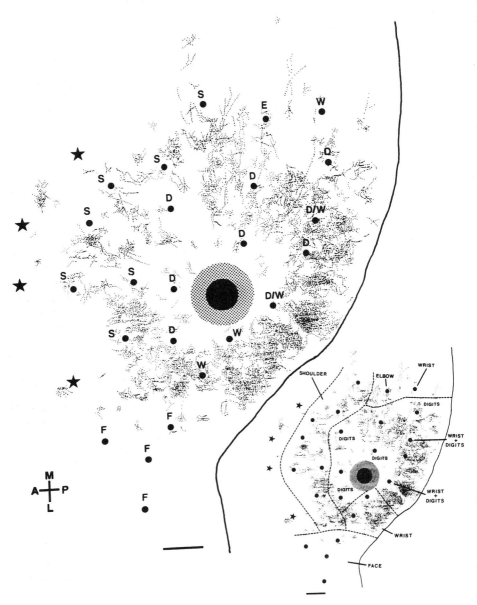

FIG 8.6 Combined electrophysiological and neuroanatomical investigation of the movement representation in the precentral gyrus of the anaesthetised macaque monkey. Surface view composite drawings made by stacking sections from flattened blocks, showing the position of electrode tracks (larger dots), the types of threshold ICMS evoked movements (letters), and the distribution of terminal fibre labelling ensuing from an injection of HRP into the centre of the digit representation (black

TABLE 8.1. Convergence of cortico-motoneuronal projections on forearm and hand motoneurones in the monkey*.

	Number tested	No. EPSP observed	Motoneurones with CM EPSPs from:		
			1 site	2 sites	3 sites
Forearm and hand	61	10	27	15	9
hand	18	1	7	6	4

*Single-pulse ICMS 20 μA pulses were applied at three different sites within the anterior bank of the central sulcus. Maximum separation of the sites was 4 mm on the cortical surface and 5 mm in the depth of the sulcal wall. Forearm: motoneurones innervating forearm muscles supplied by the median, ulnar, and deep radial nerves. Hand: motoneurones innervating intrinsic hand muscles (adapted from Lemon 1990).

cortical surface, although most were considerably smaller. Jankowska *et al.* (1975b) used near-threshold surface anodal stimuli to evoke cortico-motoneuronal EPSPs in hindlimb motoneurones of the anaesthetised macaque. Cortico-motoneuronal EPSPs could be evoked from regions 3–7 mm^2 in area; and regions projecting to motoneurones of the same muscle were not identical, and often did not overlap at all. These authors went on to show that a similar representation was revealed by weak ICMS. Fritz *et al.* (1985) recorded intracellularly from macaque cervical motoneurones and compared the cortico-motoneuronal EPSPs elicited by ICMS delivered through electrodes fixed at three sites within the hand region of area 4. Table 8.1 shows that although these stimulus sites were separated by as much as 2–4 mm on the cortical surface, and by up to 5 mm in depth within the bank of the central sulcus, cortico-motoneuronal EPSPs could be evoked in 9/61 tested cervical motoneurones (C7-T1 segments) from all three sites by single ICMS pulses at 20 μA. Four out of 18 hand motoneurones could be excited from all three sites.

8.4.2 Convergence

The multiple representation of outputs to a particular muscle or motoneurone implies a convergent input, as illustrated in Fig. 8.9, from Andersen *et al.* (1975). The convergent cortico-motoneuronal input to muscles and

and stippled circle). In this type of reconstruction, labelling in the anterior bank of the central sulcus appears as though projected on to a surface view. Terminal fibre labelling (stipple) shows distinct patchy distribution. Inset shows a figure overlain by a semischematic indication of the threshold movement zones. Monkey anaesthetised with a mixture of ketamine and barbiturate. Bars, 1 mm. (Reproduced with permission from Huntley and Jones (1991).)

Overlapping cortico−motoneuronal projections

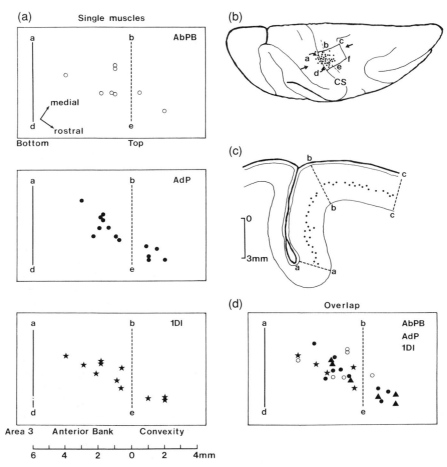

FIG 8.7 Multiple representation and overlapping representation of muscles in the motor cortex of the macaque monkey (*m. nemestrina*). Distribution of CM neurones producing PSF in the EMGs of three intrinsic hand muscles: AbPB (abductor pollicis brevis), AdP (adductor pollicis), and 1DI (first dorsal interosseous). Their location is plotted on an unfolded map of the precentral gyrus. This unfolding is illustrated in (b) and (c). (b): The area investigated is indicated by the rectangle *abcdef*. (c): Sagittal section taken between the straight arrows in (b). The gyrus was unfolded along lamina V, marked by the presence of Betz cells (dots in (c)). In the unfolded map, lines a–d and b–e represent the bottom and top of the sulcus, respectively. The location of neurones encountered in penetrations in the bank of the sulcus was calculated by measuring their position relative to the unfolded lamina V. (d): Overlap between CM cells projecting to the three muscles. Lines linking symbols indicate different muscles facilitated by the same CM cell. (Adapted from Lemon (1990).)

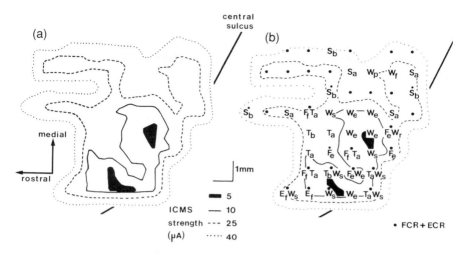

FIG 8.8   Comparison of the precentral representation of the extensor carpi radialis (ECR) muscle with the movements evoked from the same sites within cortical lamina V of the macaque monkey (*m. mulatta*). In each map, the heavy, oblique line represents the central sulcus; anterior is to the left, medial toward the top. Parts of the map overlapping the central sulcus indicate buried areas in its anterior bank. (a): Projection of the lamina V, ECR map on to the cortical surface, in the form of current threshold contours. The dark areas enclose all points from which activity was evoked in the ECR muscle with currents of less than 5 μA. Similarly, the solid lines enclose all regions with thresholds less than 10 μA, and so on. The map does not change in shape with intensities greater than 25 μA, which indicates that the 40 μA map is broadened only by current spread. (b): Projection of the movements observed from the same sites in lamina V on to the ECR contour map. Note that wrist extension (W_e) occurs only on stimulation within or immediately adjacent to the two low-threshold sites. At all other locations, the ECR muscle is activated as one of a set of stabilizing muscles, during another primary movement. Movement code: E_f, elbow flexion; F_e, finger extension; F_f, finger flexion; T_a, thumb adduction; S_a, S_b, shoulder adduction or abduction; W_e, wrist extension; W_f, wrist flexion; W_p, wrist or forearm pronation; W_s, wrist or forearm supination. Two symbols indicate a more complex movement. The filled circles (•) show all locations from which coactivation of ECR and FCR muscles was obtained. (Reproduced with permission from Humphrey (1986).)

motoneurones has been dealt with in Chapter 4 (Section 4.14); here we shall address only the cortical mapping of this convergent projection.

Variation in the threshold for exciting a given motor unit was taken by Andersen *et al.* (1975) to indicate variation in the 'texture' of the colony, and was used as evidence for a differential distribution of the PTNs projecting to the motoneurone (see Fig. 8.9). This is in keeping with the

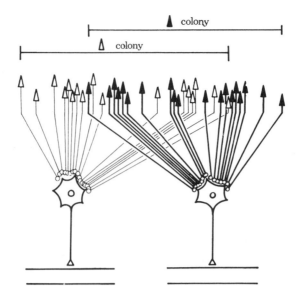

FIG 8.9 Diagram summarizing the structure of the monosynaptic CM projection to the baboon's hand. The colonies of cells projecting to two motoneurones of a single muscle are shown. This diagram emphasizes the overlap between colonies and the variation in the distribution density of the CM cells belonging to each colony; the authors used the term 'aggregations of colonies' to describe the CM input to a whole muscle. (Reproduced with permission from Andersen *et al.* (1975).)

clustering of PTNs observed in retrograde labelling studies (Jones and Wise 1977; Murray and Coulter 1981; Sessle and Wiesendanger 1982; see Fig. 2.14) and by the observations of Asanuma and Rosén (1972), who demonstrated the existence of low-threshold ICMS 'hot spots' within the monkey motor cortex.

Cheney and Fetz (1985) and Lemon *et al.* (1987) found that most of the stimulus-evoked EMG effects were much larger than those seen in spike-triggered averages from cortico-motoneuronal cells recorded at the same cortical locus (compare Fig. 8.10(a),(b)), probably because ICMS at a single locus is likely to excite several cortico-motoneuronal cells that all project to the same muscle. But there is a striking *variation* in amplitude of poststimulus effects from different sites, again suggesting an uneven excitation of output elements by the ICMS delivered to different parts of the total representation. The variation in poststimulus excitation of EMG activity in two thenar muscles (abductor pollicis brevis: AbPB, and flexor pollicis brevis: FPB) from different cortical sites is illustrated in Fig. 8.10(c); this variation occurred despite the fact that a cortico-

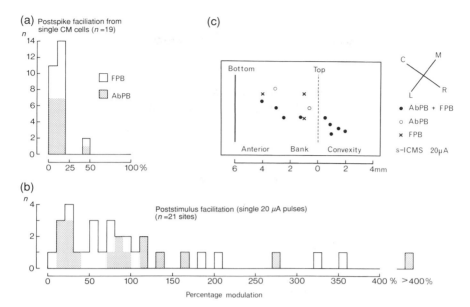

FIG 8.10 Comparison of the facilitatory effects of single cells and of ICMS in the monkey motor cortex. (a): Percentage modulation of PSF effects in two thenar muscles (AbPB and FPB) produced by 19 different CM cells. Most cells produced facilitation ranging from 8 to 20 per cent of background EMG. (b): Amplitude of poststimulus facilitation of these same muscles produced by single 20 μA ICMS pulses. Most of these effects were obtained from sites at which the cells indicated in (a) were recorded. Note the large range in the amplitude of these effects. (c): Distribution of effective ICMS points on an unfolded map of the precentral gyrus (see Fig. 8.7 for details of unfolding). (Reproduced with permission from Lemon (1990).)

motoneuronal cell projecting to either one or both of these muscles was present at almost every site tested. These cells produced PSF ranging in amplitude from 5 to 42 per cent in AbPB and FPB (Fig. 8.10(a)). In contrast, poststimulus facilitation ranged from 10 to 510 per cent of background EMG with 20μA shocks (Fig. 8.10B), and from 8 to 162 per cent with 10 μA shocks. Given the probability that ICMS may excite intra-cortical systems afferent to the output PTNs, these results may reflect the 'patchiness' of thalamocortical and cortico-cortical inputs (see Section 2.1).

Strong surface anodal stimulation can excite an entire cortico-motoneuronal colony (Phillips and Porter 1964), while ICMS usually only excites a relatively small proportion of it (Andersen *et al.* 1975). Fritz *et al.* (1985) compared the cortico-motoneuronal EPSP evoked by single-pulse ICMS with the *total* cortico-motoneuronal input, estimated by recording the monosynaptic EPSP produced by a maximal shock to the medullary pyramid. For 26 hand motoneurones, the proportion of the maximal pyramidal EPSP evoked by ICMS was 26 ± 15 per cent (range 10–63 per cent) at $50 \, \mu A$ and 9 ± 5 per cent (2–20 per cent) at $20 \, \mu A$.

There is also convergent inhibition of target motoneurones. Jankowska *et al.* (1976) showed that the areas from which disynaptic inhibition could be evoked in hindlimb motoneurones by surface anodal stimulation were also large and discontinuous. The inhibitory area partially overlapped areas from which the same motoneurone could be excited.

8.4.3 Differential outputs to different muscles

The 'differential accessibility' of the musculature of the hands, feet, tongue, and face was established in the studies of Sherrington, Woolsey, and Penfield. This can be attributed partly to the greater amplitude of the EPSPs produced by individual corticospinal cells in the motoneurones innervating these distal muscle groups (see Section 4.13), and partly to the fact that the colonies of cortico-motoneuronal cells are more numerous and extensive than for the motoneurones of the proximal limbs and trunk (Jankowska *et al.* 1975b; Phillips and Porter 1977 pp. 154–72). A third possibility, namely that there are differences in the susceptibility to electrical stimulation of the corticospinal projections to these different regions, has not yet been investigated, although this is becoming an important issue in terms of our understanding of the effects of non-invasive stimuli upon the human cortex.

In most studies in man and in macaque monkeys, the responses obtained with the lowest thresholds have been in the facial muscles or in the intrinsic muscles of the hand, and sites within the anterior bank of the sulcus have the lowest threshold for hand and finger movements (Kwan *et al.* 1978; Lemon *et al.* 1986; Huntley and Jones 1991). Although Sessle and Wiesendanger (1982) emphasized that movements of the proximal arm could be evoked with ICMS below $10 \, \mu A$, the distribution of thresholds shown in Fig. 8.11 could be taken to reflect the relative strength and numbers of cortico-motoneuronal projections to different muscles as discussed in Chapter 4. Indeed, section of the pyramidal tract generally raises the threshold of ICMS required to elicit movement (see Section 8.5 below). But this is not evidence in itself that the movements of distal muscles evoked by low-threshold, repetitive ICMS are due to monosynaptic corticospinal projections. Low-threshold effects have been observed in the conscious cat (Armstrong and Drew 1985a, b) and rat (Sapienza *et al.* 1981), in which the cortico-motoneuronal projection is sparse or absent (see Section 2.9). Since the effects of repetitive ICMS seem to require substantial temporal facilitation at both cortical and spinal levels (see above), it is likely that the ICMS threshold reflects this rather than the presence or absence

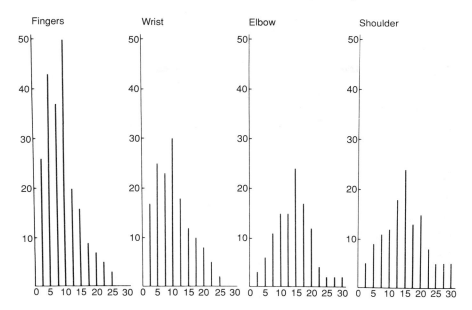

FIG 8.11 Distributions of threshold currents required to evoke forelimb movements at loci within the precentral gyrus of the macaque monkey (*m. arctoides*). The number of loci is plotted on the ordinate. The threshold currents for movements of the fingers, wrist, elbow, and shoulder are plotted separately. (Reproduced with permission from Kwan *et al.* (1978).)

of cortico-motoneuronal connections. The significance of the presumptive cortico-motoneuronal connections is more clearly seen when STA or single pulse ICMS is employed (Lemon *et al.* 1987).

8.4.4 Overlapping outputs

The extensive colonies for individual motoneurones, and the 'aggregations of colonies' projecting to different muscles, make it impossible to 'fit' the cortical representation of the entire musculature into the limits of area 4 without considerable overlap. In fact, some degree of overlap in the cortical representation of movements, muscles and motoneurones has been a feature of most of the mapping studies referred to above. In the classic study of Chang *et al.* (1947), surface stimulation of the monkey cortex sometimes produced 'solitary' contraction of individual muscles, although these authors commented that 'solitary responses are by no means the typical response to cortical stimulation'. A more common observation was that such stimulation (60 Hz a.c.) tended to produce contractions of different strengths in a variety of muscles. The ICMS study of Kwan *et al.*

(1978) revealed some segregation of zones from which shoulder, elbow, wrist, and, particularly, finger movements could be evoked, but as Fig. 8.5 demonstrates, the movement map of primary motor cortex produced by Kwan *et al.* (1978) is as conspicuous for its overlap as for the 'nested' arrangement suggested in the description provided by the authors. The overlapping regions of the orofacial representation are shown in Fig. 8.12 from Huang *et al.* (1988), who investigated 969 different microelectrode penetrations in 10 unanaesthetised macaques. An almost complete overlap of regions for movements of the face, jaw, and tongue was found, and ICMS in 53 per cent of all penetrations produced 'mixed' movement responses of these structures. The posteromedial border of this orofacial region overlapped with that for finger movements, and both categories of movement were found within the same penetration on many occasions. The lateral border was unresponsive to ICMS below 30 μA, and corresponded to a border region beyond which there were no large pyramidal cells in lamina V. The situation may be different in the baboon, where there appears to be an inexcitable zone of cortex between the hand and face representations (Samulack *et al.* 1990). Huntley and Jones (1991) found that the profuse connections linking different parts of the arm and hand area of the macaque cortex did not traverse the arm/face border to any significant extent.

All of the studies which have investigated cortico-motoneuronal projections to *motoneurones* have reported overlap. Jankowska *et al.* (1975b) showed that the overlap in the macaque hindlimb cortex for motoneurones of the same muscle was sometimes as great as for motoneurones innervating different muscles. Andersen *et al.* (1975) found almost complete overlap between the areas occupied by the colonies supplying single motor units in intrinsic hand and long forearm muscles of the baboon. Overlap of the cortico-motoneuronal projections to different hand *muscles* shown in Fig. 8.7 is indicated by superimposition of the plots for the three different muscles (see Figure 8.7(d)).

Part of the overlap observed in STA studies could result from the divergent output from single corticospinal neurones (see Section 4.12). A further cause of overlap is the presence in a cell cluster of cortico-motoneuronal neurones with different muscle fields. In most cases, neighbouring cortico-motoneuronal cells have common output targets (Asanuma *et al.* 1979; Cheney and Fetz 1985; Cheney *et al.* 1985) and for this reason these muscles will receive a strong convergent facilitation from ICMS delivered within the cluster. However, for cell clusters projecting to the hand it is not uncommon to find adjacent cells which facilitate different muscles. Each neurone has its own characteristic muscle field. Some muscles are common targets for each member of a cell cluster, and these muscles receive the *predominant* output of the cluster, as revealed by single pulse ICMS (Lemon *et al.* 1987).

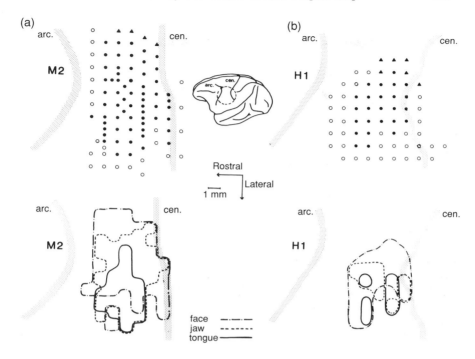

FIG 8.12 Pattern of face, jaw, and tongue representation in primary motor cortex of 2 macaque monkeys (*m. fascicularis*). Top half of (a) and (b) is schematic drawing of cortical region explored by ICMS in monkeys M2 and H1; dotted circle in inset diagram shows approximate location of area explored. Sites marked with symbols indicate point of entry of ICMS electrode penetrations. ○, no ICMS response detected; ●, face, jaw or tongue movements; ▲, forelimb or trunk movements. Lower half of (a) and (b) depicts the same cortical area as shown in corresponding top half with contour lines enclosing penetrations in which movements of face, jaw and tongue were obtained by ICMS. arc , arcuate sulcus; cen , central sulcus. (Reproduced with permission from Huang *et al.* (1988).)

In the example shown in Fig. 8.13, two PTNs recorded by the same microelectrode showed a clear cross-correlation of their spontaneous activity (Fig. 8.13(a)). Despite this synaptic linkage, PTN 1 facilitated all four muscles shown, while PTN 2 produced PSF in only two of them (Fig. 8.13(b)). ICMS at this site produced large effects in the 'common' muscles, adductor pollicis (AdP) and abductor digiti minimi (AbDM), and weaker effects in the other muscles (Lemon 1990). The heterogeneous nature of cell clusters in the hand area is revealed by the fact that while single cortico-motoneuronal neurones often facilitated only one or two

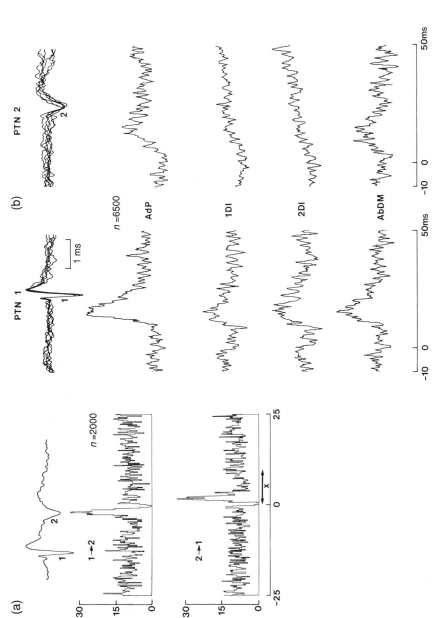

FIG 8.13 Heterogeneous outputs of neighbouring CM cells in monkey motor cortex. (a): Two PTNs recorded via the same electrode showed a clear cross-correlation in their activities. (b): their output effects differed, however: PTN 1 produced PSF in the STAs of all four hand muscles illustrated, while PTN 2 facilitated only two of them (AdP and AbDM). 6500 spike events used to compile STAs in each case. (Reproduced with permission from Lemon (1990).)

muscles, ICMS at the site of these neurones usually facilitated additional muscles, as shown in Fig. 8.14 (Lemon 1988). The 'muscle field' of the cortico-motoneuronal cell illustrated in Fig. 8.14(a) consisted of three intrinsic thumb muscles, but single ICMS (10 μA) at the site of this cell recruited two additional hand muscles (1DI and AbDM; Fig. 8.14(d)), while repetitive ICMS (7μA) facilitated EMG from six muscles and suppressed the forearm flexor, FCU (Fig. 8.14(e)). The results from this type of experiment for 10 loci at which cortico-motoneuronal cells were recorded are shown in Fig. 8.15. Additional muscles were almost always recruited by ICMS even with weak, single ICMS (< 10μA); but this phenomenon was most striking with repetitive or tetanic ICMS below 10μA.

Multiple representation and overlap of outputs in feline motor cortex has also been reported in studies using chronically implanted electrodes in conscious cats (Nieoullon and Rispal-Padel 1976; Armstrong and Drew 1984c).

8.5 PYRAMIDAL AND PARAPYRAMIDAL OUTPUT MAPS

The contribution of the corticofugal pathways to the form of the output map has been looked at in experiments mapping the effects of cortical stimulation before and after section of the pyramidal tract. These studies have shown that the cortical representation of outputs revealed by low-threshold stimuli is to a large extent dependent on the integrity of the pyramidal tract, a finding which, in the primate at least, reflects the co-extensive distribution of the electrically excitable cortex with large corticospinal or corticobulbar neurones (Sessle and Wiesendanger 1982; Weinrich and Wise 1982; Huang *et al.* 1988). It has been demonstrated in both the cat and the monkey that chronic section of the pyramidal tract abolishes the short-latency EMG responses evoked by low-threshold ICMS within the primary motor cortex (Felix and Wiesendanger 1971; Asanuma *et al.* 1981; Armstrong and Drew 1984c, 1985a). Lewis and Brindley (1965) also found that the threshold for evoking movements by surface faradic stimulation (100 Hz a.c.) of the baboon cortex was raised following acute section of the pyramids.

The topography of the output map is changed by pyramidotomy. Lewis and Brindley (1965) reported a profound decrease in the number of different movements that could be elicited; some ipsilateral movements were found. Mitz and Humphrey (1986), examined in detail the movements evoked by ICMS in the precentral gyrus of two Rhesus monkeys before and 6 weeks after unilateral pyramidotomy. In one animal with an almost complete destruction of the left pyramid, it proved almost impossible to find any low threshold sites from which arm or hand movements could be elicited (only 6 sites produced movement with ICMS trains of less than

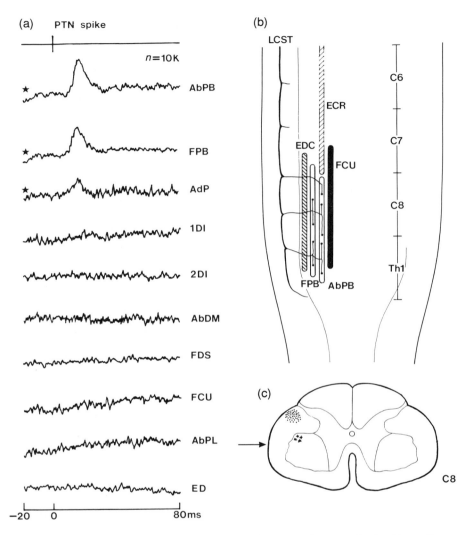

FIG 8.14   (a): distribution of postspike facilitation from a single CM cell to muscles of the hand and forearm in the monkey. Spike-triggered averages of EMG recorded concurrently from ten muscles and averaged with respect to 10 000 spikes from a pyramidal-tract neurone (PTN), which discharged at time zero. All data were recorded while the monkey performed a precision-grip task between thumb and index finger. Asterisks indicate averages with postspike facilitation: AbPB, FPB, and AdP. (b): Schematic horizontal section, at the level indicated by the arrow in (c), through the lower cervical cord showing a relatively restricted output from the axon of a single CM cell running in the lateral corticospinal tract (LCST), and with collaterals contacting motoneurone cell columns innervating two thumb muscles (FPB and AbPB), but not EDC, ECR, or FCU. (d): Poststimulus averages of EMG

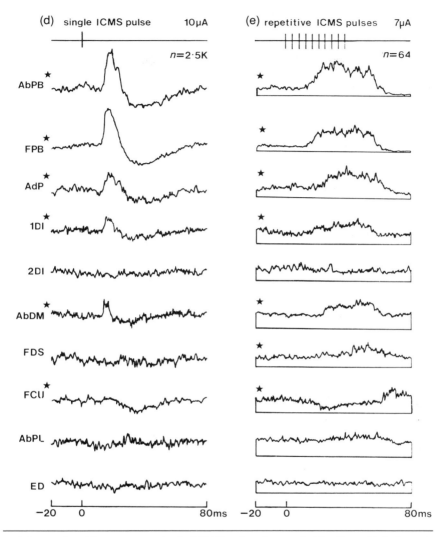

activity made with respect to single ICMS pulses (strength 10 μA) applied through
the microelectrode at the site at which the pyramidal-tract neurone in (a) was
recorded. Facilitation followed by suppression occurred in five muscles (AbPB,
FPB, AdP, 1DI, and AbDM), while FCU showed only suppression. (e): responses
to repetitive ICMS stimuli (ten shocks at 300 Hz, strength 7 μA) at the same site.
Seven muscles showed responses. Abbreviations (intrinsic hand muscles): AbPB and
FPB, abductor and flexor pollicis brevis; AdP, adductor pollicis; 1DI and 2DI, first
and second dorsal interosseous; AbDM, abductor digiti minimi; forearm muscles:
FDS, flexor digitorum superficialis; FCU, flexor carpi ulnaris; AbPL, abductor
pollicis longus; ED, extensor digitorum communis. (Reproduced with permission
from Lemon (1988).)

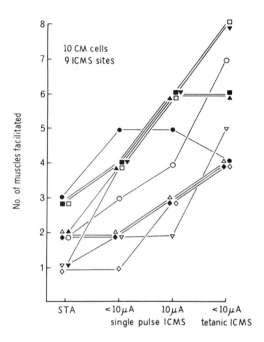

FIG 8.15   The number of muscles facilitated by 10 different CM cells (each represented by a different symbol), is plotted on the extreme left. The number of muscles facilitated by single ICMS shocks of 4–8 μA applied to the sites of these CM cells has been plotted in the second column ($< 10\ \mu$A). The number facilitated by 10 μA single shocks (third column) and by repetitive shocks of < 10 A (extreme right) are also shown. Note the recruitment of additional muscles by ICMS of increasing strength. (Reproduced with permission from Lemon *et al.* (1987).)

60 μA). Much stronger ICMS, using electrodes with large tips, did produce movements, although these required a greater amount of both spatial and temporal summation. But the topography of the parapyramidal or 'extrapyramidal' map so revealed was similar to that before section. These authors reported an expansion in the cortical area from which forearm pronation/supination movements could be elicited (cf. Woolsey *et al.* 1952). In the cat, evoked movements were largely restricted to the more proximal musculature (Asanuma *et al.* 1981).

As was discussed in Phillips and Porter (1977; p. 48), Woolsey *et al.* (1972) studied the movement responses produced by stimulation of the motor cortex of the macaque monkey more than a year after complete section of the pyramidal tract on one side. Not only were the thresholds for motor responses elevated on the operated side, but the responses obtained from stimulation of this cortex never involved the distal joints of the forelimb and hindlimb. Hence the points on the cortex of the normal side from which movements about these distal joints were most readily obtained were represented on the operated side by points from which movements about proximal joints were now obtained with stronger stimuli, as though the representations of these proximal movements had expanded. Although Lewis and Brindley (1965) styled the effects they could obtain from the cortex after pyramidal tract section as describing the map of 'extrapyramidal' outputs from the cerebral cortex, it is preferable to recognize that a number of different populations of cortical efferent neurones could be activated by these stimuli and contribute to the motor responses obtained. Indeed the so-called 'extrapyramidal' projections, issuing from widespread regions of the cortex and projecting to the pontine nuclei and striatum, may make only a limited contribution to, or have no effect at all on, such motor responses because their normal connections involve them in re-entrant activation of PTNs. More important may be the parapyramidal neurones (Phillips and Porter 1977, p. 107) which are located within the motor cortex but whose axons or collaterals leave the internal capsule, cerebral peduncle, or pontine pyramidal bundles without ever reaching the medullary pyramid, where they could be sectioned (see Sections 2.5, 2.6). These projections could activate brainstem nuclei and exert indirect influences on spinal motor centres as indicated in Fig. 1.12 (p. 26).

8.6 INPUT MAPS WITHIN THE MOTOR CORTEX

The afferent input from receptors in the periphery to different regions of the sensory cortex is now recognized as an important factor in determining the shape of the map. Unlike neurones found in the sensory areas, motor cortex neurones do not respond very well to sensory stimuli in the anaesthetised state, and the full wealth of the somatosensory input to area 4 can really be appreciated only in the conscious animal, where a large proportion of neurones is found to be responsive to such stimuli (see Chapter 6). Here we consider those aspects of the sensory map which reinforce the features of the output map discussed above.

8.6.1 Input–output relations at the single neurone level

There is good evidence that most motor cortex neurones receive their afferent input from a restricted peripheral zone, and that this zone is generally smallest for units with inputs from more distal regions. It is also well-established that, for many neurones, there is a close relationship between the afferent input zone and the motor output function deduced from their natural discharge in association with movement performance (see Phillips and Porter 1977, pp. 237–264). This important principle was first demonstrated by showing that ICMS in the vicinity of neurones responding to passive stimulation of a particular region of the cat's forelimb usually activated muscles and produced joint movement in the same forelimb region (Asanuma *et al.* 1968; Sakata and Miyamoto 1968). The principle has been shown to apply to single neurones whose natural discharge was associated with movement of a particular joint and which received inputs from passive rotation of that joint (Lemon *et al.* 1976). It has also been demonstrated that cortical neurones whose activity was strongly modulated only during naturally performed independent finger movements had small receptive fields on the hand, many of them from localized regions of the glabrous skin (Lemon 1981a). Cheney and Fetz (1984) went further and demonstrated that about half of the cortico-motoneuronal cells facilitating wrist flexor or extensor muscles during active, voluntary movement responded to passive stretch of these same muscles when this was imposed by a torque motor attached to the manipulandum. Lemon (1992) found that all CM neurones that produced PSF in an intrinsic thumb muscle responded either to tactile stimulation of the thumb or to passive movement of that digit.

8.6.2 Multiple representation and overlap

Thus both single unit recording and microstimulation suggest a good correlation between sensory input and motor output territories at the level of the single cortical neurone. This implies that the input map should exhibit many features of the output map described above, and this is indeed the case. Neurones responding to stimulation of the same body part are found in quite separate cortical zones, often with discontinuities between the different zones. The extensive mapping of inputs by Wong *et al.* (1978), showed a 'nested' arrangement of inputs that closely matched that described for ICMS-evoked movements (see Fig. 8.5). But, as with the motor map, one is as struck by the overlap as by the segregation of afferent inputs. This point is again demonstrated by re-plotting the original data of Wong *et al.* (1978) on to a single map, shown in Fig. 8.16.

Strick and Preston (1982a, b) reported that, in the squirrel monkey, there were two representations of the hand that could be identified by ICMS. These authors found a segregation of peripheral input to these two representations, with neurones in a rostral region responding almost exclusively to 'deep' inputs (joint manipulation and muscle palpation), while neurones in a more caudal region responded chiefly to cutaneous inputs. In the macaque monkey, there is evidence for differences in both the thalamic projections and functional organization of the rostral (convexity) and caudal (sulcal) hand representations (see Section 6.5). A separation of deep and

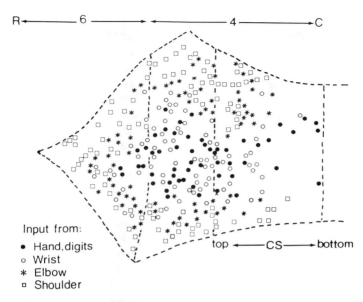

FIG 8.16 Multiple representation and overlap of somatosensory inputs to the motor cortex of the macaque monkey (*m. arctoides*). The location of neurones responding either to cutaneous stimuli or to passive joint movement have been plotted on an unfolded map of the precentral gyrus, with the bottom of the central sulcus (CS) lying to the right (see Fig. 8.5 for details). Neurones responsive to inputs from the hand are located in a central core region occupying the bank of the sulcus and the most caudal part of the convexity of the gyrus. These neurones are surrounded by nested rings of neurones responding to wrist, elbow, and shoulder. Note the multiple representation of these inputs. The separation between the nested rings is certainly not complete, and there is considerable overlap of input. Compare with output map from the same study shown in Fig. 8.5. (Redrawn from Figs. 4 and 6 of Wong *et al.* (1978).)

cutaneous submodalities into respectively rostral and caudal areas was reported by Tanji and Wise (1981) for the hindlimb region of the macaque cortex. Their results are shown in Fig. 8.17. Evidence for a dual input/output motor representation of the forelimb in the cat motor cortex has also been reported by Pappas and Strick (1981a), Yumiya and Ghez (1984) and Armstrong and Drew (1985a).

Several authors have found evidence for overlap in the afferent projections to neighbouring neurones: neurones recorded within a few 100 μm of each other in the same electrode penetration sometimes received inputs from different parts of the limb (Lemon and Porter 1976a; Wong *et al.* 1978; Lemon 1981b). Although it could be argued that some of these pairs

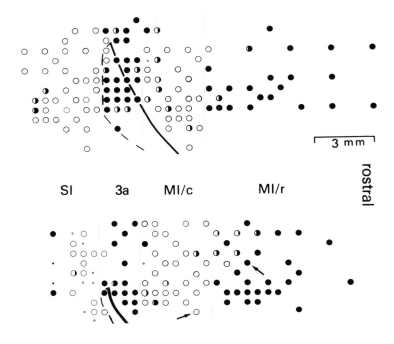

Fɪɢ 8.17 Submodality segregation in the leg representation of the sensorimotor cortex in the conscious macaque monkey (*m. fascicularis*). Data from 2 monkeys shown. Dotted lines separate the physiologically defined cortical regions. Filled circles indicate penetrations where non-cutaneous units were found; open circles show the location of cutaneous units. Partially filled or partially open circles indicate penetrations with a non-cutaneous unit-to-cutaneous unit ratio of 2:1 (filled) or 1:2 (open). Half-filled circles show where classes are more evenly mixed. (Reproduced with permission from Tanji and Wise (1981).)

of neurones may have been situated in adjacent cortical columns, with different properties and connections, which were traversed by the electrode track, it is also likely that the proximity of such neurones did allow them to interact strongly through the close association of their intertwined processes. Lemon (1981b) studied the properties of 135 'cell groups': groups of neurones, 2 to 9 in number and recorded within 500 μm of each other. Two thirds of the groups had afferent input from the same zone of the monkey's arm or hand, and showed very similar activity during a complex task involving all upper limb muscles (see Fig. 8.18). But a significant proportion (35 per cent) of the cell groups contained neurones receiving input from more than one arm zone, which could be contiguous, such as elbow and shoulder (22 per cent of groups) or discontinuous, such as shoulder and hand (13 per cent). Individual neurones in these groups

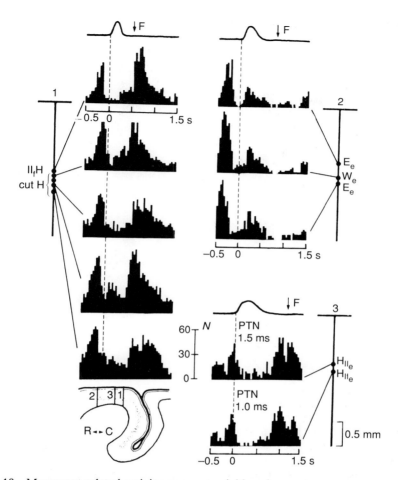

FIG 8.18 Movement-related activity amongst neighbouring motor cortex neurones in the macaque monkey. Peri-response histograms show activity during a trained task which required the monkey to first pull a spring-loaded lever and then collect a food reward from a small food well. Onset of lever movement is at time zero and mean lever displacement is indicated above the histograms. Contact of the monkey's hand with the food rewards is indicated by the arrow F. Three groups of cells were encountered within three penetrations (1–3). Their source of sensory input and activity during the task was very similar. The location and receptive fields of the neurones are indicated. In the first group, all of the 5 cells responded to natural stimulation of the hand (H): one to flexion of the index finger (II_f), and the rest to cutaneous (cut) stimuli. In the second group, the cells responded to elbow or to wrist extension (E_e, W_e). In the third group, both cells were identified PTNs whose antidromic latencies are shown; they both responded to index extension (II_e). Histograms represent cumulative activity of each neurone for sixteen successive lever pulls for a period of 0.5 s before and 1.5 s after beginning of lever movement. Histogram binwidth 40 ms. Scale shows number (N) of spikes/bin. The three groups shown were recorded in three different monkeys. (Reproduced with permission from Lemon (1981b).)

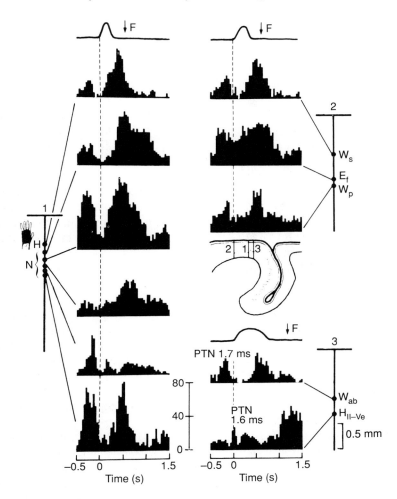

FIG 8.19 Contrasting patterns of behaviour in neurones of the same cell group. For details of histograms see Fig. 8.18. N, no apparent response to natural stimulation. W_s and W_p: wrist supination and pronation. W_{ab}: radial deviation of the wrist. Despite the close proximity of these neurones, they showed quite different sources of input and activity. (Reproduced with permission from Lemon (1981b).)

displayed quite contrasting patterns of activity during movement (see Fig. 8.19).

Thus these cell groups or clusters were heterogeneous in both their input zones and their output targets. The substrate for multiple representation of inputs may be the extensive ramifications of axons carrying input to the motor cortex which has been referrred to above (see Section 8.2).

These input systems make synaptic contacts in a selective and focused manner within each distribution territory.

8.7 DYNAMIC FEATURES OF THE OUTPUT MAP

All the above descriptions assume a relatively stable, hard-wired motor output map. Indeed, early studies of the output map emphasized its stability (Craggs and Rushton 1976). Schmidt and McIntosh (1979) were able to test this directly by determining the movements evoked from microwire electrodes permanently implanted to a depth of 1.5 mm within the motor cortex of macaques. Since these electrodes could record from one and the same neurone for many days, it is probable that there was very little drift of the electrode after recovery from the implantation operation. Several cases were documented in which responses from the same muscle could be elicited from the same electrode site over long periods (up to 28 days). Kwan *et al.* (1978) also reported that, in general, penetrations made between 3 and 18 months apart at identical cortical sites yielded similar responses to ICMS.

But these results do not prove that the output map is immutable. The property of plasticity of the representation is now a well-established feature of cortical maps in the visual and somatosensory areas. Brown and Sherrington (1912) referred to the 'instability of a cortical point' and showed that stimulation of the cortex was itself capable of altering the responses evoked from a given cortical locus (see Phillips and Porter 1977, p. 37; Nudo *et al.* 1990). Given the complexity of the intra-areal map described above, convincing evidence of a reshaping of the cortical map is best obtained by looking at the boundaries of the areal map, for instance at the face–arm border. In the rat, a number of studies by Donoghue, Sanes, and their colleagues have demonstrated shifts in this boundary. Maps were constructed by delivering ICMS in large numbers of penetrations made throughout the sensorimotor cortex in rats sedated with ketamine. Sanes *et al.* (1990) found that when the motor cortex was mapped after chronic forelimb amputation there was an expansion of the area devoted to shoulder movements, but no significant increase in the area of the vibrissal representation. Chronic transection of the facial nerve had more dramatic effects, resulting in a significant expansion in the forelimb territory (see Fig. 8.20). No obvious differences were observed between the motor maps of rats operated either 1 week or 5 months previously. Indeed when pre- and post-transection mapping was carried out in rats subjected to *acute* facial nerve section, similar shifts in the map were detected within hours of nerve injury (Donoghue *et al.* 1990). In these animals, ICMS (<60 μA) within the vibrissal region never produced any activation of contralateral forelimb EMG. But within 1 to 4 hrs of

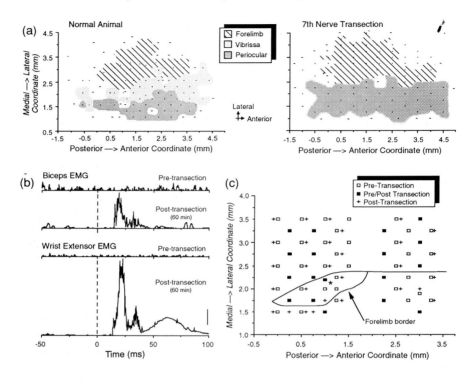

FIG 8.20   M1 reorganization with nerve transection. (a): Surface views of the rat frontal cortex illustrating the major functional regions in M1 in a normal animal (left panel) and experimental animal with a facial nerve transection (right panel). Each dot indicates an electrode penetration site at which movement was evoked at stimulation currents $\leqslant 60\ \mu$A. The shadings indicate contiguous subzones within M1 representing different body parts (see key). In the normal animal the vibrissa zone is interposed between the laterally placed forelimb zone and the medially placed periocular zone. In the experimental animal, with a facial nerve transection 123 days before the map was generated, the former vibrissa zone is 'occupied' by a medial expansion of the forelimb zone and a lateral expansion of the periocular zone. (b): Muscle responses before and soon after nerve transection. Evoked EMG from stimulation in the normal vibrissa zone at the site marked by an asterisk in (c). Prior to facial nerve transection (pretransection traces), no EMG response could be evoked in either biceps or wrist extensor muscles. Within 60 min (post-transection traces), EMG from both biceps and wrist extensor (muscles was evoked from this site. (c): M1 output map before and after facial nerve transection. The medial extent of the M1 forelimb zone was determined before (open and filled squares) and after (filled squares and crosses) the facial nerve was transected. The post-transection mapping was completed within 3 hours, and the forelimb border shifted medially for a total expansion of $\sim 1\ \text{mm}^2$ of the forelimb area. (Reproduced with permission from Sanes and Donoghue (1991).)

transection, these stimuli were effective in producing contraction in biceps or in wrist extensor muscles; the forelimb area increased by between 1 and 2 mm^2. This is a very small shift, particularly when we remember the spread of current that is possible when using repetitive ICMS; but it represents a very considerable expansion of the forelimb area in a normal rat (2.4 mm^2).

Given the indirect and trans-synaptic action of repetitive ICMS (see Section 8.2), a possible explanation of these findings is that there has been a rapid reorganization of synaptic interconnections between the vibrissal and forelimb regions, which has occurred in response to the functional changes in afferent input to these regions caused by the nerve injury. This would include the important input that is normally directed to the cortex continuously from the vibrissae. A forelimb representation might be unmasked by the reshaping of the excitatory and particularly of the inhibitory connections provided by these afferents. Subsequently, Jacobs and Donoghue (1991) demonstrated that the shifts produced by nerve injury can be mimicked by small injections of the GABA antagonist, bicuculline, into the motor cortex.

A recent study by Hall *et al.* (1990) has suggested that significant reorganization can occur in the human motor cortex. Four amputees were investigated, two congenital and two with traumatic amputations. Magnetic stimulation of the cortex in these patients revealed that the stump muscles on the amputated side were more readily excited from the contralateral cortex than were the same muscles on the intact side. In addition, the number of scalp positions from which the stump muscles could be excited was greater than for the intact arm, suggesting that a greater cortical area was now devoted to the representation of the stump. These findings were true for both congenital amputees, and for one patient who lost his arm at an early age (10 years). A patient who had lost his arm at 55 showed no evidence of cortical reorganization when examined in this way.

All of the above results speak in favour of a dynamic organization of the output map, although the changes observed to date have all followed drastic intervention on the part of either nature or the experimenter. It would be of particular interest to know if dynamic changes in the organization of the output map occur during the emergence of a motor function — the acquisition of skill and precision in a motor task or the learning of a new motor performance. The methods using long term recording from well characterized and functionally identified PTNs using permanently implanted microwires (Schmidt and McIntosh 1979) offers the opportunity for examining the involvement of particular neurones in defined regions of the motor map during periods of learning. Moreover, because the technique is ideal for simultaneously monitoring the input/output properties and the responses of a number of neurones situated in several locations, relative changes in their relationships to movement performance can be assessed. In this way attempts could be made to understand the functional significance of the dynamic changes which may be observed for movement performance and for the learning of new motor skills.

8.8 MECHANISMS FOR DYNAMIC CHANGE

We have presented evidence for the structural and physiological organization of connected elements in the motor cortex, changes in which could allow for dynamic, plastic alterations in function to be documented. Whether or not neuronal sprouting, or the unmasking of existing synapses from a prevailing inhibition or biochemical suppression, is involved in the expansion of output territories which can be observed under these experimental conditions is still largely unknown. A number of investigators have attempted to study long lasting changes in neuronal behaviour which could provide a basis for such modifications. Baranyi and Szente (1987) demonstrated long-lasting changes in EPSPs evoked in cat motor cortex neurones from stimulation of the VL thalamus, pyramidal tract (recurrent EPSPs), corpus callosum or a peripheral nerve. These EPSPs were shown to be facilitated for long periods (40–60 min) if they were paired with either antidromic, orthodromic, or current-induced action potentials of the neurone in the motor cortex, and these effects were shown to depend on postsynaptic modifications of the cortical neurone. Asanuma and his colleagues demonstrated that tetanic stimulation of the somatosensory cortex could produce long-term potentiation (LTP), lasting for more than 30 min, in the amplitude of cortico-cortical EPSPs evoked in motor cortex neurones from the sensory cortex (Sakamoto *et al.* 1987). These effects were not replicated for EPSPs evoked in the same cells from the VL thalamic nucleus. However, pairing the tetanic stimulation of both thalamus and sensory cortex did produce LTP of VL evoked EPSPs (Iriki *et al.* 1989). These authors suggested that LTP in the motor cortex may be important in the learning of new motor skills, and especially for the changes of synaptic efficiency that allow a learned movement to be directed by motor cortex neurones when it is no longer dependent upon sensory feedback for its control. Iriki *et al.* (1989) observed LTP in superficial cortical cells, but not in cells of the deeper layers, V and VI, including PTNs. Interestingly, Iriki *et al.* (1990) have documented dramatic and well sustained, long term facilitation of synaptic transmission from intraspinal collaterals of these same PTNs which engage spinal interneurones. The mechanisms of plastic change within the motor cortex itself will undoubtedly be the subject of extensive experimental endeavour in the future. The description of mechanisms of plastic change which may provide the basis for motor learning will be aided greatly by the study of biophysical processes which may be detected in *in vitro* slices of motor cortex.

Houk (1991) and Houk and Barto (1991) have drawn attention to the fact that adaptive changes which occur during learning and which may be detected as modifications in features of a cortical map, may nevertheless have components of those 'learned' changes distributed through many connected systems. These authors point out that theories of motor learning must be constrained by neuroanatomical findings of the kind we have been documenting in this book. They will also be limited by the physiological facts of synaptic actions, generated within connected networks of neurones. The cellular (biophysical) and molecular (biochemical) properties of the neurones themselves may be modifiable. Changes that are observed in such documented phenomena as the altered areal features of the output map, and its regional organization, can be a reflection of modifications to the inputs to these territories, and such modifications can be produced by functional alterations at distant, connected sites. The changes are then imposed on the motor map by the inputs derived from these distant sites. Houk (1991) therefore provides a reminder of the complex and intimate relationship of the cerebellum to the motor cortex and of the well supported theories and speculations (Marr 1969; Ito 1985) of cerebellar involvement in learning. The role of the inferior olive, and of its climbing fibres ascending to the cerebellar cortex, has been implicated in motor learning. It is conceivable that adaptive changes occurring within the cerebellar cortex, dependent on inputs from the inferior olive, could influence both cortical and spinal territories which may be changed functionally during the acquisition of a new movement skill. Such concepts are clearly accessible to experimental investigation.

8.9 FUNCTIONS OF THE OUTPUT MAP

What is represented in the motor cortex output map? We must now examine whether the recent investigations of the structure of the output map have helped us to understand its function. From the descriptions given above it is no longer possible to think in terms of the output map as a simple, somatotopic representation of either joint movements or muscles. Multiple representation and overlap of outputs to different motoneurones and muscles is at variance with the observations of Asanuma (1975, 1981, 1989) who has suggested that a single muscle is represented within a single functional column within the motor cortex. The difficulty of establishing clear spatial maps within M1 has meant that while primary sensory and association areas have been successively subdivided on the basis of the separate spatial representations of aspects of their functions, M1 is still considered by many to be a single integrated cortical region. This is not to say that it is homogeneous. Rather, we suggest that the cortical outputs represented within M1 are not mapped in spatially separated zones. Outputs are mapped in a manner that is more closely related to the *functions* which they subserve. Clusters of cortical cells, concerned with the co-ordination of muscle action at different joints, need not necessarily be mapped in a manner which reflects the spatial organization of the anatomy of the limb. We should not forget that the corticospinal tract itself lacks obvious somatotopic organization of its fibres (Section 2.8); it is perhaps not so surprising that such an organization is also lacking in the primary region of cortex from which much of the tract is derived.

It may be fruitful to look for a spatial organization of neurones whose parametric relationship to different aspects of voluntary movement has been identified (Georgopoulos *et al.* 1984; Alexander and Crutcher 1990a). Unfortunately, most studies have concentrated on the nature of this parametric relationship and they have all too often ignored the spatial representation of these functions within the cortex. The problem has been compounded by the fact that in many studies, the cells from which recordings have been made have not been identified or localized histologically.

It is clear from a number of studies in which relatively simple movements have been studied, that so-called 'task-related' neurones can be recorded from large areas of the primary motor cortex (Lemon *et al.* 1976; Wong *et al.* 1979; Lamarre *et al.* 1981; Evarts *et al.* 1983; Alexander and Crutcher 1990a). This presumably reflects the multiple representation of muscles and movements referred to above in Section 8.4. Although the complex features of the output map revealed by recent studies were not stressed by earlier investigators, there was plenty of evidence for both multiple representation and overlap in their published work (e.g. Leyton and Sherrington 1917; Penfield and Boldrey 1937). While it may seem obvious that the large volume of cortex devoted to representation of movements of the hand reflects the importance of the cortex–hand relationship, what precisely is represented in this extensive territory is much less clear. On multiple representation, Hughlings Jackson reasoned that 'the small muscles of the hand will be represented by much more grey matter in the highest centres than will be the large muscles of the upper arm, because they serve in more numerous different movements' (Jackson 1932, p. 262). The huge repertoire of movements of which the primate hand is capable presumably demands more motor cortical circuitry than that required for simpler movements, such as reaching. Thus the multiple representation of a single muscle can be seen as the substrate for the many different combinations in which a particular muscle can be used, for instance during performance of different gripping tasks. Recently, Flament *et al.* (1993) demonstrated that the amplitude of responses of the 1DI muscle to magnetic stimulation of the contralateral cortex varied according to the task in which the muscle was engaged. A possible explanation of this finding is that different subpopulations of corticospinal neurones influencing the

1DI muscle were recruited during the different tasks, and that because the spatial distribution of these subpopulations varied, they were differentially susceptible to the magnetic stimulus.

Control theorists have stressed the importance of discovering how the motor system overcomes the 'degrees of freedom problem' (Bernstein 1967, p. 127). This problem arises from the potentially infinite number of ways in which a multiarticulate limb could be used to achieve a particular motor 'goal', such as reaching for a target or grasping an object. A partial solution to this problem may be provided by cortico-motoneuronal and other descending and interneuronal systems in that their patterns of synaptic connectivity must necessarily restrict the total 'library' of possible muscle synergies which may be accessed, while still providing a variety of approaches to the single motor goal.

The change in emphasis from a simple somatotopy to consider the complex features of the modern map has come at a time in which much more work is being devoted to the study of complex, multijoint movements (Georgopoulos *et al.* 1984; Jeannerod 1988). Most natural movements involve use of multiple muscles acting at many joints. The traditional view of a somatotopically organized output map within the motor cortex has previously emphasized the control of systems operating about separate joints and of relatively circumscribed and isolated output modules controlling movements of each of the hand, elbow, or shoulder. Overlap of outputs speaks against such a division and against such separate and independent output modules. Two important substrates for this overlap must be the divergent influence of a single cortico-motoneuronal neurone upon several related muscles and the heterogeneous clustering of output neurones. The organization of the intra-areal map plays down the representation of individual joints and highlights the coordination of action initiated by many muscles at different joints. Local interaction of output units with different targets is provided by the 'overlap between contiguous joint zones' (Kwan *et al.* 1978). Evidence for such interaction can be obtained by demonstrating synaptic connectivity between cortico-motoneuronal cells with different muscle fields (see Fig. 8.13).

Thus the representation of more proximal shoulder and elbow muscles could be thought of as part of the control system subserving reaching, prehension, and manipulation of objects, rather than for the organization of proximal limb movement *per se*. Long ago, Penfield and Rasmussen commented 'one might suppose that if the complicated skills of the thumb had come to be represented in the large extent of the precentral gyrus devoted to the thumb, and the movements of the arm were confined to the small segment of the motor strip devoted to the arm, that removal of the arm area would result in marked disability of the arm with little involvement of fine movements of thumb and fingers. But this is not the result — a small excision within the shoulder and elbow area, as determined by electrical stimulation, produced weakness and awkwardness in the whole upper extremity, *including the hand'* (our italics; Penfield and Rasmussen 1952, p. 218). The distribution of afferent feedback to the motor cortex is such as to provide cell clusters with information about several different regions of the moving limb (Lemon 1981b). Huang *et al.* (1988) suggest that 'the various input channels to the motor cortex, each of which transmits different sensory information, have to be redistributed to separate multiple output channels which address the same set of motor units'.

Accuracy of reach and stability of the proximal arm are essential prerequisites for the successful execution of relatively independent finger movements. One feature of this control must be the co-contraction of multiple muscles that is essential for joint stability (Smith 1981). As we have discussed earlier, Humphrey (1982, 1986) found evidence that the activity of cortical neurones recorded while monkeys controlled wrist joint position was such that it was related either to the independent activation of synergist muscles for joint movement or, for another population of cortical cells, to the co-contraction of antagonist muscles for stiffening of the joint during steady holding (see Section 5.5). These two populations of cells were mapped separately in the movement map of the motor cortex: those concerned with independent activation were located at sites where ICMS produced contractions of the wrist muscle ECR which resulted in wrist extension movements (see Fig. 8.8). Those concerned with co-contraction were found where ICMS elicited other movements in which ECR played a stabilizing role (see Fig. 8.8).

8.10 SUMMARY

Outputs from the primary motor cortex can be detected in a variety of ways, including the recording of postsynaptic potentials, modulation of spinal reflexes, activation of motor units or EMG, and the production of movements. Outputs to different parts of the body musculature are represented in the classical 'areal map': the face, arm, and leg representations. Within each of these is an 'intra-areal map', which has a number of distinctive features. Rather than a single cortical focus for a motoneurone, there are multiple representations. The same is true for each muscle and movement. These representations are large and often discontinuous. Within each areal map, the largest representation is devoted to the most distal elements (the lips, tongue, fingers, and toes), and these elements are more easily excited and with weaker electrical stimuli than are the more proximal elements. There is substantial overlap between the outputs to different motoneurones, muscles, and movements. This overlap results partly from the divergent output from single corticospinal cells and partly from the intermingling of corticospinal neurones with different targets.

It is possible that the multiple representation of outputs reflects the different combinations in which outputs to a different muscle are required for the production of different movements. The overlap of outputs probably reflects the need, when executing multijoint movements, for local synaptic interaction of outputs to different segments of the limb. These functional features of the intra-areal map cannot be represented in terms of a somatotopic re-mapping of the muscles and joints; instead, they may be represented in spatially segregated clusters of cells encoding specific parameters of movement or specific combinations of output organisation in a task-related manner. The map of outputs appears to be in register with that of inputs arriving from the limbs and face. Afferent inputs from one and the same region are again subject to multiple representation and this may reflect the need to supply each of the different output clusters with sensory information from the relevant segment of the moving limb. The convergence of information from different parts of the limb on to a single cluster of cells is again indicative of the co-ordination of outputs directed to different parts of that limb. These inputs are important for the selection and control of corticospinal output units, and some of the results obtained with electrical stimulation of the cortex should perhaps be interpreted in terms of exciting these input systems, rather than the corticospinal neurones themselves. The output map is a dynamic map and can be influenced by manipulation or removal of its output target, or by changing afferent input. Remodelling of the input–output organization of the motor cortex may be essential for the acquisition of motor skills.

9

Synthesis: corticospinal function and voluntary movement

9.1 INTRODUCTION

In this book we have tried to explore the relationship between the neuronal connectivity of the corticospinal system and functional aspects of the execution of a voluntary movement, especially of the hand. Sherrington, in his 9th Silliman Lecture (1906), identified a number of parallel evolutionary processes which together had resulted in a purposefully useful arm and hand, under the dominant control of the cerebral cortex. Skilled use of the hands is central to our cultural, creative, and technological achievements: gesture and communication, making and using of tools, writing, painting, drawing, love making, emotional enjoyment, and entertainment through the playing of musical instruments and of physical and intellectual games.

As we have seen, when compared to lower mammals, two key developments have taken place in the primate motor system. The first is the increasingly important size and role of the motor areas of the cerebral cortex and their dominance over the enlarged motor output pathways to the spinal cord. The influence of the corticospinal tract increases, in primates, at the expense of other descending pathways, such as the rubrospinal tract. Progressively, in higher mammals, the motor centres of the brain, including the lateral cerebellum and the basal ganglia, address the final common path for movement control through the cerebral cortex and the corticospinal tract, rather than through the brainstem. Descending systems from the brainstem themselves come under increasing cortical control by efferent projections from motor areas of the cerebral cortex. The second major development is the appearance of direct, cortico-motoneuronal connections providing monosynaptic linkage between the motor cortex and spinal motoneurones.

These two evolutionary developments underpinned the provision of a system for discrete motor control of the arm and hand by a part of the brain that was easily and relatively directly accessible by those other regions of the cerebral cortex specialized to deal with visual and somatosensory information relevant to voluntary movements of the hand and arm. The motor cortex was uniquely well-placed to supply the efferent, executive projections for organized cortical mechanisms subserving the key functions of visuomotor control of the hand and tactile exploration with it. As the brilliant anatomist and primatologist John Napier has pointed out, the hand has several advantages over the eye: 'it can see in the dark and it can see round corners; most important of all, it can interact with the environment, rather than just observe it' (Napier 1980, p. 22).

The parallel evolution of cortical mechanisms to analyse foveal and glabrous sensation has been claimed to demand a cerebral centre to be concerned particularly with the control the hand, and the motor cortex became the focus for movement control commands from the highest cerebral levels. The hand was required to be engaged in purposeful, skilful movements: for prehension, exploration, manipulation, and tool-making. The basic synergies of the spinal cord, evolved for the control of locomotion and support, could not provide the new forms of muscular interactions which the arm, promoted 'from a simple locomotor prop to a delicate explorer of space in manifold directions' now needed (Sherrington 1906, pp. 352–353). The development of cortico-motoneuronal connections permitted a direct cortical modulation of these spinal segmental mechanisms, and a breaking up of the rigid synergies of the spinal apparatus. By allowing direct access to the motoneurones and bypassing the organized networks of intraspinal connections, the cortico-motoneuronal system gave the cerebrum a direct influence on the final common path itself. The existence of a direct pathway from cerebral cortex to muscle that provides for motor neurones to be only one synapse removed from the intricate workings of the thinking brain itself has been fully documented.

We have seen that the cells of origin of the cortico-motoneuronal pathway are themselves in receipt of a large variety of different inputs. Injections of neuroanatomical tracers into the motor cortex reveal an organized pattern of local intrinsic circuitry, as well as labelling neurones in many other cortical areas retrogradely (Chapters 2, 7, 8). These experiments provide us with the critical evidence that allows the motor cortex and its cortico-motoneuronal output to be regarded as a summing point for the many different inputs that are necessary for efficient and effective control of a voluntary task. But it is the increasingly significant functional interactions of the visual and tactile senses with this control system that explain why a cortical location for this control system is so critically important for purposeful voluntary movement. While, with every skilled hand movement that we make, we can be aware of the enormous advantages which seem to have been conferred by this evolutionary development, we are also reminded, from time to time, of the price that must be paid for placing so many of the eggs of skilled control in the one cortical basket. The catastrophic effects of stroke on the control of voluntary movement in man is dramatic when compared to the results of damage affecting similar areas in lower mammals (Chapter 3).

9.2 MULTIPLICITY OF FUNCTIONS WITHIN THE CORTICOSPINAL TRACT

The existence of a compact bundle of fibres coursing together through the brainstem as the pyramidal tract has, since the time of François-Franck (1887), been a powerful inducement challenging scientists and theorists to discover a single function for the tract (Bucy *et al.* 1964; Paillard 1978). In Chapter 2 we described three important pieces of evidence that suggest that this single tract subserves more than a single function: the widespread origin of the tract, the patterns of termination of the different projections from different cortical regions within the spinal grey matter, and, finally, the general lack of any somatotopic organization within the fibres of the tract.

The recent work of Dum and Strick (1991) has confirmed and extended the idea that the corticospinal tract arises from multiple cortical areas. A major objective of many single-unit neurophysiological studies has been to compare the neuronal behaviour in one cortical region with that observed in other zones during the performance of one and the same experimental task. Such experiments have included the study of most of the areas giving rise to the corticospinal tract, although few observations have been limited to the corticospinal neurones within them. The functional operations of these different cortical areas have been treated in separate chapters in this book because of the evidence that the neuronal mechanisms revealed within them do exhibit distinctive differences.

Some of these differences include the timing of activity relative to movement onset in somatosensory and primary motor cortex (Section 5.2), and the preponderance of activity in premotor cortex that is related to the visual guidance or triggering of limb movement. There are differences in the timing of activities in SMA and M1 relative to preparation for and then the onset of an instructed limb movement, and in the force-related activities of M1, area 5, and the premotor cortex. There are particularly striking contrasts between the activities of SMA and premotor cortex during performance of 'internally guided' and visually guided movements, respectively. No doubt other interesting differences will come to light as a result of future experiments. This book has tried to chart some of the recent advances through which neurophysiologists focus on the critical cortical operations which are deduced to contribute defined aspects of voluntary movement. To highlight differences in the output functions, contributed by corticospinal elements from different locations, there is a pressing need for more studies which compare the activities of identified corticospinal neurones arising from different cortical areas and making identifiably different connections with spinal cord elements or other brain regions.

But this evidence for functional differences between the deduced operational actions of the cortical areas should not distract us from the features that are common to them (Kalaska and Crammond 1992). Here we can cite the encoding of arm direction, during reaching in space, by populations of neurones in areas 4, 5, and 6, and the preparatory activity occurring before an instructed movement in these same areas. Neurones in both the postcentral and the precentral cortex encode force. These observations show that rather than there being abrupt functional boundaries between the different cytoarchitectonic areas giving rise to the corticospinal tract, there is a gradient of operational activity which flows from one area to another. Moreover, a region of cerebral cortex, possibly covering several cytoarchitectural areas, clearly contains within it overlapping representations of multiple aspects of voluntary movement. In an experiment designed to examine single neurone activity during the performance of a visually guided arm movement, Godschalk *et al.* (1981) found a predominance of movement-related neuronal activity in the primary motor cortex, M1, while the predominant pattern of activity in the postarcuate area (area 6) was related to the location of the visual cue guiding the movement. But some movement-related neurones were found in area 6 and 'visual-related' neurones in area 4. Alexander and Crutcher (1990a) found that early-onset activity that preceded an instructed elbow movement was found both in motor cortex and SMA, although it was more common in the latter. While neurones active during internally and visually triggered movements predominated in the SMA and premotor cortex, respectively, neurones of both type were found in both areas.

The absence of any sharp functional dichotomy probably explains the results of lesion studies: lesions restricted to one histologically defined cortical motor area rarely produce a complete deficit of a given function or task. Such lesions usually influence performance on a number of different behavioural tests, usually with a strong effect on one particular aspect of performance. The work of Passingham and his colleagues provides the best illustration of this point (see Chapter 7).

The corticospinal tract may not be involved only in the execution of movements, but also in the learning of new movements and the development of motor skills. There have been suggestions that the corticospinal tract may be active primarily in the acquisition of new skills, and that after a skill is learned, the execution of the task may in some way be 'taken over' by subcortical pathways (Kennedy 1990). Although this may be an attractive notion, it does not explain why corticospinal outputs are active during highly overtrained tasks, as has been observed repeatedly in primate studies, or during locomotion, as is observed in the cat (Armstrong and Drew 1984a). Further, STA and stimulation studies have shown that these outputs are actively contributing to the execution of the movement task in monkeys and in humans, and not just 'monitoring' movement performance. This analysis is in line with PET studies indicating increased neuronal activity in motor cortex during both learning and execution of a new task (Seitz *et al.* 1990). Finally, should the control of learned movements have been relegated to some subcortical structures following their acquisition, the profound interference with the performance of such learned tasks and long-established movement performances following a stroke would not be explained. Thus, while there are probably important changes demonstrable in the activities of these outputs during motor learning, the learning of new motor tasks is unlikely to be the only role of corticospinal activation.

The description of the different patterns of termination of corticospinal projections arising from different cortical regions was one of the major contributions made by Hans Kuypers. The differences in termination of corticospinal axons from the postcentral, primary somatosensory area and from primary motor cortex have been given in detail in Chapter 2. In the primate, these results imply that the corticospinal projections from the postcentral gyrus are important in the control of sensory input (see Section 6.8), in contrast to the direct impact of precentral cortico-motoneuronal projections on motoneuronal activity providing for direct activation of muscles. But we need to know much more about the pattern of individual corticospinal terminations to fully reveal any functional differences that such connections might imply. This will involve more detailed intraxonal injection studies for the construction of terminal patterns of arborization, and more careful STA and single-ICMS studies in non-primary motor cortex. There is a suggestion that fibres in the corticospinal tract may be collected together in functional groups, rather than on the basis of the level of their spinal destination. This could explain the absence of any obvious somatotopic organization within the tract.

9.3 THE SIGNIFICANCE OF THE CORTICO-MOTONEURONAL SYSTEM FOR VOLUNTARY MOVEMENT

Although the evidence presented in Chapter 3 shows the strength of correlation between the development of cortico-motoneuronal connections and the performance of skilled, independent finger movements, the reader will require a convincing argument as to why a cortico-motoneuronal system should be a prerequisite for such movements. We have argued that such a system is essential to modify or even to bypass the spinal synaptic connectivity originally evolved for the use of the upper limb as a 'prop' in posture and locomotion. The spinal cord's neuronal organization is based on relatively rigid muscular synergies, and a mechanism to fractionate this is of particular importance for the muscles of the hands and digits which may need to be employed in a variety of flexible associations during voluntary movements. It is interesting that, immediately before the onset of a voluntary movement, there are marked changes in transmission through spinal reflex pathways (Baldiserra and Pierrot Deseilligny 1989; Crone and Nielsen 1989), and that these changes appear to be dependent upon whether or not the intended voluntary act requires a co-contracted or a reciprocal pattern of muscle activity (Nielsen and Kagamihara 1992).

The importance of the cortico-motoneuronal system has been underlined by the striking effects that can be produced in a large variety of human limb and trunk muscles by non-invasive brain stimulation. The latencies of these responses have indicated that, in many cases, they result from excitation of the rapidly conducting PTNs. These experiments completed an important chapter in motor neurophysiology begun with the description by Bernhard *et al.* in 1953 of short-latency motor effects produced by cortical stimulation in the monkey. Neurophysiologists have concentrated their attention on these large PTNs, the synchronous volleys and the cortico-motoneuronal effects that they produce. If the fast PTNs were alone in the establishment of direct cortico-motoneuronal connections, it might be necessary to question how such a small fraction of the entire corticospinal tract could play such an important part in the execution of skilled motor performance. It may still be the case that these fast cortico-motoneuronal cells have an importance that is out of all proportion to their numbers. However, the demonstration of the existence of a significant number of slow PTNs with cortico-motoneuronal connections affecting the intrinsic muscles of the hand (Section 4.11) suggests that there are a larger number of cortico-motoneuronal contributors than was originally considered on the basis of electrical stimulation studies. More work is needed on the slowly conducting corticospinal neurones, especially those which derive from the motor cortex. These cells may be relatively unimportant in the influence they exert at the onset of rapid movements, but they could be critical for control under more steady-state conditions or during slow manipulatory actions under visual or tactile guidance. Many slowly conducting corticospinal axons are derived from the non-primary motor areas and their contributions during voluntary movement performance need to be understood (Chapter 2).

9.4 THE ROLE OF THE CORTICO-MOTONEURONAL SYSTEM IN THE MOTOR HIERARCHY

In this final chapter we should like to emphasize the important point that a cortico-motoneuronal system provides the rest of the motor system with the capacity for independent finger movements: the cortico-motoneuronal system is itself the servant of higher levels within the motor system from which commands and directives will be issued. When these inputs are removed from the cortico-motoneuronal cells, the neurones hyperpolarize and become inactive (Matsumura *et al.* 1988); they clearly do not themselves generate the command signals for movement.

The comparative anatomy of the cortico-motoneuronal system (Chapter 3) has provided some important evidence as to its function in different primates. But, as we have pointed out above, the cortico-motoneuronal system is part of a series of parallel evolutionary developments, and its appearance late in the evolutionary day was accompanied by that of cortical, striatal, and cerebellar mechanisms that could operate upon the hand through the motor cortex and the emerging cortico-motoneuronal system. This evolutionary pattern may be considered to be reiterated in the late ontogenetic appearance of cortico-motoneuronal synapses. But again, while it may be true that maturation of these connections is essential for the normal development of relatively independent finger movements, these connections are in essence providing the means by which other important influences, concerned with the development of hand use, can operate upon the control of the hand. The 'higher level' processes which include motor learning, acquisition of skills, training, experience, emotions, and cognition (Jeannerod 1988, pp. 67–68) are enabled to operate on voluntary movement through cortico-motoneuronal connections. The importance of this functional and structural hierarchy is most clearly seen in patients who apparently possess an intact cortico-motoneuronal pathway, yet for whom normal voluntary movement is impossible because of damage to structures which would normally interact with, and express themselves through, the cortico-motoneuronal system; such patients include those suffering from Parkinsons's disease (Dick *et al.* 1984).

Conversely, damage to other levels of the hierarchy can also produce striking deficits in finger movements; for example, Jeannerod *et al.* (1984) described the inability of a patient with a well defined lesion in the parietal cortex to organize the essential sequences of movement to correctly grasp objects, unless she was allowed to do so under visual control. Brinkman and Kuypers (1973) showed deficient finger control in split brain monkeys deprived of visual input to the hemisphere contralateral to the hand being used; but these monkeys showed normal finger movements when tactile cues could be used to control the movement. These deficits are reminiscent of those described in deafferented patients, such as the classic case described by Rothwell *et al.* (1982) and referred to in Chapter 6.

9.5 POSSIBLE CONTRIBUTIONS OF THE CORTICOSPINAL SYSTEM DURING VISUOMOTOR CO-ORDINATION IN MAN

An important problem for the motor hierarchy to solve is the co-ordination of several diverse motor systems, best exemplified by visuomotor control of eye, head, and hand movements (Jeannerod 1988, pp. 41–54). The introduction of kinematic techniques has provided fascinating insights into the organization of different aspects of human voluntary movement. In a number of kinematic studies, two components of human prehension were described: transportation of the hand to, and grasp of, the object. These components must be closely co-ordinated for accurate prehension (Wing *et al.* 1986). In a recent study (Paulignan *et al.* 1990), the object to be retrieved was a dowel placed directly in front of the subject, at a distance of around 35 cm from the hand, in its initial resting position. The transportation of the hand towards the object was a rapid movement lasting around 550 ms; the wrist had a bell-shaped velocity curve peaking at around 100–150 cm.s^{-1}. This component was shown by Jeannerod (1984) to be little affected by whether or not visual feedback about the movement of the limb was available. Anticipatory grip formation took place during transportation: grip aperture first opened around 100 ms after reaching began, and then began to close at 300–340 ms. In both the transportation and grasp components there was evidence of considerable trial by trial variability in the handpath used by the subjects; this variability decreased as the hand neared the object.

Jeannerod (1988) has discussed the possible neural organization for these two components. In the Brinkman and Kuypers (1973) study, split-brain monkeys deprived of visual input to the hemisphere contralateral to the moving limb could reach accurately for objects, but could not make the correct visuomotor adjustments to their grasp that a special test board required them to make (an adaptation of that shown in Fig. 3.9). As discussed in Chapter 2, Brinkman and Kuypers' interpretation of this was that relatively independent finger movements required the activity of crossed corticospinal and cortico-motoneuronal projections, and that these projections could, in the split-brain animal, be accessed only by visual inputs under conditions of contralateral eye–hand control. The reaching or transportation component was under the control of bilaterally organized descending pathways, and could therefore be driven from either hemisphere (see Fig. 2.17). There is also evidence from split-brain patients of different control systems for the hand and for more proximal limb movements (Gazzaniga *et al.* 1967).

Efficient prehension requires a high degree of co-ordination of these two control systems. Several studies have attempted to dissociate the transport and grasp components, by changing either object location or size, to affect transport and grasp, respectively (Wallace and Weeks 1988; Paulignan *et al.* 1991; Haggard 1991). These studies have all indicated some interdependence of timing between the two control systems or channels. While there may be separate motor channels for each component, these results suggest that their co-ordination is likely to be organized at the level of the motor cortex, which gives rise to the transport and grasp channels, or at a higher level. In considering the question of co-ordination, it should not be forgotten that new evidence on the representation of motor outputs within the motor cortex suggests that the location of outputs with particular targets may well be organized for allowing very close interactions between proximal and distal segments of the limb (Section 8.9).

9.6 POSSIBLE CONTRIBUTIONS OF THE CORTICOSPINAL SYSTEM DURING ACTIVE TOUCH AND PREHENSION IN MAN

Charles Phillips, in his essay 'Active Touch', traced the history of the idea that, for normal hand function, sensation and movement are inextricably mixed (Phillips 1986, pp. 76–77). Charles Bell, writing in 1833, had stated: 'But the motion of the fingers is especially necessary to the sense of touch — embracing the object, and feeling it on all its surfaces; sensible to its solidity and to its resistance when grasped; moving round it and gliding over its surface, and, therefore, feeling every asperity' (Bell 1833, pp. 202–3).

The investigation and demonstration of active touch owes a great deal to the experiments of Roland Johansson, Goran Westling, and their colleagues. The importance of this work has been to elucidate the programme of precision grip control in everyday situations. In their initial experiments, Johansson and Westling (1984) demonstrated that, when lifting an object from a table, subjects produced an isometric grip force between thumb and index finger that was appropriate to the load to be lifted: neither too much force nor too little force was exerted. The load and grip forces increased in parallel during the lifting phase; when holding the object in air, the ratio between grip force and load force was automatically adjusted by subjects to a value that ensured that the object did not slip from their grasp. A small but significant 'safety margin' was established: the difference in the grip/load force ratio adopted by the subject and the ratio at which a slip would occur. During a task such as holding a glass as it was steadily filled with water, the increasing load force was paralleled by a co-ordinated increase in grip force, such that the safety margin remained constant (Johansson and Westling 1987b).

Johansson and Westling (1984) found that the size of this safety margin was adjusted to suit the frictional conditions at the gripping surface; with a slippery object, surfaced with silk, grip force was increased to about twice the value exerted upon a rough object, surfaced with sandpaper.

Both the rapid response to object slips and the adaptation to frictional conditions appeared to depend upon signals from tactile afferents supplying cutaneous mechanoreceptors in the tips of the thumb and index finger. Anaesthetizing these areas abolished these important responses, and slippage of the object occurred. Subjects eventually adapted to conditions of impaired sensory feedback, by increasing their grip forces substantially, thus preventing any further slips.

To discover the nature of the afferent signals contributing to control of precision grip, they recorded activity in cutaneous afferents in the median nerve using the microneurographic technique (Westling and Johansson 1987). Even small slips were reliably signalled by rapidly adapting RA I, RA II, and slowly adapting SA I receptors (Johansson and Westling 1987a). These signals appeared to trigger a sharp increase in grip force, so that the safety margin was restored. The delay between slip of the object (detected by an accelerometer mounted on it) and the onset of increased EMG activity was in the region of 65 ms, much shorter than the subjects' reaction time. Since these automatic responses have the same latency as other long-latency reflex responses of proposed transcortical origin (see Section 6.7), it may well be that these rapid and powerful responses to slip may also be transcortical in nature (Johansson 1991). Subjects were not always aware that these automatic responses had occurred. It is significant that these responses were very much larger than those obtained, for instance, by electrical stimulation of the digital sensory nerves. This illustrates that the relevance of the sensory input to the task being performed is extremely important in influencing the type and size of the response obtained. Peripheral events are appropriately signalled by a temporal pattern of nerve impulses in particular, spatially organized afferents from a population of relevant receptors. This is a common characteristic of the sensorimotor system (Prochazka 1989; see Section 6.8). 'These circumstances indicate that a neuronal mechanism identifies and selectively disregards stimuli of no relevance to the current motor task' (Johansson 1991, p. 349).

Johansson and Westling (1988) have also shown that the reflex responses to a given input are not invariant, but depend very much on the instructions given to the subject and on the degree of anticipatory control: a sudden increase in load of the object (triggered by an experimenter dropping a ball unexpectedly into a cup attached to the object) produced a large reflex response. But the response was very much smaller if the subject dropped the ball; in this case there were significant changes in grip force *before* the load was increased, which presumably made such large reflex changes inappropriate.

It must be said that there is no direct evidence yet for a contribution of the cortico-motoneuronal system to the different functional aspects of precision grip described above. However, the existence, in the monkey, of cortico-motoneuronal cells with muscle fields restricted to a few hand muscles, together with the rapid responses of such cells to sensory feedback from the skin, would provide an ideal mechanism for the rapid adaptation of grip force to meet new conditions at the periphery. It is also of interest that motor cortex neurones are particularly insensitive to 'irrelevant' inputs during movement (Lemon 1979; Jiang *et al.* 1990, 1991). Of particular interest is a recent observation by Edin *et al.* (1992) that during precision grip of objects in which the frictional forces on the surfaces encountered by the index finger and thumb are different, there is evidence for independent control of tangential forces exerted by the two digits. The finding that some cortico-motoneuronal cells appear to code finger and thumb forces independently (Maier *et al.* 1993), provides further circumstantial evidence for cortico-motoneuronal contributions to fine precision grip in monkeys and in man.

9.7 RELATIONS OF THE CEREBELLUM AND BASAL GANGLIA TO CORTICOSPINAL FUNCTION IN VOLUNTARY MOVEMENT

We have described in earlier chapters of this book how the corticospinal projections from the cerebral cortex come under the influence of a very large number of inputs which are demonstrably involved in contributing to voluntary movement. Recent PET studies of regional cerebral blood flow (rCBF) during the performance of voluntary arm and hand movements by human subjects demonstrate the involvement of motor cortex, supplementary motor area (SMA), and premotor cortex (Roland *et al.* 1980a; Fox *et al.* 1985; Raichle 1987; Deiber *et al.* 1991). Anatomical and functional studies in monkeys, which provide the background for interpretation of changes in premotor and supplementary motor neuronal activity during voluntary movement performance, have already been described in Chapter 7.

PET studies have also been able to illuminate local changes in the cerebellum and basal ganglia during voluntary movement. Clinicopathological correlations have, of course, historically associated damage or disease affecting the cerebellar hemisphere with intention tremor and the inability to control the rate, range and force of voluntarily initiated actions (Holmes 1939). From our earlier descriptions of the connections between the cerebellum and the motor cortex, whose outputs have been correlated with aspects of timing, direction, and force in movement performance, it could be concluded that the cerebellum may exert its influence on movement in part by way of actions relayed through corticospinal outputs. Moreover, the involuntary movements which are characteristic of particular basal ganglia diseases are well documented (Wilson 1914; Marsden 1987). Hence it should have been no surprise to Roland *et al.* (1982) to detect specific changes in rCBF in the putamen, globus pallidus, and ventrolateral thalamus when their subjects were performing a normal movement task using the fingers of one hand (Fig. 5.13, p. 243). It remains for the unique aspects of the contributions of these brain regions to the operations of intracortical networks and to the modulation of corticospinal outputs to be evaluated, and for the mechanisms by which the cerebellum and basal ganglia influence corticospinal involvement in voluntary movement to be understood.

Considerable opportunity exists to dissect the separable components of language and speech in human studies, and to seek correlation of the sites of rCBF changes with aspects of language—the recognition of single words, articulation, and the mental generation of words in the absence of external cues or prompts (Petersen *et al.* 1988; Wise *et al.* 1991a, b). Such studies can contribute to our understanding of the regional functional anatomy of the human brain in connection with a uniquely human voluntary action—speech. They also allow for insights to be obtained concerning the regional organization within the brain of learning, and remembering, as well as of correlates of the acquisition of the motor skills of articulation involved in pronouncing foreign or unfamiliar words.

Colebatch, *et al.* (1990a) used PET to study rCBF in patients exhibiting essential tremor while at rest, when postural tremor was evident, and during repetitive passive movements of the wrist. Normal subjects were also studied at rest, while maintaining the same postures without tremor and while imitating tremor voluntarily. Right-sided postural tremor of the arm was accompanied by greater flow than at rest in both cerebellar hemispheres, as well as in the left sensorimotor cortex and both premotor regions. When passive movements of the relaxed right wrist were imposed by the observer, an increase in rCBF was revealed in similar cerebral cortical areas. However, the cerebellum showed no change. When normal subjects imitated tremor of the right wrist with the arm extended, there was increased flow in both cerebellar hemispheres accompanied by the other cortical changes, including those in the supplementary motor areas and thalamus, which had been described previously by Roland *et al.* (1982). These changes always appeared as the accompaniments of a repetitive sequence of voluntary movements. Hence it must be concluded, from the study of responses to imposed movements, that the cerebellar involvement, and the rCBF changes revealed there, are not in response to the afferent signals generated either by tremor or by repetitive movements. Cerebellar activation must be associated with output drives. In essential tremor, it is conceivable that oscillations of activity in pathways affected by olivocerebellar connections impose their influence on outputs from the motor cortex through the thalamus, without the control of 'voluntary' activity which, otherwise, would be reflected in blood flow changes in supplementary motor areas. Supplementary motor area activation occurred when tremor was mimicked by normal subjects. Under these conditions the movements were cerebrally driven as a voluntary motor activity.

A number of references have been made earlier to the possible involvement of the cerebellum in generating or conditioning the sustained, plastic changes which have been demonstrated in the organization of the corticospinal outputs associated with 'motor learning'—the acquisition of new motor skills and the refinement of voluntary movement performances (Ito 1985). Seitz *et al.* (1990) measured rCBF during the course of learning a complicated sequence of voluntary finger movements in an attempt to identify the structures in the brain which showed functional neuronal change during the acquisition of the motor skill. Comparisons were made between the measures of regional flow at rest, during the initial stages of learning of the finger touching task illustrated in Fig. 5.13, during the advanced stages of learning, and then during the skilled performance of the task when maximum speed, accuracy, and precision had been acquired. They concluded that motor learning was accompanied, as it progressed, by decreases in activity in limbic and other structures, and by increases in activity in corticocerebellar and corticostriatal circuits which are also associated with the performance of the acquired skilled movements. In these experiments, the rate at which the sequence was performed was not controlled; some of the changes in rCBF may have resulted from the different numbers of slowly performed novel sequences and rapidly performed learned sequences that were included in the sample time.

Whatever the structures and the mechanisms involved, the primate brain exhibits the most remarkable plastic adaptations in situations requiring new motor strategies to be learned in order to perform essential movement tasks. While there is overwhelming evidence that major disturbances to muscle innervation, such as those produced by nerve-crossing experiments in mammals, are accompanied by no significant changes in patterns of spinal reflex organization (Eccles 1959), dramatic 'functional' modification of the central nervous system's influence on these stable 'hard wired' connections must occur to explain an animal's ability to achieve near-normal motor performance utilizing incorrect and inappropriate peripheral innervation of limb muscles after nerve regeneration. In humans, this high level of adaptability of the brain's machinery for control of co-ordinated muscle contractions allows restoration of function in denervated muscle by transposition and implantation of a foreign nerve (as in the treatment of facial palsy). It also provides for successful, effective utilization of transposed muscles or tendons in the production of appropriate useful movements of the fingers of an injured hand (Moberg 1972). Moberg's observations that muscle re-innervation after peripheral nerve lesions must be accompanied by some appropriate restoration of sensory function in order to lead to effective recovery of finger movements, would be consistent with the interactions between sensory and motor events which has been discussed above in connection with 'active touch'.

Brinkman *et al.* (1983) operated on young monkeys and produced major bilateral re-arrangements in the peripheral innervation of the distal forearm and hand by cross-union of predominantly flexor with predominantly extensor nerves. Following the period of nerve regeneration and 'incorrect' re-innervation, these animals regained the ability to perform natural, self paced voluntary movements of their hands and fingers, including the ability to perform relatively independent finger movements in a manner almost indistinguishable from normal. Recovery was excellent and hand and finger movements were performed near perfectly after ulnar-radial cross anastomosis. Moderately well controlled finger movements were acquired after median-radial cross anastomosis. As has been observed in attempts to produce useful function after nerve damage in humans by hand surgery, restoration of function in muscles normally innervated by the median nerve is difficult to achieve. In spite of this, the experiments demonstrate conclusively the adaptive capabilities of the primate central nervous system and the capacity of the primate brain to undergo plastic change. These changes allow the central controlling commands impinging on a stable complex of spinal connections to be so modified that a precise flexion movement may be produced by activation in the spinal cord of the newly connected extensor motoneurones which now innervate the motor units whose contractions are required (Porter 1985). Appropriate fractionation of muscle use is achieved. It is clearly possible that the cerebellum plays a part in the production of these plastic changes in the brain's output systems, in a manner similar to that which has been proposed for the cerebellum's role in the modification of both the gain and the phase of vestibulo-ocular reflexes when these are modified by the wearing of prismatic spectacles (Gonshor and Melvill Jones 1976).

9.8 DISTURBANCES OF CORTICOSPINAL FUNCTION AND VOLUNTARY MOVEMENT

Denny-Brown and Botterell (1948) described the modifications of motor function that were produced by lesions in area 4. It is now recognized that such lesions, while removing the intrinsic networks which are the targets for so many extrinsic projections to the motor cortex and a significant proportion of the cells of origin of the output projections which will contribute corticospinal influences, leave intact corticospinal projections from premotor, supplementary, and cingulate motor as well as from postcentral sensory areas. Nevertheless, an initial hemiplegic paralysis resulted. This rapidly resolved as recovery of movements about the proximal joints occurred leaving a residual disorder affecting movements about the distal joints. At first, both postural reactions and stretch reflexes, including the tendon jerk, were depressed. These reactions also recovered gradually and eventually the stretch reflexes reached a hyperactive stage.

The neurological sequelae of vascular lesions involving other regions of the cerebral cortex or of the internal capsule are well documented in standard neurological textbooks. After acute ischaemic brain damage, clinical recovery of aspects of neurological function is often observed. We have emphasized already that recovery of voluntary motor control may be more complete for muscles acting about the proximal joints of the limb than for those acting distally. Denny-Brown (1950) stated: 'It is commonplace to find that the patient with partial paralysis following a cortical lesion can extend or flex any one finger only by extending or flexing all fingers'. The capacity to fractionate the use of distally acting muscles is diminished when the outflow projections through the corticospinal tract are affected. The muscular weakness in movements, even of distal joints, has a characteristic distribution which is more evident in some groups of muscles (Colebatch and Gandevia 1989).

The mechanism of recovery of function after vascular lesions affecting voluntary movement could involve increased activation of neural connections spared by the ischaemic event, sprouting of collaterals previously not involved in the connectivity essential for that voluntary movement, or the utilization of ipsilateral projections from the non-damaged hemisphere. Recently, Frackowiak *et al.* (1991) used PET to study changes in the functional organization of the brain in patients recovering from anatomically defined capsular infarcts. The anatomical lesion was revealed by computed x-ray tomography (CT) scans or by magnetic resonance imaging (MRI) and, in all patients studied, the damage was confined to the striatocapsular region, without directly involving the cerebral cortex.

During separate periods of examination of rCBF, these patients performed repetitive movements of the fingers of the normal, unaffected hand and of the previously paretic, recovered hand so that, in each patient, rCBF changes accompanying movements of the normal hand were regarded as the 'control' values. When the fingers of the unaffected hand were being moved, the pattern of the changes in rCBF was most evident in the contralateral sensorimotor cortex and the ipsilateral cerebellar hemisphere. Statistically significant bilateral increases in rCBF also occurred in the supplementary motor area (SMA) and the supramarginal gyrus when the unaffected hand was used. The major finding in this study was that, when the recovered hand, contralateral to the infarct, was being used, the pattern of change in rCBF involved significant increases in the sensorimotor cortex and the cerebellar hemispheres on both sides, in addition to bilateral increases in rCBF in SMA, the supramarginal gyrus and the insular and premotor cortices. Hence it was deduced that ipsilateral motor pathways must be involved in the recovery from motor disability caused by a capsular infarct. The reorganization of corticospinal pathways after brain damage can now be detected by non invasive magnetic stimulation of the brain (Benecke *et al.* 1991; Farmer *et al.* 1990b; Capaday *et al.* 1991).

9.9 VOLUNTARY MOVEMENTS OF THE HANDS FOR LANGUAGE
AND COMMUNICATION: LATERALIZATION OF FUNCTIONS

In most cultures, oral communication between individuals is assisted and
enriched by gestures. Emphasis and embellishment of spoken language
can be provided by voluntary movements of the hands and arms, not only
in the theatre, but also in everyday conversation. In addition, a whole
linguistic system has been developed which allows deaf people to com-
municate with gestures. The gestures (signs) give meaning to visual forms
which are created by voluntary movements of the hands and arms in space
and time. The sign language is used not only in everyday conversation but
in intellectual argument, in creative communication, in scientific debate,
and in the expression of feelings through poetry, humour, or drama.
American Sign Language (ASL), we learn from Bellugi *et al.* (1989, 1990),
is 'a primary linguistic system that has been passed down from one generation of deaf people to the next'. It shares underlying principles of organization with spoken languages. However, the physical expression of those
principles utilises the formal devices that are available through the performance of gestures in three-dimensional space and with an appropriate
tempo, combined with the visual recognition and interpretation of the
subtleties and complexities of the motor performance (the handshapes
themselves, the arm movements that are made, their temporal organization
and the spatial locations within which the gestures occur). Analysis of sign
languages reveals that those that have developed independently (American
Sign Language and British Sign Language, for example) are mutually
incomprehensible — unrelated sign languages 'reveal not only differences
in lexicon and grammar, but even systematic phonetic differences that
may cause native signers from one sign language to have an 'accent' in a
newly learned sign language' (Bellugi *et al.* 1989).

Detailed study of the American Sign Language using powerful three-
dimensional computergraphic analysis of the movement gestures captured
cinematographically, and their temporal features, combined with measurements of perceptual and linguistic elements of the communication itself,
have allowed a description of the way in which syntax and grammar, for
example, are handled in this language. According to Bellugi *et al.* (1989),
'In sign language, space itself bears linguistic meaning'. In his introduction
to Poizner *et al.*'s (1987) fascinating book with the challenging title: What
the hands reveal about the brain, John C. Marshall stated: 'Communicating
in a visual language, quite unrelated to spoken English and expressed in
a transitory medium even more difficult to notate than classical ballet,
a sign language poet could not hope that his or her work would be
printed for posterity. Prior to widespread use of cinematography, the
deaf literary artist was thus deprived of the permanent record of cultural
tradition.'

Bellugi *et al.* (1990) have now used their detailed cinematographic and analytic tools to examine the nature of the deficits in sign language ability which are consequent upon damage to the brain in deaf signers. Deaf people are no less likely than those who can hear and speak to suffer major brain damage from stroke, cerebral disease or head injuries. With modern diagnostic methods such as CT scans, able to provide a delineation of the extent of cerebral damage following a stroke, the deficits observed in the performance of sign language and the decomposition of the structure of this language itself could be correlated, in deaf stroke victims, with regions of anatomical and functional specialization defined for the brains of those possessed of the ability to hear and speak. Deaf patients, who had always communicated in sign language, and who had suffered either a right- or left-sided stroke, were assessed using a battery of tests designed to measure their sign language capacity, their spatial cognitive abilities, and their motor function in spatial tasks. The results of such studies emphasize several features of the brain's organization for the control of voluntary movement of the hand which are pertinent to the topic of this book.

Lateralization of the language functions of the brain to the left hemisphere has been a principle of neurology since the initial establishment of the concept of localization of function by Broca in the 1860s (see Chapter 1). Knowledge of spatial relationships and the organization of spatial aspects of human behaviour, including voluntary movement of the hands and arms within this visuospatial environment, has been known for a similarly long period to depend, in considerable measure, on normal function of the right cerebral hemisphere. What happens to deaf patients, dependent for communication upon the use of gestures organized in a spatial domain, which space itself is an element of language, when afflicted by a left- or right-sided stroke?

Bellugi *et al.* (1990) studied a number of such patients. Left hemisphere damage led to clear sign language aphasias. 'One left hemisphere damaged signer (GD) was agrammatic for ASL [American Sign Language]. After her stroke, her signing was severely impaired; it was halting and effortful, and reduced to single sign utterances, shorn of the syntactic and morpho-logical markings of ASL.' The form of the disorder recognized in the sign language decomposition depended upon the location of the brain damage. Lesions principally affecting the left frontal or the left parietal regions produced different effects. Left frontal lesions severely limited sign language and reduced it to simple, non-fluent utterances. Left parietal lesions could produce significant disturbances in sign comprehension and many errors in sign production which, while perhaps remaining fluent in performance, could be grammatically inappropriate and jargon-like. Here we recognize that the local and regional organization of the left hemisphere in the deaf, as well as in those who can hear, must have a genetic predisposition to become specialized for language development.

This specialization does not depend on sound and hearing or on the acquisition of speech. This specialization for language is available, we presume through the motor cortex and its cortico-motoneuronal connections, to be expressed by means of the voluntary control of the hands and arms in gesture-visual communication.

Even though the right hemisphere has a major role to play in the organization of, and knowledge of, spatial relationships, and in spite of the essential spatial nature of sign language, right hemisphere strokes did not render deaf users of sign language aphasic. After right hemisphere damage, these patients exhibited fluent, virtually error-free communication with a good range of grammatical forms and no defects in the accurate performance of their signs. It is particularly of note that, even though patients with right-sided lesions frequently neglected the left side of their extra-personal space in non-language tasks, they correctly included signs within this left space in their spatially organized sign language, and exhibited no impairment in the grammatical aspects of their communication, which depended on voluntary movements within this left space. Bellugi *et al.* (1989) describe their observations: 'Across a range of tasks, including drawing, spatial construction, spatial attention, judgement of line orientation, facial discrimination, right-lesioned signers showed the classical visuospatial impairments seen in hearing patients with right hemisphere damage . . . Even the right-lesioned signer who was an artist before her stroke showed disorganisation, failure to indicate perspective, and neglect of left hemispace in her drawings afterwards.' Yet she had no defects in her sign language.

We have referred earlier to the task-specific nature of the particular behaviours that have been observed in neurophysiological experiments, analysing neurones and their functional connections in monkeys and in man (Chapter 5). It appears that even the specialized role of a region of cerebral cortex may be dependent on the context within which its task is to be performed. The specialized function of the right hemisphere for managing spatial relationships is revealed when knowledge of those spatial relationships or the expressive description of them by voluntary action such as drawing, is required. However, language is the specialized function of the left hemisphere. For deaf users of sign language, in which spatial relationships are essential elements of that language, the spatial requirements of syntax are the province of the left hemisphere, and voluntary movements within that space, for language purposes, are under left hemisphere control.

Within this book we have referred in many places to the capacities of modern imaging techniques and non-invasive stimulation studies to illuminate the anatomical substrates involved in voluntary movement performance in human subjects. They can be used to depict functional maps of the human brain or to assess functional competence in defined neuronal systems. The use of these techniques, and the more fine-grained elaborations that we may expect to become available in the future, to study motor performances in speech, in sign language, and in other purposeful voluntary actions is likely to advance our understanding of the brain's motor functions in quite dramatic ways. It is to be hoped that these studies will not only allow us better to describe and explain the effects of brain damage on voluntary movement performance, but, in the long term, to help by providing remedial assistance and scientifically determined rehabilitation strategies for restoration of neurological function.

The era of non-invasive investigation is just dawning, and at this time we can offer our readers only a fascinating glimpse of the power of these new techniques to give new insights and real understanding of the human brain and its involvement in the management of voluntary movement. These techniques are already being used to diagnose the location of damage to the motor system in patients, to assess the patient's prospects of recovery, to stimulate new approaches to therapeutic treatments, and to guide the interventions that may assist an individual's rehabilitation. But we should not forget that much of our ability to interpret and comprehend the new pictures of brain performance, that the non invasive techniques offer, is based upon decades of animal research which have provided the essential details of the anatomy, physiology, and behaviour of the integrated motor system within the brain. It is now becoming clear that many of these results are of great value in understanding the changes that follow damage to the motor system, and that they have provided the sound scientific framework upon which further understanding can be built.

References

[Numbers in brackets indicate page on which the reference is cited]

Abbs, J. H. and Cole, K. J. (1987). Neural mechanisms of motor equivalence and goal achievement. In *Higher mechanisms of brain function* (eds. S. Wise and E. V. Evarts), pp. 15–43. Wiley, New York. [314]

Abeles, M. (1991). *Corticonics. Neural circuits of the cerebral cortex.* Cambridge University Press. [162]

Abzug, C. M., Maeda, M., Peterson, B. W., and Wilson, V. J. (1974). Cervical branching of lumbar vestibulospinal axons. *J. Physiol.* **243**, 499–522. [147]

Adrian, E. D. and Moruzzi, G. (1939). Impulses in the pyramidal tract. *J. Physiol.* **97**, 153–199. [249]

Ageranioti, S. A. and Chapman, C. E. (1989). Gating of cutaneous inputs during an active tactile discrimination task versus passive receptive field testing in the monkey. *Soc. Neurosci. Abstr.* **15**, 314. [270]

Aguilar, M. J. (1969). Recovery of motor function after unilateral infarction of the basis pontis. *Am. J. Phys. Med.* **48**, 279–288. [116]

Albe-Fessard, D. and Liebeskind, J. (1966). Origine des messages somato-sensitifs activant les cellules du cortex moteur chez le singe. *Exp. Brain Res.* **1**, 127–146. [254]

Albe-Fessard, D., Lamarre, Y., and Pimpaneau, A. (1966). Sur l'origine fusoriale de certaines afférences somatiques atteignant le cortex moteur du singe. *J. Physiol. (Paris)* **58**, 443–444. [254]

Alexander, G. E. and Crutcher, M. D. (1990a). Preparation for movement: neural representations of intended direction in three motor areas of the monkey. *J. Neurophysiol.* **64**, 133–150. [230, 290, 344, 351]

Alexander, G. E. and Crutcher, M. D. (1990b). Neural representations of the target (goal) of visually guided arm movements in three motor areas of the monkey. *J. Neurophysiol.* **64**, 164–178. [230]

Allen, G. I. and Tsukahara, N. (1974). Cerebrocerebellar communication systems. *Physiol. Rev.* **54**, 975. [58]

Allum, J. H. J., Hepp-Reymond, M.-C., and Gysin, R. (1982). Cross-correlation analysis of interneuronal connectivity in the motor cortex of the monkey. *Brain Res.* **231**, 325–334. [45]

Alstermark, B. and Kümmel, H. (1990a). Transneuronal transport of wheat germ agglutinin conjugated horseradish peroxidase into last order spinal inter-neurones projecting to acromio- and spinodeltoideus motoneurones in cat. 1. Location of labelled interneurones and influence of synaptic activity on the transneuronal transport. *Exp. Brain Res.* **80**, 83–95. [130]

Alstermark, B. and Kümmel, H. (1990b). Transneuronal transport of wheat germ agglutinin conjugated horseradish peroxidase into last order spinal inter-neurones projecting to acromio- and spinodeltoideus motoneurones in cat. 2. Differential labelling of interneurones depending on movement type. *Exp. Brain Res.* **80**, 96–103. [130, 132]

Alstermark, B. and Sasaki, S. (1986). Integration in descending motor pathways controlling the forelimb in the cat. 14. Differential projection to fast and slow motoneurones from excitatory C3–C4 propriospinal neurones. *Exp. Brain Res.* **63**, 530–542. [189]

Alstermark, B., Lundberg, A., Norrsell, U., and Sybirska, E. (1981). Integration in descending motor pathways controlling the forelimb in the cat. 9. Differential behavioural defects after spinal cord lesions interrupting defined pathways from higher centres to motoneurones. *Exp. Brain Res.* **42**, 299–318. [117, 118]

Alstermark, B., Pinter, M., and Sasaki, S. (1983a). Brainstem relay of disynaptic pyramidal EPSPs to neck motoneurons in the cat. *Brain Res.* **259**, 147–150. [61]

Alstermark, B., Pinter, M., and Sasaki, S. (1983b). Convergence on reticulospinal neurons mediating contralateral pyramidal disynaptic EPSPs to neck motoneurons. *Brain Res.* **259**, 151–154. [61]

Alstermark, B., Lundberg, A., and Sasaki, S. (1984). Integration in descending motor pathways controlling the forelimb in the cat. 12. Interneurones which may mediate descending feed-forward inhibition and feed-back inhibition from the forelimb to C3–C4 propriospinal neurones. *Exp. Brain Res.* **56**, 308–322. [132]

Alstermark, B., Górska, T., Johannisson, T., and Lundberg, A. (1986). Effects of dorsal column transection in the upper cervical segments on visually guided forelimb movements. *Neurosci. Res.* **3**, 462–466. [119]

Alstermark, B., Lundberg, A., Pettersson, L.-G., Tantisera, B., and Walkowska, M. (1987). Motor recovery after serial spinal cord lesions of defined descending pathways in cats. *Neurosci. Res.* **5**, 68–73. [119]

Alstermark, B., Isa, T., Lundberg, A., Petterson, L.-G., and Tantisira, B. (1990a). The effect of low pyramidal lesions on forelimb movements in the cat. *Neurosci. Res.* **7**, 71–75. [119]

Alstermark, B., Kümmel, H., Pinter, M., and Tantisera, B. (1990b). Integration in descending motor pathways controlling the forelimb in the cat. 17. Axonal projection and termination of C3–C4 propriospinal neurones in the C6–Th1 segments. *Exp. Brain Res.* **81**, 447–461. [130, 132]

Alstermark, B., Isa, T., and Tantisira, B. (1991). Integration in descending motor pathways controlling the forelimb in the cat. 18. Morphology and termination of collaterals from C3–C4 propriospinal neurones in the segment of origin. *Exp. Brain Res.* **84**, 561–568. [132]

Amassian, V. E. and Berlin, L. (1958). Early cortical projections of group I afferents in the forelimb muscle nerves of the cat. *J. Physiol.* **143**, 61P. [249]

Amassian, V. E. and Ross, R. J. (1978). Developing role of sensorimotor cortex and pyramidal tract neurons in contact placing in kittens. *J. Physiol. (Paris)* **74**, 165–184. [103]

Amassian, V. E. and Weiner, H. (1966). Monosynaptic and polysynaptic activation of pyramidal tract neurons by thalamic stimulation. In *The thalamus* (eds. D. P. Purpura and M. D. Yahr), pp. 256–281. Columbia University Press, New York. [49]

Amassian, V. E., Stewart, M., Quirk, G. J., and Rosenthal, J. L. (1987). Physiological basis of motor effects of a transient stimulus to cerebral cortex. *Neurosurg.* **20**, 74–93. [305]

Andersen, P., Hagan, P. J., Phillips, C. G., and Powell, T. P. S. (1975). Mapping by microstimulation of overlapping projections from area 4 to motor units of the baboon's hand. *Proc. R. Soc. London, Ser. B.* **188**, 31-60. [187, 313, 317, 319, 321, 322, 323, 326]

Antinucci, F. and Visalberghi, E. (1986). Tool use in Cebus apella: A case study. *Int. J. Primatol.* **7**(4), 351-363. [94]

Aoki, M., Fujito, Y., Satomi, H., Kurosawa, Y., and Kasaba, T. (1986). The possible role of collateral sprouting in the functional restitution of corticospinal connections after spinal hemisection. *Neurosci. Res.* **3**, 617-627. [112]

Araki, T., Endo, K., Kawai, Y., Ito, K., and Shigenaga, Y. (1976). Supraspinal control of slow and fast spinal motoneurones of the cat. *Prog. Brain Res.* **44**, 413-432. [189]

Armand, J. (1982). The origin, course and terminations of corticospinal fibers in various mammals. *Prog. Brain Res.* **57**, 329-360. [77, 79, 83, 84, 85, 86, 88, 315]

Armand, J. and Kuypers, H. G. J. M. (1980). Cells of origin of crossed and uncrossed corticospinal fibers in the cat. *Exp. Brain Res.* **40**, 23-34. [83]

Armand, J., Holstege, G., and Kuypers, H. G. J. M. (1985). Differential corticospinal projections in the cat. An autoradiographic tracing study. *Brain Res.* **343**, 351-355. [79, 86]

Armand, J., Kably, B., and Jacomy, H. (1991). Lesion-induced plasticity of the pyramidal tract during development in the cat. In *Tutorials in motor neuroscience* (eds. J. Requin & G. E. Stelmach), pp. 625-640. Kluwer Academic Publishers. [99, 100]

Armstrong, D. M. (1965). Inhibitory actions on pyramidal neurones. B.Sc. thesis. Oxford University. [238]

Armstrong, D. M. and Drew, T. (1984a). Discharges of pyramidal tract and other motor cortical neurones during locomotion in the cat. *J. Physiol.* **346**, 471-495. [210, 238, 351]

Armstrong, D. M. and Drew, T. (1984b). Locomotor-related neuronal discharges in cat motor cortex compared with peripheral receptive fields and evoked movements. *J. Physiol.* **346**, 497-517. [160, 238]

Armstrong, D. M. and Drew, T. (1984c). Topographical localization in the motor cortex of the cat for somatic afferent responses and evoked movements. *J. Physiol.* **350**, 33-54. [248, 259, 317, 329]

Armstrong, D. M. and Drew, T. (1985a). Electromyographic response evoked in muscles of the forelimb by intracortical stimulation in the cat. *J. Physiol.* **367**, 309 326. [312, 317, 324, 329, 335]

Armstrong, D. M. and Drew, T. (1985b). Forelimb electromyographic responses to motor cortex stimulation during locomotion in the cat. *J. Physiol.* **367**, 327-351. [324]

Asanuma, C., Thach, W. T., and Jones, E. G. (1983). Distribution of cerebellar terminations and their relation to other afferent terminations in the ventral lateral thalamic region of the monkey. *Brain Res. Rev.* **5**, 237-265. [263]

Asanuma, H. (1975). Recent developments in the study of the columnar arrangement of neurons within the motor cortex. *Physiol. Rev.* **55**, 143-156. [343]

Asanuma, H. (1981). The pyramidal tract. In *Handbook of physiology—the nervous system II* (eds. J. M. Brookhart and V. B. Mountcastle), pp. 703–733. American Physiological Society, Bethesda, Maryland. [312, 343]

Asanuma, H. (1989). *The motor cortex*. Raven, New York. [343]

Asanuma, H. and Arissian, K. (1984). Experiments on functional role of peripheral input to motor cortex during voluntary movements in the monkey. *J. Neurophysiol.* 52, 212–227. [110, 261]

Asanuma, H. and Arnold, A. P. (1975). Noxious effects of excessive currents used for intracortical stimulation. *Brain Res.* 96, 103–107. [305]

Asanuma, H. and Keller, A. (1991). Neurobiological basis of motor learning and memory. *Concepts in Neurosci.* 2, 1–30. [56]

Asanuma, H. and Rosén, I. (1972). Topographical organisation of cortical efferent zones projecting to distal forelimb muscles in the monkey. *Exp. Brain. Res.* 14, 243–256. [48, 313, 322]

Asanuma, H. and Sakata, H. (1967). Functional organization of a cortical efferent system examined with focal depth stimulation in cats. *J. Neurophysiol.* 30, 35–54. [48, 306, 312, 313]

Asanuma, H., Stoney, S. D., and Abzug, C. (1968). Relationship between afferent input and motor outflow in cat motorsensory cortex. *J. Neurophysiol.* 31, 670–681. [249, 334]

Asanuma, H., Fernandes, J., Schiebel, M. E., and Schiebel, A. B. (1974). Characteristics of projections from the nucleus ventralis lateralis to the motor cortex in cats. An anatomical and physiological study. *Exp. Brain Res.* 20, 315–330. [50, 310]

Asanuma, H., Arnold, A., and Zarzecki, P. (1976). Further study on the excitation of pyramidal tract cells by intracortical microstimulation. *Exp. Brain Res.* 26, 443–461. [305, 306, 314]

Asanuma, H., Zarzecki, P., Jankowska, E., Hongo, T., and Marcus, S. (1979). Projection of individual pyramidal tract neurons to lumbar motor nuclei of the monkey. *Exp. Brain Res.* 34, 73–89. [178, 179, 326]

Asanuma, H., Larsen, K., and Yumiya, H. (1980). Peripheral input pathways to the monkey motor cortex. *Exp. Brain Res.* 38, 349–355. [261]

Asanuma, H., Babb, R. S., Mori, A., and Waters, R. S. (1981). Input–output relationships in cat's motor cortex after pyramidal section. *J. Neurophysiol.* 46, 694–703. [329, 332]

Ashby, P. and Wiens, M. (1989). Reciprocal inhibition following lesions of the spinal cord in man. *J. Physiol.* 414, 145– 157. [205]

Ashby, P. and Zilm, D. (1982a). Relationship between EPSP shape and cross-correlation profile explored by computer simulation for studies on human motoneurons. *Exp. Brain Res.* 47, 33–40. [133, 134, 135, 192]

Ashby, P. and Zilm, D. (1982b). Characteristics of postsynaptic potentials produced in single human motoneurons by homonymous group 1 volleys. *Exp. Brain Res.* 47, 41–48. [133]

Bach-y-Rita, P. (1981). Brain plasticity as a basis for the development of rehabilitation procedures for hemiplegia. *Scand. J. Rehab. Med.* 13, 73–80. [113]

Baker, M. A., Tyner, C. F., and Towe, A. L. (1971). Observations on single neurons recorded in the sigmoid gyri of awake, non-paralysed cats. *Exp. Neurol.* 32, 388–403. [249]

Baker, J. R., Bremner, F. D., Cole, J. D., and Stephens, J. A. (1988). Short-term synchronization of intrinsic hand muscle motor units in a 'Deafferented' man. *J. Physiol.* **396**, 155P. [177]

Baldissera, F. and Pierrot-Deseilligny, E. (1989). Facilitation of transmission in the pathway of non-monosynaptic Ia excitation to wrist flexor motoneurones at the onset of voluntary movement in man. *Exp. Brain Res.* **74**, 437–439. [136, 137, 353]

Baldissera, F., Hultborn, H., and Illert, M. (1981). Integration in spinal neuronal systems. In *Handbook of physiology — the nervous system II* (eds. J. M. Brookhart and V. B. Mountcastle), pp. 509–595. American Physiological Society, Bethesda, Maryland. [27, 132, 143, 202, 207]

Bannister, C. M. and Porter, R. (1967). Effects of limited direct stimulation of the medullary pyramidal tract on spinal motoneurons in the rat. *Exp. Neurol.* **17**, 265–275. [86]

Baranyi, A. and Szente, M. B. (1987). Long-lasting potentiation of synaptic transmission requires postsynaptic modifications in the neocortex. *Brain Res.* **423**, 378–384. [342]

Bard, P. (1938). Studies on the cortical representation of somatic sensibility. *Harvey Lect.* **33**, 143–169. [117]

Barnard, J. W. and Woolsey, C. N. (1956). A study of localization in the cortico-spinal tracts of monkey and rat. *J. Comp. Neurol.* **105**, 25–50. [83, 115]

Barron, D. H. (1934). The results of unilateral pyramidal section in the rat. *J. Comp. Neurol.* **60**, 45–56. [119]

Bates, C. A. and Killackey, H. P. (1984). The emergence of discretely distributed pattern of corticospinal projection neurones. *Dev. Brain Res.* **13**, 265–273. [97]

Bawa, P., and Lemon, R. N. (1993). Recruitment of motor units in response to transcranial magnetic stimulation in man. *J. Physiol.* (in press). [190, 193]

Beevor, C. E. and Horsley, V. (1890). A record of the results obtained by electrical excitation of the so-called motor cortex and internal capsule in an Organ-Outan (Simia satyrus). *Phil. Trans. R. Soc. London, Ser. B.* **181**, 129–158. [6]

Belhaj Saif, A., Fourment, A. and Maton, B. (1990). Post-spike facilitation of elbow muscle activity by area 4 cells in monkey isometric contraction. *Europ. J. Neurosci.* suppl. 3, 1290. [189]

Bell, C. (1833). *The hand: Its mechanism and vital endowments as evincing design*, The Bridgewater Treatises, IV. Pickering, London. [356]

Bellugi, U., Poizner, H., and Klima, E. S. (1989). Language, modality and the brain. *Trends in Neurosci.* **12**, 380–388. [363]

Bellugi, U., Poizner, H., and Klima, E. S. (1990). Mapping brain function for language: evidence from sign language. In *Signal and sense: local and global order in perceptual maps* (eds. G. M. Edelman, W. E. Gall, and W. M. Cowan), pp. 521–543. Wiley-Liss, New York. [363, 364]

Benecke, R., Meyer, B.-U., and Freund, H.-J. (1991). Reorganisation of descending motor pathways in patients after hemispherectomy and severe hemispheric lesions demonstrated by magnetic brain stimulation. *Exp. Brain Res.* **83**, 419–426. [100, 115, 116, 362]

Bennett, K. M. B. (1992). Corticomotoneuronal control of precision grip tasks. Thesis, Cambridge University. [175, 179, 181, 182, 237]

Bennett, K. M. B. and Lemon, R. N. (1991). The activity of monkey cortico-motoneuronal (CM) cells is related to their pattern of post-spike facilitation of intrinsic hand muscles. *J. Physiol.* **435**, 53. [174]

Bennett, K. M. B., Lemon, R. N., and Werner, W. (1989). Indirect excitation of corticospinal neurones by intracortical stimulation in the conscious monkey. *J. Physiol.* **418**, 103. [204, 306]

Bentivoglio, M. and Rustioni, A. (1986). Corticospinal neurons with branching axons to the dorsal column nuclei in the monkey. *J. Comp. Neurol.* **253**, 260–276. [61, 66]

Berardelli, A., Sabra, A. F., and Hallett, M. (1983). Physiological mechanisms of rigidity in Parkinson's disease. *J. Neurol. Neurosurg. Psychiat.* **46**, 45–53. [271]

Berkley, K. (1983). Spatial relationships between the terminations of somatic sensory motor pathways in the rostral brainstem of cats and monkeys. II. Cerebellar projections compared with those of the ascending somatic sensory pathways in lateral diencephalon. *J. Comp. Neurol.* **220**, 229–251. [261]

Bernhard, C. G. and Bohm, E. (1954). Cortical representation and functional significance of the corticomotoneuronal system. *Arch. Neurol. Psychiat.* **72**, 473–502. [146]

Bernhard, C. G., Bohm, E. and Petersén, I. (1953). Investigations on the organization of the corticospinal system in monkeys (Macaca Mulatta). *Acta Physiol. Scand.* **29**, suppl. 106, 79–105. [94, 146, 353]

Bernstein, N. (1967). *The co-ordination and regulation of movements*. Pergamon, Oxford. [345]

Biber, M. P., Kneisley, L. W., and LaVail, J. H. (1978). Cortical neurons projecting to the cervical and lumbar enlargements of the spinal cord in young and adult monkeys. *Exp. Neurol.* **59**, 492–508. [97]

Bishop, A. (1964). Use of the hand in lower primates. In *Evolutionary and genetic biology of primates* (ed. J. Buettner-Janusch), Vol. 2, pp. 133–225. Academic Press, New York. [93]

Bishop, P. O., Jeremy, D., and Lance, J. W. (1953). Properties of pyramidal tract. *J. Neurophysiol.* **16**, 537–550. [52, 165]

Bodian, D. (1975). Origin of specific types in the motoneuron neuropil of the monkey. *J. Comp. Neurol.* **159**, 225–244. [153]

Boivie, J., Grant, G., Albe-Fessard, D., and Levante, A. (1975). Evidence for a projection to the thalamus from the external cuneate nucleus in the monkey. *Neurosci. Letts.* **1**, 3–8. [261]

Boniface, S. J., Mills, K. R., and Schubert, M. (1991). Responses of single motoneurons to magnetic brain stimulation in healthy subjects and patients with multiple sclerosis. *Brain* **114**, 643–662. [190]

Bortoff, G. A. and Strick, P. L. (1990). Termination of corticospinal efferents within the cervical cord of New World primates. *Soc. Neurosci. Abstr.* **16**, 729. [94]

Botteron, G. W. and Cheney, P. D. (1989). Corticomotoneuronal postspike effects in averages of unrectified EMG activity. *J. Neurophysiol.* **62**, 1127–1139. [155]

Bregman, B. S. and Goldberger, M. E. (1982). Anatomical plasticity and sparing of function after spinal cord damage in neonatal cats. *Science* **217**, 553–555. [100, 112]

Bregman, B. S. and Goldberger, M. E. (1983). Infant lesion effect: III. Anatomical correlates of sparing and recovery of function after spinal cord damage in newborn and adult cats. *Devel. Brain Res.* **9**, 137–154. [100]

Bremner, F. D., Baker, J. R. and Stephens, J. A. (1991a). Correlation between the discharge of motor units recorded from the same and from different finger muscles in man. *J. Physiol.* **432**, 355–380. [175]

Bremner, F. D., Baker, J. R., and Stephens, J. A. (1991b). Variation in the degree of synchronization exhibited by motor units lying in different finger muscles in man. *J. Physiol.* **432**, 381–399. [175]

Brink, E., Harrison, P. J., Jankowska, E., McCrea, D. A. and Skoog, B. (1983a). Post-synaptic potentials in a population of motoneurones following activity of single interneurones in the cat. *J. Physiol.* **343**, 341–359. [130]

Brink, E., Jankowska, E., McCrea, D. A., and Skoog, B. (1983b). Inhibitory interactions between interneurones in reflex pathways from group Ia and group Ib afferents in the cat. *J. Physiol.* **343**, 361–373. [130, 131]

Brinkman C. (1974) Split-brain monkeys: cerebral control of contralateral and ipsilateral arm, hand and finger movements. Thesis, Erasmus University, Rotterdam. [110, 111]

Brinkman, C. (1981). Lesions in supplementary motor area interfere with a monkey's performance of a bimanual coordination task. *Neurosci. Letts.* **27**, 267–270. [292, 293]

Brinkman, C. (1984). Supplementary motor area of the monkey's cerebral cortex: short- and long-term deficits after unilateral ablation and the effects of subsequent callosal section. *J. Neurosci.* **4**, 918–929. [292, 293]

Brinkman, J. and Kuypers, H. G. J. M. (1973). Cerebral control of contralateral and ipsilateral arm, hand and finger movements in the split-brain Rhesus monkey. *Brain* **96**, 653– 674. [74, 112, 354, 355]

Brinkman, C. and Porter, R. (1979). Supplementary motor area in the monkey: Activity of neurons during performance of a learned motor task. *J. Neurophysiol.* **42**, 681–709. [277, 279, 280, 281, 282, 283, 290, 300]

Brinkman, C. and Porter, R. (1983). Supplementary motor area and premotor area of monkey cerebral cortex: functional organization and activities of single neurons during performance of a learned movement. In *Motor control mechanisms in health and disease* (ed. J. E. Desmedt), pp. 393–420. Raven, New York. [299]

Brinkman, J., Bush, B. M., and Porter, R. (1978). Deficient influences of peripheral stimuli on precentral neurones in monkeys with dorsal column lesions. *J. Physiol.* **276**, 27–48. [110, 260]

Brinkman, J., Porter, R., and Norman, J. (1983). Plasticity of motor behavior in monkeys with crossed forelimb nerves. *Science* **220**, 438–440. [361]

Brinkman, J., Colebatch, J. G., Porter, R., and York, D. H. (1985). Responses of precentral cells during cooling of post-central cortex in conscious monkey. *J. Physiol.* **368**, 611–625. [263]

Broca, P. P. (1861) quoted from Goldstein, K. (1953) In *The founders of neurology* (ed. Webb Haymaker), pp. 259–263. Thomas, Springfield, Illinois. [2]

Brock, L. G., Coombs, J. S., and Eccles, J. C. (1952). The recording of potentials from motoneurones with an intracellular electrode. *J. Physiol.* **117**, 431–460. [126]

Brodal, P. (1978). The corticopontine projection in the rhesus monkey. Origin and principles of organization. *Brain* **101**, 251–283. [58]

Brodal, A., Taber, E., and Walberg, F. (1960). The raphe nuclei of the brain stem in the cat. II. Efferent connections. *J. Comp. Neurol.* **114**, 239–259. [61]

Brodmann, K. (1906). Beiträge zur histologischen Lokalisation der Grosshirnrinde. Fünfte Mitteilung: Über den allgemeinen Baulan des Cortex pallii bei den Mammaliern und Zwei homologe Rindenfelder im besondern. *J. Psychol. Neurol.* (Lpz) **25**, 275–400. [13, 15]

Brooks, V. B. and Stoney, S. D. (1971). Motor mechanisms: the role of the pyramidal system in motor control. *Ann. Rev. Physiol.* **33**, 265–277. [249]

Brooks, V. B., Rudomin, P., and Slayman, C. L. (1961a). Sensory activation of neurons in the cats' cerebral cortex. *J. Neurophysiol.* **24**, 286–301. [249]

Brooks, V. B., Rudomin, P., and Slayman, C. L. (1961b). Peripheral receptive fields of neurons in the cats' cerebral cortex. *J. Neurophysiol.* **24**, 302–325. [249]

Brouwer, B. and Ashby, P. (1990). Corticospinal projections to upper and lower limb spinal motoneurons in man. *Electroenceph. Clin. Neurophysiol.* **76**, 509–519. [192, 193]

Brown, A. G. (1981). *Organization in the spinal cord.* Springer Berlin. [124]

Brown, A. G. and Fyffe, R. E. W. (1978). The morphology of group Ia afferent fibre collaterals in the spinal cord of the cat. *J. Physiol.* **274**, 111–127. [124, 153]

Brown, A. G. and Fyffe, R. E. W. (1981). Direct observations on the contacts made between Ia afferent fibres and α-motoneurones in the cat's lumbosacral spinal cord. *J. Physiol.* **313**, 121–140. [139, 153]

Brown, L. T. (1971). Projections and termination of the corticospinal tract in rodents. *Exp. Brain Res.* **13**, 432–450. [82, 86]

Brown, M. C., Lawrence, D. G., and Matthews, P. B. C. (1968). Antidromic inhibition of presumed motoneurones by repetitive stimulation of the ventral root in the decerebrate cat. *Experienta* **24**, 1210. [30]

Brown, T. G. and Sherrington, C. S. (1912). On the instability of a cortical point. *Proc. R. Soc. London, Ser. B.* **85**, 250–277. [20, 25, 339]

Bruce, I. C. and Tatton, W. G. (1980a). Sequential output–input maturation of kitten motor cortex. *Exp. Brain Res.* **39**, 411–419. [103]

Bruce, I. C. and Tatton, W. G. (1980b). Synchronous development of motor cortical output to different muscles in the kitten. *Exp. Brain Res.* **40**, 349–353. [103]

Bruce, I. C. and Tatton, W. G. (1981). Descending projections to the cervical spinal cord in the developing kitten. *Neurosci. Lett.* **25**, 227–231. [98]

Bucy, P. C., Keplinger, J. E., and Siqueira, E. B. (1964). Destruction of the 'Pyramidal Tract' in man. *J. Neurosurg.* **21**, 385–398. [115, 350]

Buller, N. P., Garnett, R., and Stephens, J. A. (1980). The reflex responses of single motor units in human hand muscles following muscle afferent stimulation. *J. Physiol.* **303**, 337–349. [135]

Burke, D., Hicks, R. G., and Stephen, J. P. H. (1990) Corticospinal volleys evoked by anodal and cathodal stimulation of the human motor cortex. *J. Physiol.* **425**, 283–299. [190]

Burke, R. E. (1968). Group Ia synaptic input to fast and slow twitch motor units of cat triceps surae. *J. Physiol.* **196**, 605–630. [127]

Burke, R. E. (1981). Motor units: anatomy, physiology, and functional organization. In *Handbook of physiology — the nervous system II* (eds. J. M. Brookhart and V. B. Mountcastle), pp. 345–422. American Physiological Society, Bethesda, Maryland. [29]

Burke, R. E., Walmsley, B., and Hodgson, J. A. (1979). HRP anatomy of group Ia afferent contacts on alpha motoneurones. *Brain Res.* **160**, 347–352. [138, 139]

Buser, P. (1966). Subcortical controls of pyramidal activity. In *The thalamus* (eds. D. P. Purpura and M. D. Yahr), pp. 323–347. Columbia University Press. New York. [249]

Buys, E. J., Lemon, R. N., Mantel, G. W. H., and Muir, R. B. (1986). Selective facilitation of different hand muscles by single corticospinal neurones in the conscious monkey. *J. Physiol.* **381**, 529–549. [148, 169, 173, 174, 181, 236]

Caliebe, F., Häussler, J., Illert, M., and Nath, D. (1991). X-ray investigations in the cat of the target-reaching and food-taking movements. *Eur. J. Neurosci.* suppl. 4, **304**. [91]

Campbell, A. W. (1905). *Histological studies on the localization of cerebral function*. Cambridge University Press. [4, 10, 12, 13, 14, 15, 16, 24]

Capaday, C., Forget, R., Fraser, R., and Lamarre, Y. (1991). Evidence for a contribution of the motor cortex to the long-latency stretch reflex of the human thumb. *J. Physiol.* **440**, 243–255. [268, 362]

Carlson, M. (1984). Development of tactile discrimination capacity in Macaca mulatta. I. Normal infants. *Dev. Brain Res.* **16**, 69–82. [104]

Casale, E. J., Light, A. R., and Rustioni, A. (1988). Direct projection of the corticospinal tract to the superficial laminae of the spinal cord in the rat. *J. Comp. Neurol.* **278**, 275–286. [86]

del Castillo, J. and Katz, B. (1954). Quantal components of the end-plate potential. *J. Physiol.* **124**, 560–573. [138]

Castro, A. J. (1972). Motor performance in rats. The effects of pyramidal tract section. *Brain Res.* **44**, 313–323. [119]

Castro, A. J. (1975). Ipsilateral corticospinal projections after large lesions of the cerebral hemisphere in neonatal rats. *Exp. Neurol.* **46**, 1–8. [99]

Castro, A. J. (1978). Analysis of corticospinal and rubrospinal projections after neonatal pyramidotomy in rats. *Brain Res.* **144**, 155–158. [99]

Catsman-Berrevoets, C.E., and Kuypers, H. G. J. M. (1976). Cells of origin of cortical projections to dorsal column nuclei, spinal cord and bulbar medial reticular formation in the rhesus monkey. *Neurosci. Letts.* **3**, 245–252. [61]

Catsman-Berrevoets, C. E. and Kuypers, H. G. J. M. (1978). Differential laminar distribution of corticothalamic neurons projecting to the VL and the center median. An HRP study in the cynomolgus monkey. *Brain Res.* **154**, 359–365. [56]

Catsman-Berrevoets, C. E., Kuypers, H. G. J. M. and Lemon, R. N. (1979). Cells of origin of the frontal projections to magnocellular and parvocellular red nucleus and superior colliculus in cynomolgus monkey. An HRP study. *Neurosci. Letts.* **12**, 41–46. [56, 58, 63]

Cavallari, P., Edgley, S. A., and Jankowska, E. (1987). Post-synaptic actions of midlumbar interneurones on motoneurones of hind-limb muscles in the cat. *J. Physiol.* **389**, 675–699. [130]

Chang, H., Ruch, T. G., and Ward, A. A. (1947). Topographical representation of muscles in motor cortex of monkeys. *J. Neurophysiol.* **11**, 39–56. [313, 314, 325]

Chao, E. Y. S., An, K.-N., Cooney, W. P., and Linscheid, R. L. (1989). *Biomechanics of the hand*, pp. 31–72. World Scientific Publishing, Singapore. [94]

Chapman, C. E. and Wiesendanger, M. (1982). Recovery of function following unilateral lesions of the bulbar pyramid in the monkey. *Electroenceph. & Clin. Neurophysiol.* **53**, 374–387. [113]

Chapman, C. E., Jiang, W., and Lamarre, Y. (1988). Modulation of lemniscal input during conditioned arm movements in the monkey. *Exp. Brain Res.* **72**, 316–334. [66, 269]

Cheema, S., Whitsel, B. L., and Rustioni, A. (1983). The corticocuneate pathway in the cat: Relations among terminal distribution patterns, cytoarchitecture and single neuron functional properties. *Somatosensory Res.* **1**, 169–205. [61]

Cheema, S., Fyffe, R., Light, A., and Rustioni, A. (1984a). Arborizations of single cortifugal axons in the feline cuneate nucleus stained by iontophoretic injection of horseradish peroxidase. *Brain Res.* **290**, 158–164. [61, 66]

Cheema, S. S., Rustioni, A., and Whitsel, B. L. (1984b). Light and electron microscopic evidence for a direct corticospinal projection to superficial laminae of the dorsal horn in cats and monkeys. *J. Comp. Neurol.* **225**, 276–290. [86]

Cheney, P. D. and Fetz, E. E. (1980). Functional classes of primate cortico-motoneuronal cells and their relation to active force. *J. Neurophysiol.* **44**, 773–791. [216, 217, 218, 219, 220, 221, 224, 225, 228, 236]

Cheney, P. D. and Fetz, E. E. (1984). Corticomotoneuronal cells contribute to long-latency stretch reflexes in the rhesus monkey. *J. Physiol.* **349**, 249–272. [236, 255, 257, 265, 334]

Cheney, P. D. and Fetz, E. E. (1985). Comparable patterns of muscle facilitation evoked by individual corticomotoneuronal (CM) cells and by single intra-cortical microstimuli in primates. Evidence for functional groups of CM cells. *J. Neurophysiol.* **53**, 786–804. [23, 148, 306, 313, 322, 326]

Cheney, P. D., Kasser, R., and Holsapple, J. (1982). Reciprocal effect of single cortico-motoneuronal cells on wrist extensor and flexor muscle activity in the primate. *Brain Res.* **247**, 164–168. [202, 204]

Cheney, P. D., Fetz, E. E., and Palmer, S. S. (1985). Patterns of facilitation and suppression of antagonist forelimb muscles from motor cortex sites in the awake monkey. *J. Neurophysiol.* **53**, 805–820. [162, 203, 326]

Cheney, P. D., Fetz, E. E., and Mewes, K. (1991). Neural mechanisms underlying corticospinal and rubrospinal control of limb movements. *Prog. Brain Res.* **87**, 213–252. [173, 181, 194, 203, 207, 210]

Chollet, F., DiPiero, V., and Wise, R. J. S. (1991). The functional anatomy of motor recovery after stroke in humans: a study with positron emission tomography. *Ann. Neurol.* **29**, 265–276. [116]

Clough, J. F. M., Kernell, D., and Phillips, C. G. (1968). The distribution of monosynaptic excitation from the pyramidal tract and from primary spindle afferents to motoneurones of the baboon's hand and forearm. *J. Physiol.* **198**, 145–166. [128, 187, 190]

Clough, J. F. M., Phillips, C. G., and Sheridan, J. D. (1971). The short latency projection from the baboon's motor cortex to fusimotor neurones of the forearm and hand. *J. Physiol.* **216**, 257–279. [206]

Cole, J. D. (1991). *Pride and the daily marathon*. Duckworth, London. [248]

Cole, J. D. and Gordon, G. (1976). Differences in timing of corticocuneate and corticogracile actions. In *Sensory functions of the skin in primates* (ed. Y. Zotterman), pp. 231–240. Pergamon, Oxford. [61]

Colebatch, J. G. and Gandevia, S. C. (1989). The distribution of muscular weakness in upper motor neuron lesions affecting the arm. *Brain* **112**, 749–763. [116, 362]

Colebatch, J. G., Findley, L. J., Frackowiak, R. S. J., Marsden, C. D., and Brooks, D. J. (1990a). Preliminary report: activation of the cerebellum in essential tremor. *Lancet* **336**, 1028–1030. [359]

Colebatch, J. G., Rothwell, J. C., Day, B. L., Thompson, P. D., and Marsden, C. D. (1990b). Cortical outflow to proximal arm muscles in man. *Brain* **113**, 1843–1856. [192, 193]

Colebatch, J. G., Sayer, R. J., Porter, R., and White, O. B. (1990c). Responses of monkey precentral neurones to passive movements and phasic muscle stretch: relevance to man. *Electroenceph. Clin. Neurophysiol.* **75**, 44–55. [257, 258]

Colebatch, J. G., Deiber, M.-P., Passingham, R. E., Friston, K. J., and Frackowiak, R. S. J. (1991). Regional cerebral blood flow during voluntary arm and hand movements in human subjects. *J. Neurophysiol.* **65**, 1392–1401. [244]

Cope, T. C., Fetz, E. E., and Matsumura, M. (1987). Cross-correlation assessment of synaptic strength of single Ia fibre connections with triceps surae motoneurones in cats. *J. Physiol.* **390**, 161–188. [135, 183, 185, 186]

Costello, M. B. and Fragaszy, D. M. (1988). Prehension in cebus and saimiri: 1. Grip type and hand preference. *American J. Primatol.* **15**, 235–245. [94]

Coulter, J. D. (1974). Sensory transmission through lemniscal pathway during voluntary movement in the cat. *J. Neurophysiol.* **34**, 831–845. [66, 269]

Coulter, J. D. and Jones, E. G. (1977). Differential distribution of corticospinal projections from individual cytoarchitectonic fields in the monkey. *Brain Res.* **129**, 335–340. [73, 76]

Cowan, J. M. A., Day, B. L., Marsden, C. D., and Rothwell, J. C. (1986). The effect of percutaneous motor stimulation on H reflexes in the muscles of the arm and leg in man. *J. Physiol.* **377**, 333–347. [200, 202]

Coxe, W. S. and Landau, W. M. (1965). Observations upon the effect of supplementary motor cortex ablation in the monkey. *Brain Res.* **88**, 763–773. [294]

Cragg, B. G. (1975). The density of synapses and neurons in normal, mentally defective and ageing human brains. *Brain* **98**, 81–90. [38]

Craggs, M. D. and Rushton, D. N. (1976). The stability of the electrical stimulation map of the motor cortex of the anaesthetized baboon. *Brain* **99**, 575–600. [315, 339]

Creutzfeldt, O. D., Lux, H. D., and Nacimiento, A. C. (1964). Intracelluläre Reizung corticaler Nervenzellen. *Pflug. Arch. Physiol.* **281**, 129–151. [51]

Crevel, H. van and Verhaart, W. J. C. (1963). The 'exact' origin of the pyramidal tract. A quantitative study in the cat. *J. Anat.* **97**, 495–515. [67, 73, 77]

Crone, C. and Nielsen, J. (1989). Spinal mechanisms in man contributing to reciprocal inhibition during voluntary dosiflexion of the foot. *J. Physiol.* **416**, 255–272. [353]

Crutcher, M. D. and Alexander, G. E. (1990). Movement-related neuronal activity selectively coding either direction or muscle pattern in three motor areas of the monkey. *J. Neurophysiol.* **64**, 151–163. [211, 216, 219, 230]

Cullheim, S. and Kellerth, J.-O. (1978). A morphological study of the axons and recurrent axon collaterals of cat α-motoneurones supplying different hind-limb muscles. *J. Physiol.* **281**, 285–299. [129]

Curtis, D. R. and Ryall, R. W. (1966). The synaptic excitation of Renshaw cells. *Exp. Brain Res.* **2**, 81–96. [29]

Damasio, A. R. and van Hoesen, G. W. (1980). Structure and function of the supplementary motor area. *Neurology* **30**, 359. [294]

Danek, A., Bauer, M., and Fries, W. (1990). Tracing of neuronal connections in the human brain by magnetic resonance imaging in vivo. *Europ. J. Neurosci.* **2**, 112–115. [116]

Darian-Smith, I., Goodwin, A., Sugitani, M., and Heywood, J. (1985). Scanning a textured surface with the fingers: Events in sensorimotor cortex. In *Hand function and the neocortex* (eds. A. W. Goodwin and I. Darian-Smith) EBR suppl. 10, pp. 17–43. Springer, Berlin. [260]

Darian-Smith, I., Darian-Smith, C., Galea, M., and Pepperell, R. (1991). Thalamocortical connections with sensorimotor areas in the mature and newborn macaque monkey. In *Motor control: concepts & issues* (eds. D. R. Humphrey and H.-J. Freund), pp. 181–197. Wiley–Interscience, Chichester. [97]

Darling, W. G. and Cole, K. J. (1990). Muscle activation patterns and kinetics of human index finger movements. *J. Neurophysiol.* **63**, 1098–1108. [94]

Datta, A. K. and Stephens, J. A. (1990). Synchronization of motor unit activity during voluntary contraction in man. *J. Physiol.* **422**, 397–419. [175]

Datta, A. K., Farmer, S. F., and Stephens, J. A. (1991). Central nervous pathways underlying synchronization of human motor unit firing studied during voluntary contractions. *J. Physiol.* **432**, 401–425. [176, 177]

Davidoff, R. A. (1989). The dorsal columns. *Neurol.* **39**, 1377–1385. [110]

Davies, J. G. McF., Kirkwood, P. A., and Sears, T. A. (1985). The detection of monosynaptic connexions from inspiratory bulbospinal neurones to inspiratory motoneurones in the cat. *J. Physiol.* **368**, 33–62. [162]

Day, B. L. and Marsden, C. D. (1982). Accurate repositioning of the human thumb against unpredictable loads is dependent upon peripheral feedback. *J. Physiol.* **327**, 393–407. [264]

Day, B. L., Rothwell, J. C., Thompson, P. D., Dick, J. P. R., Cowan, J. M. A., Berardelli, A., and Marsden, C. D. (1987). Motor cortex stimulation in intact man. II. Multiple descending volleys. *Brain* **110**, 1191–1209. [190]

Day, B. L., Dressler, D., Maertens de Noordhout, A., Marsden, C. D., Nakashima, K., Rothwell, J. C., and Thompson, P. D. (1989). Electric and magnetic stimulation of human motor cortex: surface EMG and single motor unit responses. *J. Physiol.* **412**, 449–473. [190, 192]

Day, B. L., Riescher, H., Struppler, A., Rothwell, J. C., and Marsden, C. D. (1991). Changes in the response to magnetic and electrical stimulation of the motor cortex following muscle stretch in man. *J. Physiol.* **433**, 41–57. [266, 268]

Deecke, L. (1987). Bereitschaftspotential as an indicator of movement preparation in supplementary motor area and motor cortex. In *Motor areas of the cerebral cortex* (eds. G. Bock, M. O'Connnor, and J. Marsh), Vol. 132, pp. 231–245. CIBA Foundation Symp., Wiley, Chichester. [290]

Deecke, L., Scheid, P., and Kornhuber, H. H. (1969). Distribution of the readiness potential, pre-motion positivity, and motor potential of human cerebral cortex preceding voluntary finger movements. *Exp. Brain Res.* **7**, 158–168. [289]

DeFelipe, J., Conley, M., and Jones, E. G. (1986). Multiple long-range focal collateralization of axons arising from corticocortical cells in monkey sensory-motor cortex. *J. Neurosci.* **6**, 3749–3766. [40, 49, 253, 310]

DeGail, P., Lance, J. W., and Neilson, P. D. (1966). Differential effects on tonic and phasic reflex mechanisms produced by vibration of muscles in man. *J. Neurol. Neurosurg. Psychiat.* **29**, 1–11. [270]

Deiber, M.-P., Passingham, R. E., Colebatch, J. G., Friston, K. J., Nixon, P. D., and Frackowiak, R. S. J. (1991). Cortical areas and the selection of movement: a study with positron emission tomography. *Exp. Brain Res.* **84**, 393–402. [240, 288, 302, 358]

Denny-Brown, D. (1950). Disintegration of motor function resulting from cerebral lesions. *J. Nerv. Ment. Dis.* **112**, 1–45. [109, 362]

Denny-Brown, D. (1966). *The cerebral control of movement*. Liverpool University Press. [34, 110, 315]

Denny-Brown, D. and Botterell, E. H. (1948). The motor functions of the agranular frontal cortex. *Res. Publ. Assoc. Nerv. Ment. Dis.* **27**, 235–345. [109, 361]

Deschênes, M. and Hammond, C. (1980). Physiological and morphological identification of ventrolateral fibers relaying cerebellar information to the cat motor cortex. *Neurosci.* **5**, 1137–1141. [49]

Deschênes, M., Labelle, A., and Landry, P. (1979a). A comparative study of ventrolateral and recurrent excitatory postsynaptic potentials in large pyramidal tract cells in the cat. *Brain Res.* **160**, 37–46. [49]

Deschênes, M., Labelle, A., and Landry, P. (1979b). Morphological characterization of slow and fast pyramidal tract cells in the cat. *Brain Res.* **178**, 251–274. [38, 54]

Dick, J. P. R., Cowan, J. M. A., Day, B. L., Beradelli, A., Kachi, T., Rothwell, J. C., and Marsden, C. D. (1984). The corticomotoneurone connection is normal in Parkinson's disease. *Nature* **310**, 407–409. [354]

Donoghue, J. P. and Wise, S. P. (1982). The motor cortex of the rat: cytoarchitecture and microstimulation mapping. *J. Comp. Neurol.* **212**, 76–88. [312, 317]

Donoghue, J. P., Suner, S., and Sanes, J. N. (1990). Dynamic organization of primary motor cortex output to target muscles in adult rats. II. Rapid reorganization following motor nerve lesions. *Exp. Brain Res.* **79**, 492–503. [339]

Donoghue, J. P., Leibovic, S., and Sanes, J. N. (1992). Organization of the forelimb area in primate motor cortex: Representation of individual digit, wrist, and elbow muscles. *Exp. Brain Res.* **89**, 1–19 [312, 315]

Duffy, F. and Burchfiel, J. (1971). Somatosensory system: organizational hierarchy from single units in monkey area 5. *Science* **172**, 273–275. [28]

Dum, R. P. and Strick, P. L. (1991). The origin of corticospinal projections from the premotor areas in the frontal lobe. *J. Neurosci.* **11**, 667–689. [67, 68, 70, 71, 72, 73, 75, 274, 276, 280, 284, 350]

Dusser de Barenne, J.G., and McCulloch, W. S. (1938). Functional organization in the sensory cortex of the monkey (macaca mulatta). *J. Neurophysiol.* **1**, 69–85. [273]

Eccles, J. C. (1957). *The physiology of nerve cells.* Johns Hopkins University Press, Baltimore, Maryland. [126]

Eccles, J. C. (1959). Plasticity at the simplest levels of the nervous system. In *The centennial lectures of E. R. Squibb & Son*, pp. 217–244. Putnam & Sons, New York. [360]

Eccles, J. C. (1964). *The Physiology of synapses.* Academic Press, New York. [29]

Eccles, J. C. (1982). The initiation of voluntary movements by the supplementary motor area. *Arch. Psychiatr. Nervenkr.* **231**, 423–441. [291]

Eccles, J. C., Fatt, P., and Koketsu, K. (1954). Cholinergic and inhibitory synapses in a pathway from motor-axon collaterals to motoneurones. *J. Physiol.* **126**, 524–562. [131]

Eccles, J. C., Eccles, R. M., and Lundberg, A. (1957). The convergence of monosynaptic excitatory afferents on to many different species of alpha motoneurons. *J. Physiol.* **137**, 22–50. [27, 128]

Eccles, J. C., Eccles, R. M., Iggo, A., and Lundberg, A. (1960). Electrophysiological studies on gamma motoneurons. *Acta Physiol. Scand.* **50**, 32–40. [30]

Eccles, R. M. and Lundberg, A. (1958). Integrative patterns of Ia synaptic actions on motoneurones of hip and knee muscles. *J. Physiol.* **144**, 271–298. [127, 128]

Edgley, S. A., Eyre, J. A., Lemon, R.N., and Miller, S. (1990). Excitation of the corticospinal tract by electromagnetic and electrical stimulation of the scalp in the macaque monkey. *J. Physiol.* **425**, 301–320. [104, 158, 189, 190, 268]

Edgley, S. A., Eyre, J. A., Lemon, R. N., and Miller, S. (1992). Direct and indirect activation of corticospinal neurones by electrical and magnetic stimulation in the anaesthetized macaque monkey. *J. Physiol.* **446**: 224P. [190]

Edin, B., Westling, G., and Johansson, R. S. (1992). Independent control of human finger tip forces at individual digits during precision lifting. *J. Physiol.* **450**, 547–564. [358]

Edwards, F. R., Redman, S. J., and Walmsley, B. (1976a). Statistical fluctuations in charge transfer at Ia synapses on spinal motoneurones. *J. Physiol.* **259**, 665–688. [139]

Edwards, F. R., Redman, S. J., and Walmsley, B. (1976b). Non-quantal fluctuations and transmission failures in charge transfer at Ia synapses on spinal motoneurones. *J. Physiol.* **259**, 689–704. [139]

Elger, C. E., Speckmann, E.-J., Caspers, H., and Janzen, R. W. C. (1977). Corticospinal connections in the rat. I. Monosynaptic and polysynaptic responses of cervical motor neurons to epicortical stimulation. *Exp. Brain Res.* **28**, 385–404. [86]

Ellaway, P. H. (1971). Recurrent inhibition of fusimotor neurones exhibiting background discharges in decerebrate and the spinal cat. *J. Physiol.* **216**, 419–439. [30]

Ellaway, P. H. and Murphy, K. S. K. (1985). The origins and characteristics of cross-related activity between gammamotoneurones in the cat. *Qut. J. Exp. Physiol.* **70**, 219–232. [186, 200]

Elliott, J. M. and Connolly, K. J. (1984). A classification of manipulative hand movements. *Develop. Med. Child. Neurol.* **26**, 283–296. [94, 95]

Endo, K., Araki, T., and Yagi, N. (1973). The distribution and pattern of axon branching of pyramidal tract cells. *Brain Res.* **57**, 484–492. [62]

Espinoza, E. and Smith, A. M. (1990). Purkinje cell simple spike activity during grasping and lifting objects of different textures and weights. *J. Neurophysiol.* **64**, 698–714. [259]

Evarts, E. V. (1964). Temporal patterns of discharge of pyramidal tract neurons during sleep and waking in the monkey. *J. Neurophysiol.* **27**, 152–171. [236]

Evarts, E. V. (1965). Relation of discharge frequency to conduction velocity in pyramidal tract neurons. *J. Neurophysiol.* **28**, 216–228. [210]

Evarts, E. V. (1966). Pyramidal tract activity associated with a conditioned hand movement in the monkey. *J. Neurophysiol.* **29**, 1011–1027. [213, 214, 235]

Evarts, E. V. (1967). Representation of movements and muscles by pyramidal tract neurons of the precentral motor cortex. In *Neurophysiological basis of normal and abnormal motor activities* (eds. M. D. Yahr and D. P. Purpura), pp. 215–251. Raven, New York. [228]

Evarts, E. V. (1968). Relation of pyramidal tract activity to force exerted during voluntary movement. *J. Neurophysiol.* **31**, 14–27. [219, 220, 228, 263]

Evarts, E. V. (1969). Activity of pyramidal tract neurons during postural fixation. *J. Neurophysiol.* **32**, 375–385. [219]

Evarts, E. V. (1972). Contrasts between activity of precentral and postcentral neurons of cerebral cortex during movement in the monkey. *Brain Res.* **40**, 25–31. [215, 216, 218]

Evarts, E. V. (1973). Motor cortex reflexes associated with learned movement. *Science* **179**, 501–503. [255, 260]

Evarts, E. V. (1981). Role of motor cortex in voluntary movements in primates. In *Handbook of physiology—the nervous system II* (eds. J. M. Brookhart and V. B. Mountcastle), pp. 1083–1120. American Physiological Society, Bethesda, Maryland. [210]

Evarts, E. V. (1986). Motor cortex output in primates. In: *Cerebral cortex* (eds. E. G. Jones and A. Peters), Vol. 5 pp. 217–241. Plenum, New York. [210]

Evarts, E. V. and Tanji, J. (1974). Gating of motor cortex reflexes by prior instruction. *Brain Res.* **71**, 479–494. [268]

Evarts, E. V. and Tanji, J. (1976). Reflex and intended responses in motor cortex pyramidal tract neurons of monkey. *J. Neurophysiol.* **39**, 1069–1080. [255, 260, 265]

Evarts, E. V., Fromm, C., Kröller, J., and Jennings, V. A. (1983). Motor cortex control of finely graded forces. *J. Neurophysiol.* **49**, 1199–1215. [219, 220, 221, 222, 227, 344]

Eyre, J. A., Miller, S., and Ramesh, V. (1991). Constancy of central conduction delays during development in man: investigation of motor and somatosensory pathways. *J. Physiol.* **434**, 441–452. [104, 108]

Farmer, S. F., Bremner, F. D., and Stephens, J. A. (1990a). Evidence for a central nervous origin of motor unit coherence in man. *J. Physiol.* **430**, 55P. [200]

Farmer, S. F., Ingram, D. A., and Stephens, J. A. (1990b). Mirror movements studied in a patient with Klippel-Feil syndrome. *J. Physiol.* **428**, 467–484. [113, 177, 178, 362]

Feldman, M. L. (1984). Morphology of the neocortical pyramidal neuron. In *Cerebral cortex* (eds. A. Peters and E. G. Jones) Vol. 1, pp. 123–200. Plenum, New York. [38, 40]

Felix, D. and Wiesendanger, M. (1971). Pyramidal and non-pyramidal motor cortical effects on distal forelimb muscles of monkeys. *Exp. Brain Res.* **12**, 81–91. [104, 329]

Ferrier, D. (1875). Experiments on the brain of monkeys. *Proc. R. Soc. Lond.* **23**, 409–430. [304]

Ferrier, D. (1876). *The Functions of the brain.* Smith Elder, London. [3]

Fetz, E. E. (1992). Are movement parameters recognizably coded in activity of single neurons? *Behav. Brain Sci.* **15**, 679–690. [211, 216, 234]

Fetz, E. E. and Baker, M. A. (1969). Response properties of precentral neurons in awake monkeys. *The Physiologist* **12**, 223P. [254]

Fetz, E. E. and Cheney, P. D. (1978). Muscle fields of primate corticomotoneuronal cells. *J. Physiol. (Paris)* **74**, 239–245. [210]

Fetz, E. E. and Cheney, P. D. (1980). Postspike facilitation of forelimb muscle activity by primate corticomotoneuronal cells. *J. Neurophysiol.* **44**, 751–772. [157, 161, 162, 164, 167, 168, 181, 189, 197, 218, 227]

Fetz, E. E. and Cheney, P. D. (1987). Functional relations between primate motor cortex cells and muscles: fixed and flexible. In *Motor areas of the cerebral cortex* (eds. G. Bock, M. O'Connor, and J. Marsh) Vol. 132, pp. 98–117. CIBA Foundation Symp., Wiley, Chichester. [204, 236]

Fetz, E. E. and Finocchio, D. V. (1971). Operant conditioning of specific patterns of neural and muscular activity. *Science* **174**, 431–435. [235]

Fetz, E. E. and Finocchio, D. V. (1972). Operant conditioning of isolated activity in specific muscles and precentral cells. *Brain Res.* **40**, 19–24. [235]

Fetz, E. E. and Gustafsson, B. (1983). Relation between shapes of post-synaptic potentials and changes in firing probability of cat motoneurones. *J. Physiol.* **341**, 387–410. [31, 135, 185]

Fetz, E. E. and Shupe, L. E. (1990). Neural network models of the primate motor system. In *Advanced neural computers* (ed. R. Eckmiller), pp. 43–50. Elsevier, Amsterdam. [234]

Fetz, E. E., Cheney, P. D., and German, D. C. (1976). Corticomotoneuronal connections of precentral cells detected by post-spike averages of EMG activity in behaving monkeys. *Brain Res.* **114**, 505–510. [155]

Fetz, E. E., Finocchio, V., Baker, M. A., and Soso, M. J. (1980). Sensory and motor responses of precentral cortex cells during comparable passive and active joint movements. *J. Neurophysiol.* **43**, 1070–1089. [216, 218, 254, 256]

Fetz, E. E., Cheney, P .D., Mewes, K., and Palmer, S. (1989). Control of forelimb muscle activity by populations of corticomotoneuronal and rubromotoneuronal cells. *Prog. Brain Res.* **80**, 437–449. [164, 169, 194, 204]

Fetz, E. E., Toyama, K., and Smith, W. (1990). Synaptic interactions between cortical neurons. In *Cerebral cortex* (eds. E. G. Jones and A. Peters) Vol. 9, pp. 1–47. Plenum, New York. [45, 46, 48, 53]

Finkel, A. S. and Redman, S. J. (1985). Optimal voltage clamping with single microelectrodes. In *Voltage and patch clamping with microelectrodes* (eds. T. G. Smith, H. Lecar, S. J. Redman, and P. W. Gage), pp. 95–120. American Physiological Society, Bethesda, Maryland. [52]

Fisher, C. M. (1992). Concerning the mechanism of recovery in stroke hemiplegia. *Can. J. Neurol. Sci.* **19**, 57–63. [116]

Flament, D., Fortier, P. A. and Fetz, E. E. (1992a). Response patterns and post-spike effects of peripheral afferents in dorsal root ganglia of behaving monkeys. *J. Neurophysiol.* **67**, 875–889. [129, 207]

Flament, D., Goldsmith, P., and Lemon, R. N. (1992b). The development of corticospinal projections to tail and hindlimb motoneurons studied in infant macaques using magnetic brain stimulation. *Exp. Brain. Res.* **90**, 225–228. [104]

Flament, D., Hall, E.J., and Lemon, R.N. (1992c). The development of cortico-motoneuronal projections investigated using magnetic brain stimulation in the infant macaque. *J. Physiol.* **447**, 755–768. [104, 105, 234]

Flament, D., Goldsmith, P., Buckley, J. C., and Lemon, R. N. (1993). Task-dependence of EMG responses in first dorsal interosseous muscle to magnetic brain stimulation in man. *J. Physiol.*, **464**, 361–378. [344]

Foehring, R. C., Schwindt, P. C., and Crill, W. E. (1989). Norpinephrine selectively reduces slow calcium and sodium-mediated potassium currents in cat neocortical neurons. *J. Neurophysiol.* **61**, 245–256. [52]

Foerster, O. (1936). The motor cortex in man in light of Hughlings Jackson's doctrines. *Brain* **59**, 135–159. [24, 25]

Forrsberg, H., Eliasson, A. C., Kinoshita, H., Johansson, R. S., and Westling, G. (1991). Development of human precision grip-I — Basic coordination of force. *Exp. Brain Res.* **85**, 451–457. [107]

Fournier, E., Meunier, S., Pierrott-Deseilligny, E., and Shindo, M. (1986). Evidence for interneuronally mediated Ia excitatory effects to human quadriceps motoneurones. *J. Physiol.* **377**, 143–169. [31, 135]

Fox, P. T., Fox, J. M., Raichle, M. E., and Burde, R. M. (1985). The role of cerebral cortex in the generation of voluntary saccades: a positron emission tomography study. *J. Neurophysiol.* **54**, 348–369. [242, 287, 288, 358]

Frackowiak, R. S. J., Weiller, C., and Chollet, F. (1991). The functional anatomy of recovery from brain injury. In *Exploring brain functional anatomy with positron tomography* CIBA Foundation Symposium 163 (eds. D. Chadwick & J. Whelan), pp. 235–244. Wiley, Chichester. [362]

Fragaszy, D. M. (1983). Preliminary quantitative studies of prehension in squirrel monkeys (saimiri sciureus). *Brain Behav. Evol.* **23**, 81–92. [94]

François-Franck, C. E. (1887). *Leçons sur les fonctions motrices du cerveau.* Doin, Paris. [79, 350]

Frank, K. and Fuortes, M. G. F. (1955). Potentials recorded from the spinal cord with microelectrodes. *J. Physiol.* **130**, 625–654. [126]

Friedlander, M. J., Sayer, R. J., and Redman, S. J. (1989). Evaluation of long term potentiation of small compound and unitary EPSPs at the hippocampal CA3-CA1 synapse. *J. Neurosci.* **10**, 814–825. [56]

Friedman, D. P. and Jones, E. G. (1981). Thalamic input to areas 3a and 2 in monkeys. *J. Neurophysiol.* **45**, 59–85. [263]

Friedman, M. M., Gould, R., Baker, J., and Williams, M. A. (1986). Computer assisted evaluation of electron microscopic autoradiography using two 'crossfire' analytical methods. *Proc. Roy. Microsc. Soc.* **21**, 279. [155]

Fries, W., Danek, A., Bauer, W. M., Witt, Th. N., and Leinsinger, G. (1990). Hemiplegia after lacunar stroke with pyramidal degeneration shown in vivo.

In *Neurologische Frührehabilitation* (eds. K. von Wild and H.-H. Janzik), pp. 11–17. Zuckscgwerdt, Munich. [116]

Fritsch, G. and Hitzig, E. (1870). Uber die elektrische Erregbarkeit des Gross-hirns. *Archs Anat. Physiol. Wiss. Med.* **37**, 300–332. (Translation by Bonin, G. Von. In *The cerebral cortex*, pp. 73–96. Thomas, Springfield, Illinois). [304]

Fritz, N., Illert, M., Kolb, F. P., Lemon, R. N., Muir, R. B., van der Burg, J., Wiedemann, E., and Yamaguchi, T. (1985). The cortico-motoneuronal input to hand and forearm motoneurones in the anaesthetized monkey. *J. Physiol.* **366**, 20P. [137, 158, 187, 189, 195, 319, 323]

Fritz, N., Illert, M., de la Motte, S., Reeh, P., and Saggau, P. (1989). Pattern of monosynaptic Ia connections in the cat forelimb. *J. Physiol.* **419**, 321–351. [129]

Fromm, C. and Evarts, E. E. (1981). Relation of size and activity of motor cortex pyramidal tract neurons during skilled movements in the monkey. *J. Neurosci.* **1**, 453–460. [218]

Fuller, J. H. and Schlag, J. D. (1976). Determination of antidromic excitation by the collision test: problems of interpretation. *Brain Res.* **112**, 283–298. [213]

Fuster, J. M. (1973). Unit activity in prefrontal cortex during delayed response performance: neuronal correlates of transient memory. *J. Neurophysiol.* **36**, 61–78. [299]

Futami, T., Shinoda, Y., and Yokota, J. (1979). Spinal axon collaterals of cortico-spinal neurons identified by intracellular injection of horseradish peroxidase. *Brain Res.* **164**, 279–284. [148]

Fyffe, R. E. W. (1991). Spatial distribution of recurrent inhibitory synapses on spinal motoneurons in the cat. *J. Neurophysiol.* **65**, 1134–1149. [131, 143]

Fyffe, R. E. W. and Light, A. R. (1984). The ultrastructure of group Ia afferent fiber synapses in the lumbrosacral spinal cord of the cat. *Brain Res.* **300**, 201–209. [141]

Gall, F. J. and Spurzheim, J. C. (1810). *Anatomie et physiologie du système nerveux en général et du cerveau particulier, avec des observations intellectuelles et morales de l'homme et des animaux, par la configuration de leur tête*. Schoell, Paris. [9]

Gandevia, S. C. and Plassman, B. L. (1988). Responses in human intercostal and truncal muscles to motor cortical and spinal stimulation. *Resp. and Physiol.* **73**, 325–338. [192]

Gandevia, S. C. and Rothwell, J. C. (1987). Activation of the human diaphragm from the motor cortex. *J. Physiol.* **384**, 109–118. [192]

Garnett, R. and Stephens, J. A. (1980). The reflex responses of single motor units in human first dorsal interosseous muscle following cutaneous afferent stimulation. *J. Physiol.* **303**, 351–364. [135]

Gatter, K. C. and Powell, T. P. S. (1978). The intrinsic connections of the cortex of area 4 of the monkey. *Brain* **101**, 513–541. [45, 49]

Gazzaniga, M. S., Bogen, J. E., and Sperry, R. W. (1967). Dyspraxia following division of the cerebral commissures. *Arch. Neurol.* **16**, 606–612. [355]

Gelfan, S. (1964). Neuronal interdependence. *Prog. Brain Res.* **11**, 238–260. [130]

Georgopoulos, A. P. (1987) Cortical mechanisms subserving reaching In *Motor areas of the cerebral cortex* (eds. G. Bock, M. O'Connor, and J. Marsh) Vol. 132, pp. 125–141. CIBA Foundation Symp. Wiley, Chichester. [231]

Georgopoulos, A. P. (1988). Neural integration of movement: role of motor cortex in reaching. *FASEB* **2**(2), 2849–2857. [230, 233, 234]

Georgopoulos, A. P., Kalaska, J. F., Caminiti, R., and Massey, J. T. (1982). On the relations between the direction of two-dimensional arm movements and cell discharge in primate motor cortex. *J. Neurosci.* **2**, 1527–1537. [231, 233]

Georgopoulos, A. P., Caminiti, R., Kalaska, J.F., and Massey, J. T. (1983). Spatial coding of movement: A hypothesis concerning the coding of movement direction by motor cortical populations. In *Neuronal coding of motor performance* (eds. J. Massion, J. Paillard, W. Schultz, and M. Wiesendanger) *Exp. Brain Res.* suppl. 7, pp. 327–336. Springer, Berlin. [231, 233]

Georgopoulos, A. P., Kalaska, J. F., Crutcher, M. D., Caminiti, R. and Massey, J. T. (1984). The representation of movement direction in the motor cortex: Single cell and population studies. In *Dynamic aspects of neocortical function* (eds. G. M. Edelman, W. E., Gall and W. M. Cowan), pp. 501–524. Wiley, Chichester. [344, 345]

Georgopoulos, A. P., Lurito, J. T., Petrides, M., Schwartz, A. B., and Massey, J. T. (1989). Mental rotation of the neuronal population vector. *Science* **243**, 234–236. [219, 231]

Ghez, C. and Pisa, M. (1972). Inhibition of afferent transmission in cuneate nucleus during voluntary movement in the cat. *Brain Res.* **40**, 145–151. [66, 269]

Ghez, C. and Shinoda, Y. (1978). Spinal mechanisms of the functional stretch reflex. *Exp. Brain Res.* **32**, 55–68. [265]

Ghosh, S. and Porter, R. (1988a). Morphology of pyramidal neurones in monkey motor cortex and the synaptic actions of their intracortical axon collaterals. *J. Physiol.* **400**, 593–615. [40, 43, 44, 47]

Ghosh, S. and Porter, R. (1988b). Corticocortical synaptic influences on morphologically identified pyramidal neurones in the motor cortex of the monkey. *J. Physiol.* **400**, 617–629. [50]

Ghosh, S., Brinkman, C., and Porter, R. (1987). A quantitative study of the distribution of neurons projecting to the precentral motor cortex in the monkey (m. fascicularis). *J. Comp. Neurol.* **259**, 424–444. [50, 252, 253, 274]

Ghosh, S., Fyffe, R. E. W., and Porter, R. (1988). Morphology of neurons in area 4 of the cat's cortex studied with intracellular injection of HRP. *J. Comp. Neurol.* **269**, 290–312. [38, 40, 41, 42, 43, 47, 49]

Gilbert, C. D. and Wiesel, T. N. (1979). Morphology and intracortical projections of functionally characterised neurones in the cat visual cortex. *Nature* **280**, 120–125. [38]

Gilman, S., Marco, L. A., and Ebel, H. C. (1971). Effects of medullary pyramidotomy in the monkey. II. Abnormalities of spindle afferent responses. *Brain* **94**, 515–530. [205]

Giuffrida, R. and Rustioni, A. (1989). Glutamate and aspartate immunoreactivity in corticospinal neurons of rats. *J. Comp. Neurol.* **288**, 154–164. [55]

Godschalk, G., Lemon, R. N., Nijs, H. J. T., and Kuypers, H. G. J. M. (1981). Behaviour of neurons in monkey peri-arcuate and precentral cortex before and during visually guided arm and hand movements. *Exp. Brain Res.* **44**, 113–116. [299, 300, 301, 351]

Godschalk, M., Lemon, R. N., Kuypers, H. G. J. M., and Ronday, H. K. (1984).

Cortical afferents and efferents of monkey post-arcuate area: an anatomical and electrophysiological study. *Exp. Brain Res.* **56**, 410–424. [73, 75, 274, 297, 298]

Godschalk, M., Lemon, R. N., Kuypers, H. G. J. M., and van der Steen, J. (1985). The involvement of monkey premotor cortex neurones in preparation of visually cued arm movements. *Behav. Brain Res.* **18**, 143–157. [299]

Goldberg, G. (1985). Supplementary motor area structure and function: review and hypothesis. *Behav. Brain Sci.* **8**, 567–615. [290]

Goldman-Rakic, P. S. (1987). Motor control function of the prefrontal cortex. In *Motor areas of the cerebral cortex* (eds. G. Bock, M. O'Connor, and J. Marsh) Vol. 132, pp. 187–197. CIBA Foundation Symp. Wiley, Chichester. [296]

Goldman-Rakic, P. S. and Selemon, L. D. (1986). Topography of projections in non human primates and implications for functional parcellation of the neostriatum. In *Cerebral Cortex* (eds. A. Peters and E. G. Jones) Vol. 5, pp. 447–466. Plenum, New York. [56]

Goldring, S. and Ratcheson, R. (1972). Human motor cortex: sensory input data from single neuron recording. *Science* **175**, 1493–1495. [210, 235, 239]

Goldstein, K. (1953). Pierre Paul Broca. In *The Founders of Neurology* (ed. W. Haymaker), pp. 259–263. Thomas, Springfield, Illinois. [2]

Gonshor, A. and Melvill-Jones, G. (1976). Extreme vestibulo-ocular adaptation induced by prolonged optical reversal of vision. *J. Physiol.* **256**, 381–414. [361]

Goodwin, G. M., McCloskey, D. I., and Matthews, P. B. C. (1972). The contribution of muscle afferents to kinaesthesia shown by vibration induced illusions of movement and by the effects of paralysing joint afferents. *Brain* **95**, 705–748. [270]

Gordon, G. and Miller, S. (1969). Identification of cortical cells projecting to the dorsal column nuclei of the cat. *Quart. J. Exp. Physiol.* **54**, 85–98. [66]

Gorska, T. and Sybirska, E. (1980). Effects of pyramidal lesions on forelimb movements in the cat. *Acta Neurobiol.* **40**, 343–359. [117, 119]

Gould, H. J., Cusick, C. G., Pons, T. P., and Kaas, J. H. (1986). The relationship of corpus callosum connections to electrical stimulation maps of motor, supplementary motor, and the frontal eye fields in owl monkeys. *J. Comp. Neurol.* **247**, 297–325. [50, 312, 315]

Graf von Keyserlingk, D. and Schramm, U. (1984). Diameter of axons and thickness of myelin sheaths of the pyramidal tract fibres in the adult human medullary pyramid. *Anat. Anz., Jena.* **157**, 97–111. [82]

Granit, R. and Kaada, B. R. (1952). Influence of stimulation of central nervous structures on muscle spindles in cat. *Acta Physiol. Scand.* **27**, 130–160. [205]

Grantyn, A. and Berthoz, A. (1987). Reticulo-spinal neurons participating in the control of synergic eye and head movements during orienting in the cat. *Exp. Brain Res.* **66**, 339–354. [146]

Grantyn, A., Ong-Meang, J. V., and Berthoz, A. (1987). Reticulo- spinal neurons participating in the control of synergic eye and head movements during orienting in the cat. II. Morphological properties as revealed by intra-axonal injections of horseradish peroxidase. *Exp. Brain Res.* **66**, 355–377. [146]

Grigg, P. and Preston, J. B. (1971). Baboon flexor and extensor fusimotor neurons and their modulation by motor cortex. *J. Neurophysiol.* **34**, 428–436. [206]

Grillner, S. (1969). Supraspinal and segmental control of static and dynamic γ-motoneurones in the cat. *Acta. Physiologica. Scand.* Suppl. **327**, 3–34. [30]

Grillner, S. and Hongo, T. (1972). Vestibulospinal effects on motoneurones and interneurones in the lumbosacral cord. In *Basic aspects of central vestibular mechanisms* (ed. A. Brodal and O. Pompeiano) *Progress in Brain Research*, vol. 37, pp. 243–262. Elsevier, Amsterdam. [30]

Groos, W. P., Ewing, L. K., Carter, C. M., and Coulter, J. D. (1978). Organization of corticospinal neurons in the cat. *Brain Res.* **143**, 393–419. [77, 315]

Gugino, L. D., Rowinski, M. J., and Stoney, S. D. (1990). Motor outflow to cervical motoneurons from racoon motorsensory cortex. *Brain Res. Bull.* **24**, 833–837. [88]

Gustafsson, B. and McCrea, D. (1984). Influence of stretch-evoked synaptic potentials on firing probability of cat spinal motoneurons. *J. Physiol.* **347**, 431–451. [185]

ter Haar Romeny, B. M., Denier van der Gon, J. J., and Gielen, C. C. A. M. (1984). Relation between location of a motor unit in the human biceps brachii and its critical firing levels for different tasks. *Exp. Neurol.* **85**, 631–650. [129]

Haaxma, R. and Kuypers, H. G. J. M. (1975). Role of occipito-frontal cortico-cortical connections in visual guidance of relatively independent hand and finger movements in Rhesus monkey. *Brain Res.* **71**, 361–366. [301]

Hagbarth, K.-E. and Eklund, G. (1966). Motor effects of vibratory stimuli in man. In *Muscle afferents and motor control* (ed. R. Granit), pp. 177–186. Almqvist & Wiksell, Stockholm. [270]

Haggard, P. (1991). Task coordination in human prehension. *J. Motor Behav.* **23**, 25–37. [356]

Hall, E. J., Flament, D., Fraser, C., and Lemon, R. N. (1990). Non-invasive brain stimulation reveals reorganised cortical outputs in amputees. *Neurosci. Letts.* **116**, 379–386. [341]

Halsband, V. and Passingham, R. E. (1982). The role of premotor and parietal cortex in the direction of action. *Brain Res.* **240**, 368–372. [295, 296]

Halverson, H. M. (1943). The development of prehension in infants. In *Child behavior and development* (eds. R. G. Barker, J. S. Konnin, and H. F. Wright) pp. 49–65. McGraw Hill, New York. [107]

Hammond, P. H. (1956). The influence of prior instruction to the subject on an apparently involuntary neuro-muscular response. *J. Physiol.* **132**, 17–18P. [264, 268]

Hammond, P. H. (1960). An experimental study of servo action in human muscular control. In *Proceedings of the 3rd International Conference on Medical Electronics*, pp. 190–199. Institution of Electrical Engineers, London. [264]

Harding, G. W. and Towe, A. L. (1985). Fiber analysis of the pyramidal tract of the laboratory rat. *Exp. Neurol.* **87**, 503–518. [80]

Harrison, P. J., Hultborn, H., Jankowska, E., Katz, R., Storai, B., and Zytnicki, D. (1984). Labelling of interneurones by retrograde transsynaptic transport of horseradish peroxidase from motoneurones in rats and cats. *Neurosci. Letts.* **45**, 15–19. [130]

Hasse, J. and van Der Meulen, J. P. (1961). Effects of supraspinal stimulation on Renshaw cells belonging to extensor motoneurons. *J. Neurophysiol.* **24**, 510–520. [30]

Hayes, N. L. and Rustioni, A. (1979). Dual projections of single neurons are visualized simultaneously: use of enzymatically inactive (^{3}H) HRP. *Brain Res.* **165**, 321-326. [63]

Hayes, N. L. and Rustioni, A. (1981). Descending projections from brainstem and sensorimotor cortex to spinal enlargements in the cat. Single and double retrograde tracer studies. *Exp. Brain Res.* **41**, 89-107. [79]

Heath, C. J., Hore, J., and Phillips, C. G. (1976). Inputs from low threshold muscle and cutaneous afferents of hand and forearm to areas 3a and 3b of baboon's cerebral cortex. *J. Physiol.* **257**, 199-227. [251]

Hécaen, H. and Albert, M. L. (1978). *Human neuropsychology*. Wiley, New York. [34]

Heffner, R. S. and Masterton, R. B. (1975). Variation in form of the pyramidal tract and its relationship to digital dexterity. *Brain Behav. Evol.* **12**, 161-200. [81, 82, 90, 91, 119]

Heffner, R. S. and Masterton, R. B. (1983). The role of the corticospinal tract in the evolution of human digital dexterity. *Brain Behav. Evol.* **23**, 165-183. [82, 90, 91, 94]

Hepp-Reymond, M.-C. (1988). Functional organization of motor cortex and its participation in voluntary movements. In *Comparative primate biology* (eds. H. D. Seklis and J. Erwin) vol. 4, 501-624. Liss, New York. [109, 110, 112, 210, 216, 218, 219, 226, 258]

Hepp-Reymond, M.-C. and Wiesendanger, M. (1972). Unilateral pyramidotomy in monkeys: Effects on force and speed of a conditioned precision grip. *Brain Res.* **36**, 117-131. [113]

Hepp-Reymond, M.-C., Trouche, E., and Wiesendanger, M. (1974). Effects of unilateral and bilateral pyramidotomy on a conditioned rapid precision grip in monkeys (macaca fascicularis). *Exp. Brain Res.* **21**, 519-527. [113, 114]

Hepp-Reymond, M.-C., Wyss, U. R., and Anner, R. (1978). Neuronal coding of static force in the primate motor cortex. *J. Physiol.* **74**, 287-291. [219, 220, 221, 227]

Herman, D., Kang, R., MacGillis, M., and Zarzecki, P. (1985). Responses of cat motor cortex neurons to cortico-cortical and somatosensory inputs. *Exp. Brain Res.* **57**, 598-604. [260]

Hern, J. E. C., Landgren, S., Phillips, C. G., and Porter, R. (1962). Selective excitation of corticofugal neurones by surface-anodal stimulation of the baboon's motor cortex. *J. Physiol.* **161**, 73-90. [305, 306]

Hess, C. W., Mills, K. R., and Murray, N. M. F. (1987). Responses in small hand muscles from magnetic stimulation of the human brain. *J. Physiol.* **388**, 397-419. [190, 314]

Hinde, R. A., Rowell, T. E., and Spencer-Booth, Y. (1964). Behaviour of socially living rhesus monkeys in their first six months. *Proc. Zool. Soc. Lond.* **143**, 609-649. [104]

Hines, M. (1944). Significance of the precentral motor cortex. In *The precentral motor cortex* (ed. P. C. Bucy), pp. 461-494. University of Illinois. [25, 313, 314]

Hoffman, D. S. and Luschei, E. S. (1980). Responses of monkey precentral cortical cells during a controlled jaw bite task. *J. Neurophysiol.* **44**, 333-348. [219, 227]

Holmes, G. (1939). The cerebellum of man. *Brain* **62**, 1-30. [358]

Holmes, G. and May, W. P. (1909). On the exact origin of the pyramidal tracts in man and other mammals. *Brain* **32**, 1–43. [67]

Holsapple, J. W., Preston, J. B. and Strick, P. L. (1990). Origin of thalamic inputs to the 'hand' representation in the primary motor cortex. *Soc. Neurosci. Abstr.* **16**, 425. [26]

Hongo, T., Lundberg, A., Phillips, C. G., and Thompson, R. F. (1984). The pattern of monosynaptic Ia-connections to hindlimb motor nuclei in the baboon: a comparison with the cat. *Proc. Roy. Soc. Lond., Ser. B.* **221**, 261–289. [128]

Hore, J. and Porter, R. (1972). Pyramidal and extrapyramidal influences on some hindlimb motoneuron populations of the arboreal bush tailed possum *Trichosurus vulpecula. J. Neurophysiol.* **35**, 112–121. [85, 312, 313]

Hore, J., Phillips, C. G., and Porter, R. (1973). The effects of pyramidotomy on motor performance in the brush-tailed possum (*Trichosurus vulpecula*). *Brain Res.* **49**, 181–184. [85, 120]

Hore, J., Preston, J. B., Durkovic, R. G., and Cheney, P. D. (1976). Responses of cortical neurons (areas 3a and 4) to ramp stretch of hindlimb muscles in the baboon. *J. Neurophysiol.* **39**, 484–500. [254, 260]

Horne, M. K. and Porter, R. (1980). The discharges during movement of cells in the ventrolateral thalamus of the conscious monkey. *J. Physiol.* **304**, 349–372. [261]

Horne, M. K. and Tracey, D. J. (1979). The afferents and projections of the ventroposterolateral thalamus in the monkey. *Exp. Brain Res.* **36**, 129–142. [261]

Hörner, M., Illert, M., and Kümmel, H. (1990). Do forelimb motoneurones to extrinsic digit extensors display axon collaterals? *Europ. J. Neurosci.* suppl. 3, 191. [129]

Houk, J. C. (1991). Outline for a theory of motor learning. In *Tutorials in motor neuroscience* (eds. G. E. Stelmach and J. Requin) Vol. 62, pp. 253–268. Kluwer, Academic Publishers, Holland. [343]

Houk, J. C. and Barto, A. G. (1991). Distributed sensorimotor learning. *Neuronal Pop. & Behav. Tech. Report* **1**, 1–28. [343]

Houk, J. C., Dessem, D. A., Miller, L. E., and Sybirska, E. H. (1987). Correlation and spectral analysis of relations between single unit discharge and muscle activities. *J. Neurosci. Methods* **21**, 201–224. [164]

Huang, C.-S., Sirisko, M. A., Hiraba, H., Murray, G. M., and Sessle, B. J. (1988). Organization of the primate face motor cortex as revealed by intracortical microstimulation and electrophysiological identification of afferent inputs and corticobulbar projections. *J. Neurophysiol.* **59**, 796–818. [315, 326, 327, 329, 346]

Huang, C.-S., Hiraba, H., and Sessle, B. J. (1989). Input–output relationships of the primary face motor cortex in the monkey. *J. Neurophysiol.* **61**, 350–362. [313]

Huisman, A. M., Kuypers, H. G. J. M., and Verburgh, C. A. (1981). Quantitative differences in collateralization of the descending spinal pathways from red nucleus and other brain stem cell groups in rat as demonstrated with the multiple fluorescent retrograde tracer technique. *Brain Res.* **209**, 271–286. [144]

Huisman, A. M., Kuypers, H. G. J. M., and Verburgh, C. A. (1982). Differences in collateralization of the descending spinal pathways from red nucleus and other brain stem cell groups in cat and monkey. *Prog. Brain Res.* **57**, 185–217. [144, 146]

Hulliger, M. (1984). The mammalian muscle spindle and its central control. *Rev. Physiol. Biochem. Pharmacol.* **101**, 1–110. [144, 146, 205, 206, 207]

Hultborn, H. and Pierrot-Deseilligny, E. (1979). Changes in recurrent inhibition during voluntary soleus contractions in man studies by an H-reflex technique. *J. Physiol.* **297**, 229–251. [30]

Hultborn, H. and Udo, M. (1972). Convergence in the reciprocal Ia inhibitory pathway of excitation from descending pathways and inhibition from motor axon collaterals. *Acta. Physiol. Scand.* **84**, 95–108. [30, 130]

Hultborn, H., Jankowska, E., and Lindström, S. (1971). Recurrent inhibition from motor axon collaterals of transmission in the Ia inhibitory pathway to motoneurons. *J. Physiol.* **215**, 591–612. [30]

Hultborn, H., Lindström, S., and Wigström, H. (1979). On the function of recurrent inhibition in the spinal cord. *Exp. Brain Res.* **37**, 399–403. [30]

Hultborn, H., Meunier, S., Pierrot-Deseilligny, E., and Shindo, M. (1987). Changes in presynaptic inhibition of Ia fibres at the onset of voluntary contraction in man. *J. Physiol.* **389**, 757–772. [205]

Hummelsheim, H., Wiesendanger, M., Bianchetti, M., Wiesendanger, R., and Macpherson, J. (1986). Further investigations of the efferent linkage of the supplementary motor area (SMA) with the spinal cord in the monkey. *Exp. Brain Res.* **65**, 75–82. [284]

Humphrey, D. R. (1972). Relating motor cortex spike trains to measures of motor performance. *Brain Res.* **40**, 7–18. [234]

Humphrey D. R. (1979). On the cortical control of visually directed reaching: contributions by nonprecentral motor areas. In *Posture and movement: perspective for integrating sensory and motor research on the mammalian nervous system* (eds. R. E. Talbott and D. R. Humphrey), pp. 51–122. Raven, New York. [274, 275]

Humphrey, D. R. (1982). Separate cell systems in the motor cortex of the monkey for the control of joint movement and of joint stiffness. In *Kyoto symposia* (eds. P. A. Buser, W. A. Cobb and T. Okuma) EEG suppl. 36, pp. 393–408. Elsvier, Amsterdam. [346]

Humphrey, D. R. (1986). Representation of movements and muscles within the primate precentral motor cortex: historical and current perspectives. *Fed. Proc.* **45**, 2687–2699. [23, 312, 315, 317, 321, 346]

Humphrey, D. R. and Corrie, W. S. (1978). Properties of pyramidal tract neuron system within a functionally defined subregion of primate motor cortex. *J. Neurophysiol.* **41**, 216–243. [37, 63, 65, 66, 73, 82]

Humphrey, D. R. and Reed, D. J. (1983). Separate cortical systems for control of joint movement and joint stiffness: Reciprocal activation and coactivation of antagonist muscles. In *Motor control mechanisms in health and disease* (ed. J. Desmedt), pp. 347–372. Raven, New York. [228]

Humphrey, D. R. and Rietz, R. R. (1976). Cells of origin of corticorubral projections from the arm area of primate motor cortex and their synaptic actions in the red nucleus. *Brain Res.* **110**, 162–169. [65]

Humphrey, D. R. and Tanji, J. (1991). What features of voluntary motor control are encoded in the neuronal discharge of different cortical motor areas? In *Motor control: concepts & issues* (eds. D. R. Humphrey and H.-J. Freund), pp. 413–443. Wiley-Interscience, Chichester. [210]

Humphrey, D. R., Schmidt, E. M., and Thompson, W. D. (1970). Predicting measures of motor performance from multiple cortical spike trains. *Science* **179**, 758–762. [234, 235]

Humphrey, D. R., Gold, R., and Reed, D. J. (1984). Sizes, laminar and topographic origins of cortical projections to the major divisions of the red nucleus in the monkey. *J. Comp. Neurol.* **225**, 75–94. [85]

Huntley, G. W. and Jones, E. G. (1991). Relationship of intrinsic connections to forelimb movement representations in monkey motor cortex: A correlative anatomic and physiological study. *J. Neurophysiol.* **66**, 390–413. [49, 310, 315, 318, 324, 326]

Hutchins, K. D., Martino, A. M., and Strick, P. L. (1988). Corticospinal projections from the medial wall of the hemisphere. *Exp. Brain Res.* **71**, 667–672. [75, 76]

Huttenlocher, P. R. (1967). Development of cortical neuronal activity in the neonatal cat. *Exp. Neurol.* **17**, 247–262. [100]

Huttenlocher, P. R. (1970). Myelination and the development of function in immature pyramidal tract. *Exp. Neurol.* **29**, 405–415. [100, 103]

Huttenlocher, P. R. and Raichelson, R. M. (1989). Effects of neonatal hemispherectomy on location and number of corticospinal neurons in the rat. *Devel. Brain Res.* **47**, 59–69. [99]

Iles, J. F., and Pisini, J. V. (1992). Cortical modulation of transmission in spinal reflex pathways of man. *J. Physiol.* **455**, 425–446. [202]

Illert, M. and Tanaka, R. (1978). Integration in descending motor pathways controlling the forelimb in the cat. 4. Corticospinal inhibition of forelimb motoneurones mediated by short propriospinal neurones. *Exp. Brain Res.* **31**, 131–141. [30]

Illert, M., Lundberg, A. and Tanaka, R. (1976a). Integration in descending motor pathways controlling the forelimb in the cat. 1. Pyramidal effects on motoneurones. *Exp. Brain Res.* **26**, 509–519. [131, 312]

Illert, M., Lundberg, A., and Tanaka, R. (1976b). Integration in descending motor pathways controlling the forelimb in the cat. 2. Convergence on neurones mediating disynaptic corticomotoneuronal excitation. *Exp. Brain Res.* **26**, 521–540. [31, 131, 312]

Illert, M., Lundberg, A., and Tanaka, R. (1977). Integration in descending motor pathways controlling the forelimb in the cat. 3. Convergence on propriospinal neurons transmitting disynaptic excitation from the corticospinal tract and other descending tracts. *Exp. Brain Res.* **29**, 323–346. [117, 131, 132]

Illert, M., Lundberg, A., Padel, Y. and Tanaka, R. (1978). Integration in descending motor pathways controlling the forelimb in the cat. 5. Properties of and monosynaptic connections on C3-C4 propriospinal neurones. *Exp. Brain Res.* **33**, 101–130. [117, 131]

Ingvar, D. H. and Philipson, L. (1977). Distribution of cerebral blood flow in the dominant hemisphere during motor ideation and motor performance. *Ann. Neurol.* **2**, 230–237. [302]

Iriki, A., Pavlides, C., Keller, A. and Asanuma, H. (1989). Long-term potentiation in the motor cortex. *Science* **245**, 1385–1387. [342]

Iriki, A., Keller, A., Pavlides, C., and Asanuma, H. (1990). Long-lasting facilitation of pyramidal tract input to spinal interneurones. *Neuro. Report* **1**, 157–160. [56, 342]

Ito, M. (1985). Cerebellar plasticity as the basis of motor learning. In *Upper motor neuron functions and dysfunctions*, recent achievements in restorative neurology No. 1 (eds. J. C. Eccles and M. R. Dimitrijevic) pp. 222–234. Karger, Basel. [343, 360]

Iwamura, Y., Tanaka, M., and Hikosaka, O. (1980). Overlapping representation of fingers in the somatosensory cortex (area 2) of the conscious monkey. *Brain Res.* **197**, 516–520. [262]

Iwamura, Y., Tanaka, M., Sakamoto, M., and Hikosaka, O. (1983a). Functional sub-divisions representing different finger regions in area 3 of the first somatosensory cortex of the conscious monkey. *Exp. Brain Res.* **51**, 315–326. [253]

Iwamura, Y., Tanaka, M., Sakamoto, M., and Hikosaka, O. (1983b). Converging patterns of finger representation and complex response properties of neurones in area I of the first somatosensory cortex in the conscious monkey. *Exp. Brain Res.* **51**, 327–337. [262]

Iwatsubo, T., Kuzuhara, S., Kanemitsu, A., Shimada, H., and Toyokura, Y. (1990). Corticofugal projections to the motor nuclei of the brainstem and spinal cord in humans. *Neurology* **40**, 309–312. [59]

Jack, J. J. B. (1978). Some methods for selective activation of muscle afferent fibres. In *Studies in neurophysiology presented to A. K. McIntyre* (ed. R. Porter), pp. 155–176. Cambridge University Press. [127]

Jack, J. J. B., Miller, S., Porter, R., and Redman, S. (1971). The time course of minimal excitatory post-synaptic potentials evoked in spinal motoneurones by group Ia afferent fibres. *J. Physiol.* **215**, 353–380. [138, 139]

Jack, J. J. B., Redman, S. J., and Wong, K. (1981). The components of synaptic potentials evoked in cat spinal motoneurones by impulses in single group Ia afferents. *J. Physiol.* **321**, 65–96. [139]

Jackson, J. H. (1874). The anatomical and physiological localisation of movements in the brain. In *Selected writings of John Hughlings Jackson* (ed. J. Taylor), vol. I. Hodder & Stoughton, London. [2]

Jackson, J. H. (1932). *Selected writings of John Hughlings Jackson* (ed. J. Taylor), vol. II. Hodder & Stoughton, London. [344]

Jacobs, K. M. and Donoghue, J. P. (1991). Reshaping the cortical motor map by unmasking latent intracortical connections. *Science* **251**, 944–947. [45, 341]

Jane, J. A., Yashon, D., DeMyer, W., and Bucy, P. C. (1967). The contribution of the precentral gyrus to the pyramidal tract of man. *J. Neurosurg.* **26**, 244–248. [67]

Jankowska, E. (1985). Further indications for enhancement of retrograde trans-neuronal transport of WGA-HRP by synaptic activity. *Brain Res.* **341**, 403–408. [132]

Jankowska, E. (1992). Interneuronal relay in spinal pathways from proprioceptors. *Prog. Neurobiol.* **38**, 335–378. [127]

Jankowska, E. and Lundberg, A. (1981). Interneurones in the spinal cord. *Trends in Neurosci.* **4**, 230–233. [135]

Jankowska, E. and Roberts, W. J. (1972). Synaptic actions of single interneurones mediating reciprocal Ia inhibition of motoneurons. *J. Physiol.* **222**, 623–642. [130]

Jankowska, E., Padel, Y., and Tanaka, R. (1975a). The mode of activation of pyramidal tract cells by intracortical stimuli. *J. Physiol.* **249**, 617–636. [187, 195, 306, 307]

Jankowska, E., Padel, Y., and Tanaka, R. (1975b). Projections of pyramidal tract cells to α-motoneurones innervating hind-limb muscles in monkey. *J. Physiol.* **249**, 637–667. [136, 179, 189, 310, 314, 319, 324, 326]

Jankowska, E., Padel, Y., and Tanaka, R. (1976). Disynaptic inhibition of spinal motoneurones from the motor cortex in the monkey. *J. Physiol.* **258**, 467–487. [30, 162, 202, 324]

Jasper, H., Ricci, G.F., and Doane, B. (1958). Patterns of cortical neurone discharge during conditioned motor responses in monkeys. In *Neurological basis of behaviour* (eds. G. Wolstenholme and C. O'Connor). Little Brown, Boston. [210]

Jeannerod, M. (1984). The timing of natural prehension movements. *J. Motor Behav.* **16**, 235–254. [355]

Jeannerod, M. (1988). *The Neural and behavioural organisation of goal-directed movements.* Clarendon Press, Oxford. [345, 354, 355]

Jeannerod, M., Michel, F., and Prablanc, C. (1984). The control of hand movements in a case of hemianaesthesia following a parietal lesion. *Brain* **107**, 899–920. [354]

Jenny, A. B. and Inukai, J. (1983). Principles of motor organization of the monkey cervical spinal cord. *J. Neurosci.* **3**, 567–575. [123, 147, 172]

Jiang, W., Chapman, C. E., and Lamarre, Y. (1990). Modulation of somatosensory evoked responses in the primary somatosensory cortex produced by intracortical microstimulation of the motor cortex in the monkey. *Exp. Brain Res.* **80**, 333–344. [66, 269, 358]

Jiang, W., Chapman, C. E., and Lamarre, Y. (1991). Modulation of the cutaneous responsiveness of neurones in the primary somatosensory cortex during conditioned arm movements in the monkey. *Exp. Brain Res.* **84**, 342–354. [269, 358]

Johansson, R. S. (1991) How is grasping modified by somatosensory input? In: *Motor control: concepts and issues* (eds. D. R. Humphrey and H.-J. Freund), pp. 331–356. Wiley, Chichester. [357]

Johansson, R. S. and Westling, G. (1984). Roles of glabrous skin receptors and sensorimotor memory in automatic control of precision grip when lifting rougher or more slippery objects. *Exp. Brain Res.* **56**, 550–564. [120, 259, 356]

Johansson, R. S. and Westling, G. (1987a). Signals in tactile afferents from the fingers eliciting adaptive motor responses during precision grip. *Exp. Brain Res.* **66**, 141–154. [357]

Johansson, R. S. and Westling, G. (1987b). Tactile afferent input influencing motor coordination during precision grip. In: *Clinical aspects of sensory motor integration* (eds. A. Struppler and A. Weindl), pp. 3–13. Springer, Berlin. [260, 356]

Johansson, R. S. and Westling, G. (1988). Programmed and reflex actions to rapid load changes during precision grip. *Exp. Brain Res.* **71**, 72–86. [357]

Johansson, R. S., Häger, C., and Bäckström, L. (1992). Somatosensory control of precision grip during unpredictable pulling loads: III. Impairments during digital anaesthesia. *Exp. Brain Res.* **89**, 204–213. [260]

Jones, E. G. (1983) Identification and classification of intrinsic circuit elements in the neocortex. In *Dynamic aspects of neocortical function* (eds. G. Edelman *et al.*), pp. 7–40. Wiley, Chichester. [45]

Jones, E. G. (1984). Laminar distribution of cortical efferent cells. In *Cerebral cortex* (eds. A. Peters and E. G. Jones) Vol. 1, pp. 521–553. Plenum, New York. [55, 56, 57, 310]

Jones, E. G. (1986). Connectivity of the primate sensory-motor cortex. In *Cerebral cortex* (eds. E. G. Jones and A. Peters) Vol. 5, pp. 113–183. Plenum, New York. [251, 252, 261, 262]

Jones, E. G. and Burton, H. (1976). Areal differences in the laminar distribution of the thalamic afferents in cortical fields of the insular, parietal and temporal regions of primates. *J. Comp. Neurol.* **168**, 197–247. [297]

Jones, E. G. and Porter, R. (1980). What is area 3a? *Brain Res. Reviews* **2**, 1–43. [76, 251]

Jones, E. G. and Powell, T. P. S. (1969). Connexions of the somatic sensory cortex of the rhesus monkey. I. Ipsilateral cortical connexions. *Brain* **92**, 477–502. [50, 250]

Jones, E. G. and Wise, S. P. (1977). Size, laminar and columnar distribution of efferent cells in the sensory-motor cortex of monkeys. *J. Comp. Neurol.* **175**, 391–437. [37, 40, 62, 73, 322]

Jones, E. G., Burton, H., and Porter, R. (1975). Commissural and cortico-cortical 'columns' in the somatic sensory cortex of primates. *Science* **190**, 572–574. [56]

Jones, E. G., Coulter, J. D., and Hendry, S. H. C. (1978). Intracortical connectivity of architectonic fields in the somatic sensory motor and parietal cortex of monkeys. *J. Comp. Neurol.* **181**, 291–348. [251, 263]

Jones, E. G., Wise, S. P., and Coulter, J. D. (1979). Differential thalamic relationships of sensory-motor and parietal cortical fields in monkeys. *J. Comp. Neurol.* **183**, 833–882. [261]

Jones, E. G., Schreyer, D. J., and Wise, S. P. (1982). Growth and maturation of the rat corticospinal tract. *Prog. Brain Res.* **57**, 361–379. [98, 100]

Joosten, E. A. J., Gribnau, A. A. M., and Dederen, P. J. W. C. (1987). An anterograde tracer study of the developing corticospinal tract in the rat: three components. *Devel. Brain Res.* **36**, 121–130. [97, 98]

Joosten, E. A. J., van der Ven, P. F. M., Hooiveld, M. H. W., and ten Donkelaar, H. J. (1991). Induction of corticospinal target finding by release of a diffusible, chemotropic factor in cervical spinal grey matter. *Neurosci. Lett.* **128**, 25–28. [98]

Kably, B. (1989) Plasticité post-lésionnelle de la voie pyramidale au cours du développement chez le chat. Thesis, University of Marseille. [99]

Kalaska, J. F., Cohen, D. A., Hyde, M. L., and Prud'homme, M. A. (1989). Comparison of movement direction-related versus load direction-related activity in primate motor cortex, using a two-dimensional reaching task. *J. Neurosci.* **9**, 2080–2102. [219, 221, 233]

Kalaska, J. F. and Crammond, D. J. (1992). Cerebral cortical mechanisms of reaching movements. *Science* **255**, 1517–1523. [351]

Kalil, K. and Schneider, G. E. (1975). Motor performance following unilateral pyramidal tract lesions in the hamster. *Brain Res.* **100**, 170-174. [120]

Kang, Y., Endo, K., and Araki, T. (1988). Excitatory synaptic actions between pairs of neighbouring pyramidal tract cells in the motor cortex. *J. Neurophysiol.* **59**, 636-647. [47]

Kang, Y., Endo, K., and Araki, T. (1991). Differential connections by intracortical axon collaterals among pyramidal tract cells in the cat motor cortex. *J. Physiol.* **435**, 243-256. [47]

Kasser, R. J. and Cheney, P. D. (1985). Characteristics of corticomotoneuronal post-spike facilitation and reciprocal suppression of EMG activity in the monkey. *J. Neurophysiol.* **53**, 959-978. [158, 160, 168, 202, 204]

Keizer, K. and Kuypers, H. G. J. M. (1984). Distribution of corticospinal neurons with collaterals to lower brain stem reticular formation in cat. *Exp. Brain Res.* **54**, 107-120. [61, 65, 70, 77]

Keizer, K. and Kuypers, H. G. J. M. (1989). Distribution of corticospinal neurons with collaterals to the lower brain stem reticular formation in monkey (Macaca fascicularis). *Exp. Brain Res.* **74**, 311-318. [66]

Kemper, T. L., Caveness, W. F., and Yakovlev, P. I. (1973). The neuronographic and metric study of the dendritic arbors of neurons in the motor cortex of Macaca mulatta at birth and at 24 months of age. *Brain* **96**, 765-782. [38]

Kennedy, P. R. (1990). Corticospinal, rubrospinal and rubro-olivary projections: a unifying hypothesis. *Trends in Neurosci.* **13**, 474-479. [351]

Kennedy, P. R. and Humphrey, D. R. (1987). The compensatory role of the parvocellular division of the red nucleus in operantly conditioned rats. *Neurosci. Res.* **5**, 39-62. [120]

Kernell, D. and Wu, C. -P. (1967). Responses of the pyramidal tract to stimulation of the baboon's motor cortex. *J. Physiol.* **191**, 653-672. [190]

Kertesz, A. (1979). *Aphasia and associated disorders: taxonomy, localization and recovery*. Grune & Stratton, New York. [34]

Kety, S. S. and Schmidt, C. F. (1946). The effects of active and passive hyperventilation on cerebral blood flow, cerebral oxygen consumption, cardiac output, and blood pressure of normal young men. *J. Clin. Invest.* **25**, 107-119. [240]

van Keulen, L. C. M. (1979). Autogenetic recurrent inhibition of individual spinal motoneurones in the cat. *Neurosci. Lett.* **21**, 297-300. [131]

Killackey, H. P., Koralek, K-A., Chiaia, N.L., and Rhoades, R. W. (1989). Laminar and areal differences in the origin of the subcortical projection neurons of the rat somatosensory cortex. *J. Comp. Neurol.* **282**, 428-445. [63]

Kirkwood, P. A. (1979). On the use and interpretation of cross-correlation measurements in the mammalian central nervous system. *J. Neurosci. Methods* **1**, 107-132. [135, 157]

Kirkwood, P. A. and Sears, T. A. (1978). The synaptic connexions to intercostal motoneurones as revealed by the average common excitation potential. *J. Physiol.* **275**, 103-134. [186]

Kirkwood, P. A. and Sears, T. A. (1982). The effects of single afferent impulses on the probability of firing of external intercostal motoneurones in the cat. *J. Physiol.* **322**, 315-336. [186]

Knox, C. K. and Poppele, R. E. (1977). Correlation analysis of stimulus-evoked changes in excitability of spontaneously firing neurons. *J. Neurophysiol.* **40**, 616–625. [135]

Koehler, W., Windhorst, U., Schmidt, J., Meyer-Lohmann, J., and Henatsch, H. D. (1978). Diverging influences on Renshaw cell responses and monosynaptic reflexes from stimulation of capsula interna. *Neurosci. Lett.* **8**, 35–39. [30]

Koeze, T. H. (1968). The independence of corticomotoneuronal and fusimotor pathways in the production of muscle contraction by cortex stimulation. *J. Physiol.* **197**, 87–105. [205]

Koeze, T. H. (1973). Thresholds of cortical activation of baboon α- and γ-motoneurones during halothane anaesthesia. *J. Physiol.* **229**, 319–337. [206]

Koeze, T. H., Phillips, C. G., and Sheridan, J. D. (1968). Thresholds of cortical activation of muscle spindles and α motoneurones of the baboon's hand. *J. Physiol.* **195**, 419–449. [206]

Koike, H., Okada, Y., Oshima, T., and Takahashi, K. (1968a). Accommodative behavior of cat pyramidal tract cells investigated with intracellular injection of currents. *Exp. Brain Res.* **5**, 173–188. [51]

Koike, H., Okada, Y., and Oshima, T. (1968b). Accommodative properties of fast and slow pyramidal tract cells and their modification by different levels of their membrane potential. *Exp. Brain Res.* **5**, 189–201. [51]

Koike, H., Mano, N., Okada, Y., and Oshima, T. (1970). Repetitive impulses generated in fast and slow pyramidal tract cells by intracellularly applied current steps. *Exp. Brain Res.* **11**, 263–281. [51]

Koike, H., Mano, N., Okada, Y., and Oshima, T. (1972). Activities of the sodium pump in cat pyramidal tract cells investigated with intracellular injection of sodium ions. *Exp. Brain Res.* **14**, 449–462. [51]

van der Kooy, D., Kuypers, H. G. J. M., and Catsman-Berrevoets, C. E. (1978). Single mammillary body cells with divergent axon collaterals. Demonstration by a simple, fluorescent double labelling technique in the rat. *Brain Res.* **158**, 189–196. [63]

Kornhuber, H. H. (1984). Attention, readiness for action, and the stages of voluntary decision in some electrophysiological correlates in man. *Exp. Brain Res.* suppl 9, 420–429. [290]

Kornhuber, H. H. and Deecke, L. (1985) The starting function of the SMA. *Behav. Brain. Sci.* **8**, 591–592. [289]

Kozhanov, V. M. and Shapovalov, A. I. (1977). Synaptic organization of supraspinal control over propriospinal ventral horn interneurons in cat and monkey spinal cord. *Nejrofiziologija*, **9**, 177–184 (translated from Russian). Plenum, New York. [130]

Kristeva, R., Keller, E., Deecke, L., and Kornhuber, H. H. (1979). Cerebral potentials preceding unilateral and simultaneous bilateral finger movements. *Electroenceph. Clin. Neurophysiol.* **47**, 229–238. [290]

Kuang, R. Z. and Kalil, K. (1990). Branching patterns of corticospinal axon arbors in the rodent. *J. Comp. Neurol.* **292**, 585–598. [86]

Kubota, K. and Hamada, I. (1978). Visual tracking and neuron activity in the post-arcute area in monkeys. *J. Physiol.* (*Paris*) **74**, 297–312. [300]

Kucera, P. and Wiesendanger, M. (1985). Do ipsilateral corticospinal fibers participate in the functional recovery following unilateral pyramidal lesions in monkeys? *Brain Res.* **348**, 297–303. [112]

Kuno, M. (1964). Quantal components of excitatory synaptic potentials in spinal motoneurones. *J. Physiol.* **175**, 81–99. [138]

Künzle, H. (1976). Thalamic projections from the precentral motor cortex in Macaca fascicularis. *Brain Res.* **105**, 253–267. [56]

Künzle, H. (1978). An autoradiographic analysis of the afferent connections from premotor and adjacent prefrontal regions (areas 6 and 9) in Macaca fascicularis. *Brain Behav. & Evol.* **15**, 185–234. [276, 297]

Kuypers, H. G. J. M. (1958a). Cortico-bulbar connexions to the pons and lower brain stem in man. *Brain* **81**, 364–388. [59, 82]

Kuypers, H. G. J. M. (1958b). An anatomical analysis of cortico-bulbar connexions to the pons and lower brain stem in the cat. *J. Anat.* **92**, 198–218. [61, 82, 119]

Kuypers, H. G. J. M. (1958c). Some projections from the peri-central cortex to the pons and lower brain stem in monkey and chimpanzee. *J. Comp. Neurol.* **110**, 221–225. [59, 82]

Kuypers, H. G. J. M. (1962). Corticospinal connections: Postnatal development in the Rhesus monkey. *Science* **138**, 678–680. [94, 98, 104]

Kuypers, H. G. J. M. (1973). The anatomical organization of the descending pathways and their contributions to motor control especially in primates. In *New developments in EMG and clinical neurophysiology* (ed. J. E. Desmedt) Vol. 3, pp. 38–68. Karger, Basel. [83, 86]

Kuypers, H. G. J. M. (1978). The organization of the motor system in primates. In *Recent advances in primatology* (eds. D. J. Chivers and J. Herbert) Vol. 1, pp. 623–634. Academic Press, New York. [88, 144]

Kuypers, H. G. J. M. (1981). Anatomy of the descending pathways. In *Handbook of physiology – the nervous system II* (eds. J. M. Brookhart and V. B. Mountcastle), pp. 597–666. American Physiological Society, Bethesda, Maryland. [56, 57, 58, 59, 76, 84, 85, 86, 88, 94, 116, 143, 144, 160, 234]

Kuypers, H. G. J. M. and Brinkman, J. (1970). Precentral projections to different parts of the spinal intermediate zone in the rhesus monkey. *Brain Res.* **24**, 29–48. [73, 76, 112, 280, 314]

Kuypers, H. G. J. M. and Huisman, A. M. (1984). Fluorescent neuronal tracers. In: *Advances in cellular neurobiology.* (eds. S. Fedoroff and L. Hertz), pp. 307–340. Academic Press, New York. [63]

Kuypers, H. G. J. M. and Tuerk, J. (1964). Contribution of the cortical fibers within the nuclei cuneatus and gracilis in the cat. *J. Anat. Lond.* **98**, 143–162. [61]

Kuypers, H. G. J. M. and Ugolini, G. (1990). Viruses as transneuronal tracers. *Trends in Neurosci.* **13**, 71–75. [78]

Kwan, H. C., MacKay, W. A., Murphy, J. T., and Wong, Y. C. (1978). Spatial organization of precentral cortex in awake primates. II. Motor outputs. *J. Neurophysiol.* **41**, 1120–1131. [312, 313, 314, 315, 316, 324, 325, 326, 339, 345]

Kwan, H. C., Murphy, J.T., and Wong, Y. C. (1987). Interaction between neurons in precentral cortical zones controlling different joints. *Brain Res.* **400**, 259–269. [45]

Lamarre, Y., Spidalieri, G., and Lund, J. P. (1981). Patterns of muscular and motor cortical activity during a simple arm movement in the monkey. *Can. J. Physiol. Pharmacol.* **59**, 748–756. [216, 344]

Lance, J. W. and DeGail, P. (1965). Spread of phasic muscle reflexes in normal and spastic subjects. *J. Neurol. Neurosurg. Psychiat.* **28**, 328–334. [270]

Lance, J. W. and Manning, R. L. (1954). Origin of the pyramid tract in the cat. *J. Physiol.* **124**, 385–399. [238]

Landgren, S., Phillips, C. G., and Porter, R. (1962a). Minimal synaptic actions of pyramidal impulses on some alpha motoneurones of the baboon's hand and forearm. *J. Physiol.* **161**, 91–111. [146, 186, 195, 200, 314]

Landgren, S., Phillips, C. G. and Porter, R. (1962b). Cortical fields of origin of the monosynaptic pyramidal pathways to some alpha motoneurones of the baboon's hand and forearm. *J. Physiol.* **161**, 112–125. [37, 187, 317]

Landry, P., Labelle, A., and Deschênes, M. (1980). Intracortical distribution of axonal collaterals of pyramidal tract cells in the cat motor cortex. *Brain Res.* **191**, 327–336. [38]

Langley, J. N. and Sherrington, C. S. (1884) quoted from Liddell, E. G. T. (1960). *The discovery of reflexes*, pp. 105–108. Clarendon Press, Oxford. [3]

Lankamp, D. J. (1967) The fibre composition of the pedunculus cerebri (crus cerebri) in man, pp. 1–40. Thesis, Leiden University. [80]

Laplane, D., Talairach, J., Meininger, V., Bancaud, J., and Orgogozo, J. M. (1977). Clinical consequences of corticectomies involving the supplementary motor area in man. *J. Neurol. Sci.* **34**, 301–314. [294]

Larsen, B., Skinhøj, E., and Lassen, N. A. (1978). Variations in regional cortical blood flow in the right and left hemispheres during automatic speech. *Brain* **101**, 193–209. [287]

Lassek, A. M. (1948). The pyramidal tract: basic considerations of corticospinal neurons. *Res. Publ. Ass. Nerv. Ment. Dis.* **27**, 106–128. [82]

Lassek, A. M. and Karlsberg, P. (1956). The pyramidal tract of an aquatic carnivore. *J. Comp. Neurol.* **106**, 425–431. [82]

Lassek, A. M. and Rasmussen, G. L. (1940). A comparative fiber and numerical analysis of the pyramidal tract. *J. Comp. Neurol.* **72**, 417–428. [90]

Lassen, N. A. (1959). Cerebral blood flow and oxygen consumption in man. *Physiol. Rev.* **39**, 183–238. [240]

Lassen, N. A. (1985). Measurement of regional cerebral blood flow in humans with single-photon-emitting radioisotopes. *Res. Publ. Ass. Nerv. Ment. Dis.* **63**, 9–20. [242]

Lassen, N. A. and Ingvar, D. H. (1961). The blood flow of the cerebral cortex determined by radioactive krypton-85. *Experienta* **17**, 42–45. [240]

Laursen, A. M. (1971). A kinesthetic deficit after partial transection of a pyramidal tract in monkeys. *Brain Res.* **31**, 263–274. [110]

Laursen, A. M., and Wiesendanger, M. (1967). The effect of pyramidal lesions on response latency in cats. *Brain Res.* **5**, 207–220. [117]

Lawrence, D. G. and Hopkins, D. A. (1976). The development of motor control in the rhesus monkey: evidence concerning the role of corticomotoneuronal connections. *Brain* **99**, 235–254. [98, 100, 104, 106, 107, 113]

Lawrence, D. G. and Kuypers, H. G. J. M. (1968a). The functional organization of the motor system in the monkey. I. The effects of bilateral pyramidal lesions. *Brain* **91**, 1–14. [104, 109, 110, 113]

Lawrence, D. G. and Kuypers, H. G. J. M. (1968b). The functional organization of the motor system in the monkey. II. The effects of lesions of the descending brain-stem pathway. *Brain* **91**, 15–36. [110]

Lawrence, D. G., Porter, R., and Redman, S. J. (1985). Corticomotoneuronal synapses in the monkey: light microscopic localization upon motoneurons of intrinsic muscles of the hand. *J. Comp. Neurol.* **232**, 499–510. [124, 147, 148, 150, 151, 152, 154, 172, 178]

Leenen, L., Meek, J., and Nieuwenhuys, R. (1982). Unmyelinated fibers in the pyramidal tract of the rat: a new view. *Brain Res.* **246**, 297–301. [80, 82]

Lemon, R. N. (1979). Short-latency peripheral inputs to the motor cortex in conscious monkeys. *Brain Res.* **161**, 150–155. [260, 358]

Lemon, R. N. (1981a). Functional properties of monkey motor cortex neurones receiving afferent input from the hand and fingers. *J. Physiol.* **311**, 497–519. [254, 256, 258, 259, 269, 270, 334]

Lemon, R. N. (1981b). Variety of functional organization within the monkey motor cortex. *J. Physiol.* **311**, 521–540. [254, 335, 336, 337, 338, 346]

Lemon, R. N. (1984). Methods for neuronal recording in conscious animals. In *IBRO Handbook Series: Methods in Neurosciences* (ed. A. D. Smith) Vol. 4, pp. 1–162. Wiley, London. [210, 213]

Lemon, R. (1988). The output map of the primate motor cortex. *Trends in Neurosci.* **11**, 501–506. [329, 330, 331]

Lemon, R. N. (1990) Mapping the output functions of the motor cortex. In *Signal and sense: local and global order in perceptual maps* (eds. G. Edelman, E. Gall, and W. M. Cowan), pp. 315–356. Wiley, Chichester. [121, 137, 148, 158, 163, 164, 187, 188, 305, 312, 317, 319, 320, 327, 328]

Lemon, R. N. (1992). Control of the monkey's hand by the motor cortex. In *The use of tools by human and non-human primates* (eds. A. Berthelet and J. Chavaillon), pp. 51–65. Fyssen Foundation Symposium. Oxford University Press. [334]

Lemon, R. N. and van der Burg, J. (1979). Short-latency peripheral inputs to thalamic neurones projecting to the motor cortex in the monkey. *Exp. Brain Res.* **36**, 445–462. [261]

Lemon, R. N. and Mantel, G. W. H. (1989). The influence of changes in the discharge frequency of corticospinal neurones on hand muscles in the monkey. *J. Physiol.* **413**, 351–378. [179, 186, 196, 197, 199, 200, 218]

Lemon, R. N. and Porter, R. (1976a). Afferent input to movement-related pre-central neurones in conscious monkeys. *Proc R. Soc. Lond. Ser. B.* **194**, 313–339. [248, 254, 256, 257, 258, 260, 335]

Lemon, R. N. and Porter, R. (1976b). A comparison of the responsiveness to peripheral stimuli of pre-central cortical neurones in anaesthetised and conscious monkeys. *J. Physiol.* **260**, 53–54P [249].

Lemon, R. N., Hanby, J. A., and Porter, R. (1976). Relationship between the activity of precentral neurones during active and passive movements in con-scious monkeys. *Proc. R. Soc. Lond., Ser. B.* **194**, 341–373. [73, 76, 235, 236, 248, 334, 344]

Lemon, R. N., Mantel, G. W. H. and Muir, R. B. (1986). Corticospinal facilitation of hand muscles during voluntary movement in the conscious monkey. *J. Physiol.* **381**, 497–527. [157, 158, 160, 164, 167, 172, 179, 204, 213, 313, 324]

Lemon, R. N., Muir, R. B., and Mantel, G. W. H. (1987). The effects upon the activity of hand and forearm muscles of intracortical stimulation in the vicinity of corticomotor neurones in the conscious monkey. *Exp. Brain Res.* **66**, 621–637. [137, 148, 201, 202, 204, 306, 308, 313, 314, 322, 323, 325, 326, 332]

Lemon, R. N., Mantel, G. W. H., and Rea, P. A. (1990). Recording and identification of single motor units in the free-to-move primate hand. *Exp. Brain Res.* **81**, 95–106. [172]

Lemon, R. N., Bennett, K. M. B., and Werner, W. (1991). The cortico-motor substrate for skilled movements of the primate hand. In *Tutorials on motor neuroscience* (eds. G. E. Stelmach and J. Requin) Vol. 62, pp. 477–495. Kluwer Academic Publishers, Holland. [158, 160, 166, 167, 168, 169, 171, 181]

Lemon, R. N., Werner, W., Bennett, K. M. B., and Flament, D. A. (1993). The proportion of slow and fast pyramidal tract neurones producing post-spike facilitation of hand muscles in the conscious monkey. *J. Physiol.* **459**, 166P. [167]

Leonard, C. T. and Goldberger, M. E. (1987a). Consequences of damage to the sensorimotor cortex in neonatal and adult cats. I. Sparing and recovery of function. *Devel. Brain Res.* **32**, 1–14. [99]

Leonard, C. T. and Goldberger, M. E. (1987b). Consequences of damage to the sensorimotor cortex in neonatal and adult cats. II. Maintenance of exuberant projections. *Devel. Brain Res.* **32**, 15–30. [98, 99]

Leong, S. K. (1976). A qualitative electron microscopic investigation of the anomalous corticofugal projections following neonatal lesions in the albino rat. *Brain Res.* **107**, 1–8. [99]

Lewis, R. and Brindley, G. S. (1965). The extrapyramidal cortical motor map. *Brain* **88**, 397–406. [329, 333]

Leyton, S. S. F. and Sherrington, C. S. (1917). Observations on the excitable cortex of the chimpanzee, orangutan and gorilla. *Q. J. Exp. Physiol.* **11**, 135–222. [5, 6, 7, 8, 112, 313, 314, 344]

Li, C.-L. (1959). Some properties of pyramidal neurones in motor cortex with particular reference to sensory stimulation. *J. Neurophysiol.* **22**, 385–394. [210]

Liddell, E. G. T. (1960). *The discovery of reflexes*. Oxford University Press [2, 3, 5]

Liddell, E. G. T. and Phillips, C. G. (1944). Pyramidal section in the cat. *Brain* **67**, 1–100. [117]

Liddell, E. G. T. and Phillips, C. G. (1950). Thresholds of cortical representation. *Brain* **73**, 125–140. [314]

Liddell, E. G. T. and Sherrington, C. G. (1925). Further observations on myotatic reflexes. *Proc. R. Soc. Lond., Ser. B.* **97**, 267–283. [127]

Lindström, S. (1973). Recurrent control from motor axon collaterals of Ia inhibitory pathways in the spinal cord of the cat. *Acta Physiol. Scand.*, suppl. **392**, 1–43. [128]

Llinás, R. (1988). The intrinsic electrophysiological properties of mammalian neurons: insights into central nervous system function. *Science* **242**, 1654–1666. [53]

Lloyd, D. P. C. (1941). The spinal mechanism of the pyramidal system in cats. *J. Physiol.* **4**, 525–546. [127, 129, 313]

Lloyd, D. P. C. (1943). Reflex action in relation to pattern and peripheral source of afferent stimulation. *J. Neurophysiol.* **6**, 111–119. [27, 30]

Lloyd, D. P. C. (1946). Facilitation and inhibition of spinal motoneurons. *J. Neurophysiol.* **9**, 421–438. [127, 128]

Long, C. and Brown, M. E. (1964). Electromyographic kinesiology of the hand: muscles moving the long finger. *J. Bone & Joint Surg.* **46A**, 1683–1706. [94]

Lucier, G. E., Rüegg, D. C., and Wiesendanger, M. (1975). Responses of neurones in the motor cortex and in area 3a to controlled stretches of forelimb muscles in cebus monkeys. *J. Physiol.* **251**, 833–853. [254]

Lund, J. S. and Lund, R. D. (1970) The termination of callosal fibres in the paravisual cortex of the rat. *Brain Res.* **17**, 25–45. [50]

Lundberg, A. (1975). The control of spinal mechanisms from the brain. In *The nervous system* (ed. D. B. Tower) Vol. 1, pp. 253–265. Raven, New York. [31]

Lundberg, A. (1979). Multisensory control of spinal reflex pathways. *Prog. Brain Res.* **50**, 11–28. [126, 127, 132]

Lundberg, A. and Voorhoeve, P. (1962). Effects from the pyramidal tract on spinal reflex arcs. *Acta. Physiol. Scand.* **56**, 201–219. [30]

Lundberg, A., Malmgren, K., and Schomberg, E. D. (1977a). Cutaneous facilitation of transmission in reflex pathways from Ib afferents to motoneurones. *J. Physiol.* **265**, 763–780. [128]

Lundberg, A., Malmgren, K., and Schomberg, E. D. (1977b). Comments on reflex actions evoked by electrical stimulation of group II muscle afferents. *Brain Res.* **122**, 551–555. [128]

Lundberg, A., Malmgren, K., and Schomberg, E. D. (1978). Role of joint afferents in motor control exemplified by effects on reflex pathways from Ib afferents. *J. Physiol.* **284**, 327–344. [128]

Luria, A. R. (1970). *Traumatic aphasia.* Mouton, The Hague. [34]

Lüscher, H.-R. and Vardar, U. (1989). A comparison of homonymous and heteronymous connectivity in the spinal monosynaptic reflex arc of the cat. *Exp. Brain Res.* **74**, 480–492. [208]

McBride, R. L., Feringa, E. R., Garver, M. K., and Williams, J. K. (1989). Prelabeled red nucleus and sensorimotor cortex neurons of the rat survive 10 and 20 weeks after spinal cord transection. *J. Neuropath. Exp. Neurol.* **48**, 568–576. [112]

McCloskey, D. I. (1978). Kinaesthetic sensibility. *Physiol. Rev.* **58**, 763–820. [270]

McCloskey, D. I. (1985). Knowledge about muscular contractions. In *The motor system in neurobiology* (eds. E. V. Evarts, S. P. Wise, and D. Bousfield), pp. 149–153. Elsevier, Amsterdam. [271]

McCloskey, D. I. and Torda, T. A. G. (1975). Corollary motor discharges and kinaesthesia. *Brain Res.* **100**, 467–470. [270]

McCloskey, D. I., Cross, M. J., Horner, R., and Potter, E. K. (1983). Sensory effects of pulling or vibrating exposed tendons in man. *Brain* **106**, 21–37. [271]

McComas, A. J. and Wilson, P. (1968). An investigation of pyramidal tract cells in the somatosensory cortex of the rat. *J. Physiol.* **194**, 271–288. [86]

McDonald, W. I. and Sears, T. A. (1970). The effects of experimental demyelination on conduction in the central nervous system. *Brain* **93**, 583–598. [103]

McGuiness, E., Sivertsen, D., and Allman, J. M. (1980). Organization of the face representation in macaque motor cortex. *J. Comp. Neurol.* **193**, 591–608. [312, 315]

MacLean, J. B. and Leffman, H. (1967). Supraspinal control of Renshaw cells. *Exp. Neurol.* **18**, 94–104. [29]

Macpherson, J. M., Marangoz, C., Miles, T. S., and Wiesendanger, M. (1982a). Micro-stimulation of the supplementary motor area (SMA) in the awake monkey. *Exp. Brain Res.* **45**, 410–416. [75]

Macpherson, J. M., Wiesendanger, M., Marangoz, C., and Miles, T. S. (1982b). Corticospinal neurones of the supplementary motor area of the monkey. *Exp. Brain Res.* **48**, 81–88. [75, 276]

Maier, M. A., Hepp-Reymond, M. -C. and Meyer, M. (1990). EMG coactivation patterns and isometric grip force in human. *Europ. J. Neurosci.*, suppl. **3**, 65. [225]

Maier, M.A, Bennett, K. M., Hepp-Reymond, M. -C. and Lemon, R. N. (1993). Contribution of the monkey cortico-motoneuronal system to the control of force in precision grip. *J. Neurophysiol* **69**, 772–785. [225, 227, 358]

Malmgren, K. and Pierrot-Deseilligny, E. (1987). Evidence that low threshold afferents both evoke and depress polysynaptic excitation of the wrist flexor motoneurones in man. *Exp. Brain Res.* **67**, 429–432. [31]

Mandelbrot, B. (1982) *The fractal geometry of nature.* Freeman, New York. [43]

Mark, R. F. and Sperry, R. W. (1968). Bimanual coordination in monkeys. *Exp. Neurol.* **21**, 92–104. [292]

Marr, D. (1969). A theory of cerebellar cortex. *J. Physiol.* **202**, 437–470. [343]

Marsden, C. D. (1987). What do the basal ganglia tell premotor cortical areas? In *Motor areas of the cerebral cortex* (eds. G. Bock, M. O'Connor, and J. Marsh) Vol. 132, pp. 282– 295. CIBA Foundation Symp. Wiley, Chichester. [358]

Marsden, C. D., Merton, P. A. and Morton, H. B. (1972). Servo action in human voluntary movement. *Nature* **238**, 140–143. [129, 264]

Marsden, C. D., Merton, P. A., and Morton, H. B. (1973). Latency measurements compatible with a cortical pathway for the stretch reflex in man. *J. Physiol.* **230**, 58–59P. [264]

Marsden, C. D., Merton, P. A., Morton, H. B., and Adam, J. (1977a). The effect of posterior column lesions on servo-responses from the human long thumb flexor. *Brain* **100**, 185–200. [264]

Marsden, C. D., Merton, P. A., Morton, H. B., and Adam, J. (1977b). The effect of lesions of the sensorimotor cortex and the capsular pathways on servo responses from the human long thumb flexor. *Brain* **100**, 503–526. [264]

Martin, G. F., Megirian, D. and Conner, J. B. (1972). The origin, course and termination of the corticospinal tracts of the tasmanian potoroo (Potorous apicalis). *J. Anat.* **111**, 263– 281. [85]

Matelli, W., Luppino, G., and Rizzolatti, G. (1985). Patterns of cytochrome oxidase activity in the frontal agranular cortex of the macaque monkey. *Behav. Brain Res.* **18**, 125–136. [274, 300]

Matsumura, M. and Kubota, K. (1979). Cortical projections to hand-arm motor area from postarcuate area in macaque monkeys: A histological study of retrograde transport of horseradish peroxidase. *Neurosci. Letts.* **11**, 241–246. [273, 274, 297]

Matsumura, M., Cope, T., and Fetz, E. E. (1988). Sustained excitatory synaptic input to motor cortex neurons in awake animals revealed by intracellular recording of membrane potentials. *Exp. Brain Res.* **70**, 463–469. [354]

Matsunami, K. and Hamada, I. (1978). Precentral neuron activity associated with ipsilateral forelimb movements in monkeys. *J. Physiol.* **74**, 319–322. [76, 235]

Matthews, M. A. and Duncan, D. (1971). A quantitative study of morphological changes accompanying the initiation and progress of myelin production in the dorsal funiculus of the rat spinal cord. *J. Comp. Neurol.* **142**, 1–22. [100, 103]

Matthews, P. B. C. (1984). Evidence from the use of vibration that the human long-latency reflex depends upon secondary spindle afferents. *J. Physiol.* **348**, 383–415. [129, 267, 270]

Matthews, P. B. C. (1989). Long-latency stretch reflexes of two intrinsic muscles of the human hand analysed by cooling the arm. *J. Physiol.* **419**, 519–538. [267]

Matthews, P. B. C. (1991). The human stretch reflex and the motor cortex. *Trends in Neurosci.* **14**, 87–91. [265]

Matthews, P. B. C., Farmer, S. F., and Ingram, D. A. (1990). On the localization of the stretch reflex of intrinsic hand muscles in a patient with mirror movements. *J. Physiol.* **428**, 561–577. [266, 268]

Mazziotta, J. C. and Phelps, M. E. (1984). Positron computed tomographic studies of cerebral metabolic responses to complex motor tasks. *Neurology* **34**, 116. [240]

Mazziotta, J. C. and Phelps, M. E. (1985). Human neuropsychological imaging studies of local brain metabolism: strategies and results. *Res. Publ. Ass. Nerv. Ment. Dis.* **63**, 121–137. [242]

Mediratta, N. K. and Nicoll, J. A. R. (1983). Conduction velocities of corticospinal axons in the rat studied by recording cortical antidromic responses. *J. Physiol.* **336**, 545–561. [82, 86]

Mendell, L. M. and Henneman, E. (1971). Terminals of single Ia fibers: location, density and distribution within a pool of 300 homonymous motoneurons. *J. Neurophysiol.* **34**, 171–187. [128, 138, 173]

Merton, P. A., Hill, D. K., Morton, H. B., and Marsden, C. D. (1982). Scope of a technique for electrical stimulation of human brain, spinal cord, and muscle. *Lancet* ii, 597–600. [192]

Mettler, F. A. (1935a). Corticofugal fiber connections of the cortex of Macaca mulatta. The frontal region. *J. Comp. Neurol.* **61**, 509–542. [273]

Mettler, F. A. (1935b). Corticofugal fiber connections of the cortex of Macaca mulatta. The parietal region. *J. Comp. Neurol.* **62**, 263–291. [273]

Mewes, K. and Cheney, P. D. (1990). Postspike facilitation (PSF) of EMG activity from neurons in primate motor thalamus. *Soc. Neurosci. Abst.* **16**, 425. [162]

Meyer, G. (1987). Forms and spatial arrangement of neurons in the primary motor cortex of man. *J. Comp. Neurol.* **262**, 402–428. [37, 45]

Midroni, G. and Ashby, P. (1989). How synaptic noise may affect cross-correlations. *J. Neurosci. Methods* **27**, 1–12. [135]

Miller, M. W. (1987). The origin of corticospinal projection neurons in rat. *Exp. Brain Res.* **67**, 339–351. [79]

Mitz, A. R. and Humphrey, D. R. (1986). Intracortical stimulation in pyramid-otomized monkeys. *Neurosci. Letts.* **64**, 59–64. [113, 329]

Moberg, E. (1972). Fingers were made before forks. *Hand* **4**, 201–206. [360]

Molenaar, I. and Kuypers, H. G. J. M. (1978). Cells of origin of propriospinal fiber and fibers ascending to supraspinal levels. An HRP study in cat and rhesus monkey. *Brain Res.* **152**, 429–450. [86]

Moll, L. and Kuypers, H. G. J. M. (1977). Premotor cortical ablations in monkeys: contralateral changes in visually guided reaching behaviour. *Science* **198**, 317–319. [295]

Mott, F. W. and Sherrington, C. S. (1895). Experiments upon the influence of sensory nerves upon movement and nutrition of the limbs. *Proc. R. Soc. Lond., Ser B.* **57**, 481–488. [3, 247]

Mountcastle, V. B. (1978). An organizing principle for cerebral function: The unit module and the distributed system. In *The mindful brain* (eds. G. M. Edelman and V. B. Mountcastle), pp. 7-50. M. I. T. Press, Cambridge, Massachusetts. [36]

Muakkassa, K. and Strick, P. (1979). Frontal lobe inputs to primate motor cortex: Evidence for somatotopically organized premotor areas. *Brain Res.* **177**, 176-182. [73, 274, 297]

Muir, R. B. (1985). Small hand muscles in precision grip: A corticospinal prerogative? *Exp. Brain Res.* suppl. 10, 155-174. [94, 173, 225]

Muir, R. B. and Lemon, R. N. (1983). Corticospinal neurons with a special role in precision grip. *Brain Res.* **261**, 312-316. [227, 230, 236, 237]

Muir, R. B. and Porter, R. (1973). The effect of a preceding stimulus on temporal summation at corticomotoneuronal synapses. *J. Physiol.* **228**, 749-763. [195]

Müller, K., Hömberg, V., and Lenard, H. -G. (1991) Magnetic stimulation of motor cortex and nerve roots in children. Maturation of cortico-motoneuronal projections. *Electroenceph. Clin. Neurophysiol.* **81**, 63-70. [100, 107]

Munk, H. (1881). Quoted from Penfield and Welch (1951) *Über die Functionen der Grosshirnrinde. Gesammelte Mitteilungen aus den Jahren 1877-80, mit Einleitung und Anmerkungen*. Hirschwald, Berlin. [15]

Murakami, F. and Higashi, S. (1988). Presence of crossed corticorubral fibers and increase of crossed projections after unilateral lesions of the cerebral cortex of the kitten: a demonstration using anterograde transport of Phaseolus vulgaris leucoagglutin. *Brain Res.* **447**, 98-108. [99]

Murray, E. A. and Coulter, J. D. (1981). Organization of corticospinal neurons in the monkey. *J. Comp. Neurol.* **195**, 339-365. [37, 40, 71, 73, 75, 76, 315, 322]

Mushiake, H., Inase, M., and Tanji, J. (1991). Neuronal activity in the primate premotor, supplementary, and precentral motor cortex during visually guided and internally determined sequential movements. *J. Neurophysiol.* **66**, 705-718. [230]

Napier, J. (1980). *Hands*. George Allen and Unwin, London. [349]

Napier, R. (1961). Prehensibility and opposability in the hands of primates. *Symp. Zool. Soc. Lond.* **5**, 115-132. [94]

Nathan, P. W. and Sears, T. A. (1960). Effects of posterior root section on the activity of some muscles in man. *J. Neuro. Neurosurg. Psychiat.* **23**, 10-22. [247]

Nathan, P. W. and Smith, M. C. (1955). Long descending tracts in man. I. Review of present knowledge. *Brain* **78**, 248-303. [83, 86]

Nathan, P. W., Smith, M. C., and Deacon, P. (1990). The corticospinal tracts in man. Course and location of fibres at different segmental levels. *Brain* **113**, 303-324. [94]

Nelson, R. J. (1984). Responsiveness of monkey primary somatosensory cortical neurons to peripheral stimulation depends on 'motor set'. *Brain Res.* **304**, 143-148. [270]

Nielsen, J. and Kagamihara, Y. (1992). The regulation of disynaptic reciprocal Ia inhibition during co-contraction of antagonistic muscles in man. *J. Physiol.* **456**, 373-391. [205, 353]

Nieoullon, A. and Gahéry, Y. (1978). Influence of pyramidotomy on limb flexion movements induced by cortical stimulation and on associated postural adjustment in the cat. *Brain Res.* **149**, 39–52. [117]

Nieoullon, A. and Rispal-Padel, L. (1976). Somatotopic localization in cat motor cortex. *Brain Res.* **105**, 405–422. [329]

Nudo, R. J. and Masterton, R. B. (1988). Descending pathways to the spinal cord: A comparative study of 22 mammals. *J. Comp. Neurol.* **277**, 53–79. [80]

Nudo, R. J. and Masterton, R. B. (1990a). Descending pathways to the spinal cord, III: Sites of origin of the corticospinal tract. *J. Comp. Neurol.* **296**, 559–583. [67, 90]

Nudo, R. J. and Masterton, R. B. (1990b). Descending pathways to the spinal cord, IV: Some factors related to the amount of cortex devoted to the corticospinal tract. *J. Comp. Neurol.* **296**, 584–597. [90, 92]

Nudo, R. J., Jenkins, W. M., and Merzinich, M. M. (1990). Repetitive microstimulation alters the cortical representation of movement in adult rats. *Somatosens. Mot. Res.* **7**, 463–483. [339]

Oka, H., Samejima, A., and Yamamoto, T. (1985). Post-natal development of pyramidal tract neurones in kittens. *J. Physiol.* **363**, 481–499. [96, 101, 103]

Okano, K. and Tanji, J. (1987). Neuronal activities in the primate motor fields of the agranular frontal cortex preceding visually triggered and self-paced movement. *Exp. Brain Res.* **66**, 155–166. [290]

O'Leary, D. D. M. and Stanfield, B.B. (1986). A transient pyramidal tract projection from the visual cortex in the hamster and its removal by selective collateral elimination. *Dev. Brain Res.* **27**, 87–99. [97]

Oleson, J. (1971). Contralateral focal increase of cerebral blood flow in man during arm work. *Brain* **94**, 635–646. [240]

Olszewski, J. (1952). *The thalamus of the macaca mulatta: An atlas for use with the stereotaxic instrument.* Karger, Basel. [261]

Orgogozo, J. M. and Larsen, B. (1979). Activation of the supplementary motor area during voluntary movement in man suggests it works as a supramotor area. *Science* **206**, 847–850. [287]

Oscarsson, O. and Rosén, I. (1963). Projection to cerebral cortex of large muscle spindle afferents in the contralateral forelimb. *J. Physiol.* **169**, 924–945. [250]

Oscarsson, O. and Rosén, I. (1966). Short-latency projections to the cat's cerebral cortex from skin and muscle afferents in the contralateral forelimb. *J. Physiol.* **182**, 164–184. [250]

Padel, Y., Sybirska, E., Bourbonnais, D., and Vinay, L. (1988). Electrophysiological identification of a somaesthetic pathway to the red nucleus. *Behav. Brain Res.* **28**, 139–151. [262]

Paillard, J. (1978). The pyramidal tract: two million fibres in search of a function. *J. Physiol.* **74**, 155–162. [120, 350]

Palmer, E. and Ashby, P. (1992). Corticospinal projections to upper limb motoneurones in humans. *J. Physiol.* **448**, 397–412. [190, 191, 192, 193]

Palmer, S. S. and Fetz, E. E. (1985a). Discharge properties of primate forearm motor units during isometric muscle activity. *J. Neurophysiol.* **54**, 1178–1193. [172, 190]

Palmer, S. S. and Fetz, E. E. (1985b). Effects of single intracortical microstimuli in motor cortex on activity of identified forearm motor units in behaving monkey. *J. Neurophysiol.* **54**, 1194–1212. [137, 190]

Pandya, D. N. and Kuypers, H. G. J. M. (1969). Cortico-cortical connections in the Rhesus monkey. *Brain Res.* **13**, 13–36. [297]

Pandya, D. N. and Vignolo, L. A. (1971). Intra- and interhemispheric projections of the precentral, premotor and arcuate areas in the Rhesus monkey. *Brain Res.* **26**, 217–233. [297]

Pappas, C. L. and Strick, P. L. (1981a). Physiological demonstration of multiple representation in the forelimb region of cat's motor cortex. *J. Comp. Neurol.* **200**, 481–490. [317, 335]

Pappas, C. L. and Strick, P. L. (1981b). Anatomical demonstration of multiple representation in the forelimb region of cat's motor cortex. *J. Comp. Neurol.* **200**, 491–500. [317]

Passingham, R. E. (1985a). Rates of brain development in mammals including man. *Brain Behav. Evol.* **26**, 167–175. [96]

Passingham, R. E. (1985b). Premotor cortex: sensory cues and movement. *Behav. Brain Res.* **18**, 175–186. [295]

Passingham, R. E. (1987). Two cortical systems for directing movement. In *Motor areas of the cerebral cortex* (eds. G. Bock, M. O'Connor, and J. Marsh) Vol. 132, pp. 151–161. CIBA Foundation Symp. Wiley, Chichester. [291, 295]

Passingham, R. E. (1988). Premotor cortex and preparation for movement. *Exp. Brain Res.* **70**, 590–596. [296, 301]

Passingham, R. E., Perry, V. H., and Wilkinson, F. (1983). The long-term effects of removal of sensorimotor cortex in infant and adult rhesus monkeys. *Brain* **106**, 675–705. [96, 100]

Passingham, R. E., Chen, Y. C., and Thaler, D. (1989). Supplementary motor cortex and self-initiated movement. In *Neural programming* (ed. M. Ito), pp. 13–24. Karger, Basel. [290, 291]

Paulignan, Y., Mackenzie, C., Marteniuk, R. and Jeannerod, M. (1990). The coupling of arm and finger movements during prehension. *Exp. Brain Res.* **79**, 431–435. [219, 355]

Paulignan, Y., Mackenzie, C., Marteniuk, R., and Jeannerod, M. (1991). Selective perturbation of visual input during prehension movements. *Exp. Brain Res.* **83**, 502–512. [356]

Pellmar, T. C. and Somjen, G. G. (1977). Velocity of supraspinal input and conduction velocity of axons of spinal motoneurons. *Brain Res.* **120**, 179–183. [189]

Penfield, W., and Boldrey, E. (1937). Somatic motor and sensory representation in the cerebral cortex of man as studied by electrical stimulation. *Brain* **60**, 389–443. [15, 17, 18, 19, 20, 315, 344]

Penfield, W. and Rasmussen, T. (1952). *The cerebral cortex of man.* Macmillan, New York. [19, 20, 21, 24, 32, 33, 313, 314, 346]

Penfield, W. and Welch, K. (1949). The supplementary motor area, in the cerebral cortex of man. *Trans. Am. Neurol. Assoc.* **74**, 179–184. [15, 21, 22, 276]

Penfield, W. and Welch, K. (1951). The supplementary motor area of the cerebral cortex. *Arch. Neurol. Psychiat.* **66**, 289–317. [276, 294]

Peters, A. and Jones, E. G. (1984). Classification of cortical neurons. In *Cerebral cortex* (eds. E. G. Jones and A. Peters) Vol. 1, pp. 107–121. Plenum, New York. [38]

Petersen, S. E., Fox, P. T., Posner, M. I., Mintun, M., and Raichle, M. E. (1988). Positron emission tomographic studies of the cortical anatomy of a single-word processing. *Nature* **331**, 585–589. [359]

Peterson, B. W., Anderson, M. E., and Filion, M. (1974). Responses of ponto-medullary reticular neurons to cortical, tectal and cutaneous stimuli. *Exp. Brain Res.* **21**, 19–44. [61, 66]

Petras, J. M. (1968). Corticospinal fibers in New World and Old World simians. *Brain Res.* **8**, 206–208. [94]

Pettersson, L. -G. (1990). Forelimb movements in the cat; kinetic features and neuronal control. *Acta Physiol. Scand.* **140**, suppl. 594, 1–60. [117, 219]

Phillips, C. G. (1956a). Intracellular records from Betz cells in the cat. *Qut. J. Exp. Physiol.* **41**, 58–69. [50]

Phillips, C. G. (1956b). Cortical motor threshold and the thresholds distribution of excited Betz cells in the cat. *Qut. J. Exp. Physiol.* **41**, 70–84. [50]

Phillips, C.G. (1959). Actions of antidromic pyramidal volleys on single Betz cells in the cat. *Q. J. Exp. Physiol.* **44**, 1–25. [50]

Phillips, C. G. (1969). Motor apparatus of the baboon's hand. *Proc. R. Soc. Lond., Ser. B.* **173**, 141–174. [263, 265]

Phillips, C. G. (1971). Evolution of the corticospinal tract in primates with special reference to the hand. In *Proceedings of the 3rd International Congress on Primatology, Zurich.* Vol. 2, pp. 2–23. Karger, Basel. [93, 94]

Phillips, C. G. (1975). Laying the ghost of 'muscles versus movements'. *Can. J. Neurol. Sci.* **2**, 209–218. [312]

Phillips, C. G. (1981). Microarchitecture of the motor cortex in primates. In *Progress in anatomy* (ed. R. J. Harrison) Vol. 1, pp. 61 94. Cambridge University Press. [36, 310]

Phillips, C. G. (1986). *Movements of the hand.* Liverpool University Press. [356]

Phillips, C. G. and Porter, R. (1964). The pyramidal projection to motoneurones of some muscle groups of the baboon's forelimb. *Prog. Brain Res.* **12**, 222–245. [187, 189, 195, 197, 323]

Phillips, C. G. and Porter, R. (1977). *Corticospinal neurones: their role in movement.* Academic Press, London. [2, 4, 9, 23, 25, 26, 32, 51, 55, 83, 92, 112, 115, 129, 165, 177, 195, 205, 206, 210, 213, 218, 236, 248, 249, 304, 305, 314, 324, 332, 333, 334, 339]

Phillips, C. G., Powell, T.P.S., and Wiesendanger, M. (1971). Projection from low-threshold muscle afferents of hand and forearm to area 3a of baboon's cortex. *J. Physiol.* **217**, 419–446. [250, 251, 252, 260]

Picard, N. and Smith, A. M. (1992a). Primary motor cortical activity related to weight and texture of grasped objects in the monkey. *J. Neurophysiol.* **68**, 1867–1881. [256, 258, 259]

Picard, N. and Smith, A. M. (1992b) Primary motor cortical responses to perturbations of prehension in the monkey. *J. Neurophysiol.* **68**, 1882–1894. [259, 260, 270]

Pierrot-Deseilligny, E. (1989). Peripheral and descending control of neurones mediating non-monosynaptic Ia excitation to motoneurones: a presumed propriospinal system in man. *Prog. Brain Res.* **80**, 305–314. [31, 129, 135, 136]

Poizner, H., Klima, E. S., and Bellugi, U. (1987). *What the hands reveal about the brain.* M. I. T., Cambridge, Massachusetts. [363]

Porter, R. (1970). Early facilitation at corticomotoneuronal synapses. *J. Physiol.* **207**, 733–745. [195]

Porter, R. (1972). Relationship of the discharges of cortical neurones to movement in free-to-move monkeys. *Brain Res.* **40**, 39–43. [218]

Porter, R. (1984). Basal ganglia links for movement, mood and memory. In *Functions of the basal ganglia* (eds. D. Evered and M. O'Connor), pp. 103–113. Ciba Foundation Symp. Wiley, Chichester. [252]

Porter, R. (1985). Motor performance after nerve crossing in monkeys. In *Upper motor neuron functions and dysfunctions*, Recent Achievements in Restorative Neurology Vol. 1 (eds. J. C. Eccles and M. R. Dimitrijevic), pp. 272–279. Karger, Basel. [361]

Porter, R. (1987). Functional studies of the motor cortex. In *Motor areas of the cerebral cortex* (eds. G. Bock, M. O'Connor, and J. Marsh) Vol. 132, pp. 83–97. Ciba Foundation Symp. Wiley, Chichester. [23, 217]

Porter, R. (1990). Somato-sensory projections to the motor cortex. In *Information processing in mammalian auditory and tactile systems* (eds. L. M. Aitkin and M. Rowe), pp. 157–167. Liss, New York. [257]

Porter, R. and Hore, J. (1969). Time course of minimal cortico-motoneuronal excitatory postsynaptic potentials in lumbar motoneurones of the monkey. *J. Neurophysiol.* **32**, 443–451. [179, 195]

Porter, R. and Lewis, M. McD. (1975). Relationship of neuronal discharges in the precentral gyrus of monkeys to the performance of arm movements. *Brain Res.* **98**, 21–36. [218]

Porter, R. and Rack, P. M. H. (1976). Timing of the response in the motor cortex of monkeys to an unexpected disturbance of finger position. *Brain Res.* **103**, 201–213. [257, 260]

Porter, R., Ghosh, S., Lange, G. D., and Smith, T. G. Jnr. (1991). A fractal analysis of pyramidal neurons in mammalian motor cortex. *Neurosci. Letts.* **103**, 112–116. [43]

Potashner, S. J., Dymczyk, L., and Deangelis, M. M. (1988). D-aspartate uptake and release in the guinea pig spinal cord after partial ablation of the cerebral cortex. *J. Neurochem.* **50**, 103–111. [55]

Powell, T. P. S. and Mountcastle, V. B. (1959). Some aspects of the functional organization of the cortex of the postcentral gyrus of the monkey: A correlation of findings obtained in a single unit analysis with cytoarchitecture. *Bull. Johns Hopkins Hosp.* **105**, 133–162. [262]

Preston, J. B. and Whitlock, D. G. (1960). Precentral facilitation and inhibition of spinal motoneurones. *J. Neurophysiol.* **23**, 154–170. [200]

Preston, J. B. and Whitlock, D. G. (1961). Intracellular potentials recorded from motoneurons following precentral gyrus stimulation in primate. *J. Neurophysiol.* **24**, 91–100. [146, 186, 200]

Preston, J. B., Shende, M. C., and Uemura, K. (1967). The motor cortex-pyramidal system: patterns of facilitation and inhibition on motoneurons innervating limb musculature of cat and baboon and their possible adaptive significance. In *Neurophysiological basis of normal and abnormal motor activities* (eds. M. D. Yahr and D. P. Purpura), pp. 61–72. Raven, New York. [313]

Prochazka, A. (1989). Sensorimotor gain control: A basic strategy of motor systems? *Prog. Neurobiol.* **33**, 281–307. [66, 207, 269, 357]

Prochazka, A. and Wand, P. (1981). Independence of fusimotor and skeletomotor systems during voluntary movement. In *Muscle receptors and movement* (eds. A. Taylor and A. Prochaska), pp. 229–244. Macmillan, London. [207]

Raichle, M. E. (1987). Circulatory and metabolic correlates of brain function in normal humans. In *Handbook of physiology — the nervous system*, Higher

Functions of the Brain (ed. F. Plum) Vol. V, pp. 643–674. American Physiological Society, Bethesda, Maryland. [358]

Raichle, M. E., Mintun, M. A., and Herscovitch, P. (1985). Positron emission tomography with 15oxygen radiopharmaceuticals. *Res. Pub. Ass. Nerv. Ment. Dis.* **63**, 51–59. [242]

Ralston, D. D. and Ralston, H. J. (1985). The terminations of corticospinal tract axons in the macaque monkey. *J. Comp. Neurol.* **242**, 325–337. [73, 75, 155, 160]

Ralston, D. D., Milroy, A. M., and Ralston, H. J. (1987). Non-myelinated axons are rare in the medullary pyramids of the macaque monkey. *Neurosci. Letts.* **73**, 215–219. [82]

Ralston, D. D., Milroy, A. M., and Holstege, G. (1988). Ultrastructural evidence for direct monosynaptic rubrospinal connections to motoneurons in macaca mulatta. *Neurosci. Letts.* **95**, 102–106. [155]

Ramón y Cajal, S. (1909). *Histologie du système nerveux de l'homme et des vertèbrès*, Vol. 1. Maloine, Paris. [37]

Ramón y Cajal, S. (1911). *Histologie du système nerveux de l'Homme et des vertèbrès*, Vol. 2. Maloine, Paris. [37]

Redman, S. J. (1990). Quantal analysis of synaptic potentials in neurons of the central nervous system. *Physiol. Rev.* **70**, 165–198. [140, 141, 186, 194]

Redman, S. J. and Walmsley, B. (1983a). The time course of synaptic potentials evoked in cat spinal motoneurones at identified group Ia synapses. *J. Physiol.* **343**, 117–133. [139]

Redman, S. J. and Walmsley, B. (1983b). Amplitude fluctuations in synaptic potentials evoked in cat spinal motoneurones at identified group Ia synapses. *J. Physiol.* **343**, 135–145. [139, 141, 142]

Reh, T. and Kalil, K. (1981). Development of the pyramidal tract in the hamster. I. A light microscopic study. *J. Comp. Neurol.* **200**, 55–67. [98, 102]

Reh, T. and Kalil, K. (1982). Development of the pyramidal tract in the hamster. II. An electron microscopic study. *J. Comp. Neurol.* **205**, 77–88. [97, 100, 103]

Relova, J. L. and Padel, Y. (1989). Short latency somaesthetic responses in motor cortex transmitted through the spino-thalamic system, in the cat. *Exp. Brain Res.* **75**, 639–643. [261, 262]

Renaud, L. P. and Kelly, J. S. (1974). Simultaneous recordings from pericruciate pyramidal tract and non-pyramidal tract neurons: Response to stimulation of inhibitory pathways. *Brain Res.* **79**, 29–44. [45]

Renshaw, B. (1941). Influence of discharge of motoneurons upon excitation of neighbouring motoneurons. *J. Neurophysiol.* **4**, 167–183. [29]

Ribot, E., Roll, J.-P., and Vedel, J.-P. (1986). Efferent discharges recorded from single skeletomotor and fusimotor fibres in man. *J. Physiol.* **375**, 251–268. [207]

Riehle, A. and Requin, J. (1989). Monkey primary motor and premotor cortex: Single-cell activity related to prior information about direction and extent of an intended movement. *J. Neurophysiol.* **61**, 534–549. [219]

Riehle, A. and Requin, J. (1993). The predictive value for performance speed of preparatory changes in neuronal-activity of the monkey motor and premotor cortex. *Behav. Brain. Res.* **53**, 35–49. [230]

Rizzolatti, G. (1987). Functional organization of inferior area 6. In *Motor areas in the cerebral cortex* (eds. G. Bock, M. O'Connor, and J. Marsh) Vol. 132, pp. 171–181. CIBA Foundation Symp. Wiley, Chichester. [274, 300]

Rizzolatti, G., Scandolara, C., Gentilucci, M., and Camarda, R. (1981a). Response properties and behavioural modulation of 'mouth' neurons of the postarcuate cortex (area 6) in macaque monkeys. *Brain Res.* **225**, 421–424. [300]

Rizzolatti, G., Scandolara, C., Matelli, M., and Gentilucci, M. (1981b). Afferent properties of periarcuate neurons in macaque monkeys. I. Somatosensory responses. *Behav. Brain Res.* **2**, 125–146. [300]

Rizzolatti, G., Scandolara, C., Matelli, M., and Gentilucci, M. (1981c). Afferent properties of periarcuate neurons in macaque monkeys. II. Visual responses. *Behav. Brain Res.* **2**, 147–163. [300]

Rizzolatti, G. Matelli, M., and Pavesi, G. (1983). Deficits in attention and movement following the removal of post-arcuate (area 6) and pre-arcuate (area 8) cortex in macaque monkeys. *Brain Res.* **106**, 655–673. [296]

Rockel, A. J., Hiorns, R. W., and Powell, T. P. S. (1980). The basic uniformity in structure of the neocortex. *Brain* **103**, 221–244. [36]

Roland, P. E. (1984). Organization of motor control by the normal human brain. *Human Neurobiol.* **2**, 205–216. [242, 302]

Roland, P. E. (1985). Application of brain blood flow imaging in behavioural neurophysiology: Cortical field activation hypothesis. *Res. Publ. Ass. Nerv. Ment. Dis.* **63**, 87–104. [242]

Roland, P. E. (1987). Metabolic mapping of sensorimotor integration in the human brain. In *Motor areas of the cerebral cortex* (eds. G. Bock, M. O'Connor, and J. Marsh) Vol. 132, pp. 251–265. CIBA Foundation Symp. Wiley, Chichester. [240, 242, 287, 288, 302]

Roland, P. E. and Larsen, B. (1976). Focal increase in cerebral blood flow during stereognostic testing in man. *Arch. Neurol.* **33**, 551–558. [240]

Roland, P. E., Skinhøj, E., Larsen, B., and Endo, H. (1977). Perception and voluntary action: localization of basic input and output functions as revealed by regional cerebral blood flow increases in the human brain. In *Cerebral vascular disease* (eds. J. S. Meyer *et al.*) pp. 40–44. Excerpta Medica, Amsterdam. [244]

Roland, P. E., Larsen, B., Lassen, N. A. and Skinhøj, E. (1980a). Supplementary motor area and other cortical areas in organization of voluntary movements in man. *J. Neurophysiol.* **43**, 118–136. [241, 242, 243, 285, 286, 358]

Roland, P. E., Skinhøj, E., Lassen, N. A., and Larsen, B. (1980b). Differential cortical areas in man in organization of voluntary movements in extrapersonal space. *J. Neurophysiol.* **43**, 137–150. [287]

Roland, P. E., Meyer, E., Shibasaki, T., Yamamoto, Y.I., and Thompson, C. J. (1982). Regional cerebral blood flow changes in cortex and basal ganglia during voluntary movements in normal human volunteers. *J. Neurophysiol.* **48**, 467–480. [242, 244, 358, 359]

Romanes, G. J. (1951). The motor cell columns of the lumbosacral spinal cord of the cat. *J. Comp. Neurol.* **94**, 313–363. [122]

Ropper, A. H., Fisher, C.M., and Kleinman, G. M. (1979). Pyramidal infarction in the medulla: a cause of pure motor hemiplegia sparing the face. *Neurology* **29**, 91–95. [115]

Rosén, I. and Asanuma, H. (1972). Peripheral afferent inputs to the forelimb area of the monkey motor cortex: Input–output relations. *Exp. Brain Res.* **14**, 257–273. [48, 248, 254, 256]

Rossini, P. M., Caramia, M. D., and Zarola, F. (1987). Mechanisms of nervous propagation along central motor pathways: non-invasive evaluation in healthy subjects and in patients with neurological disease. *Neurosurg.* **20**, 183–191. [271]

Rothwell, J. C., Traub, M. M., Day, B. L., Obeso, J. A., Thomas, P. K. and Marsden, C. D. (1982). Manual motor performance in a deafferented man. *Brain* **105**, 515–542. [247, 264, 354]

Rothwell, J. C., Gandevia, S. C., and Burke, D. (1990). Activation of fusimotor neurones by motor cortical stimulation in human subjects. *J. Physiol.* **431**, 743–756. [206]

Rothwell, J. C., Thompson, P. D., Day, B. L., Boyd, S., and Marsden, C. D. (1991). Stimulation of the human motor cortex through the scalp. *Exp. Physiol.* **76**, 159–200. [137, 192, 193]

Rudomin, P. (1990). Presynaptic control of synaptic effectiveness of muscle spindle and tendon organ afferents in the mammalian spinal cord. In *The segmental motor system* (eds. M. D. Binder and L. M. Mendell), pp. 349–380. Oxford University Press. [207]

Russel, J. R. and DeMyer, W. (1961). The quantitative cortical origin of pyramidal axons of Macaca rhesus, with some remarks on the slow rate of axolysis. *Neurology* **11**, 96–108. [67]

Rustioni, A. and Cuénod, M. (1982). Selective retrograde transport of D-aspartate in spinal interneurons and cortical neurons of rats. *Brain Res.* **236**, 143–155. [55]

Rustioni, A. and Hayes, N. L. (1981) Corticospinal tract collaterals to the dorsal column nuclei of cats. *Exp. Brain Res.* **43**, 237–245. [66]

Ryall, R. W. (1970). Renshaw cell mediated inhibition of Renshaw cells: patterns of excitation and inhibition from impulses in motor axon collaterals. *J. Neurophysiol.* **33**, 257–270. [29]

Sahs, A. L., Hartman, E. C., and Aronson, S. M. (1979). *Stroke: cause, prevention, treatment and rehabilitation*. Castle House Publications, London. [33]

Sakai, M. (1978). Single unit activity in a border area between the dorsal prefrontal and premotor regions in the visually conditioned motor task of monkeys. *Brain Res.* **147**, 377–383. [300]

Sakai, S. T. (1990). Corticospinal projections from areas 4 and 6 in the raccoon. *Exp. Brain Res.* **79**, 240–248. [77]

Sakamoto, T., Porter, L. L., and Asanuma, H. (1987). Long-lasting potentiation of synaptic potentials in the motor cortex produced by stimulation of the sensory cortex in the cat: a basis of motor learning. *Brain. Res.* **413**, 360–364. [342]

Sakata, H. and Iwamura, Y. (1978). Cortical processing of tactile information in the first somatosensory and parietal association areas of the monkey. In *Active touch* (ed. G. Gordon), pp. 55–73. Pergamon, Oxford. [281]

Sakata, H. and Miyamoto, J. (1968). Topographic relationship between the receptive fields of the neurons in the motor cortex and in the movements elicited by focal stimulation in freely moving cats. *Jap. J. Physiol.* **18**, 489–507. [334]

Sakata, H., Takaoka, Y., Kawarasaki, A., and Shibutami, H. (1973). Somatosensory properties of neurons in the superior parietal cortex (area 5) of the rhesus monkey. *Brain Res.* **64**, 85–102. [281]

Samulack, D. D., Waters, R. S., Dykes, R. W., and McKinley, P. A. (1990). Absence of responses to microstimulation at the hand–face border in baboon primary motor cortex. *Can. J. Neurol. Sci.* **17**, 24–29. [326]

Sanes, J. N. and Donoghue, J. P. (1991). Organization and adaptability of muscle representations in primary motor cortex. *Exp. Brain Res.* suppl. (in press). [340]

Sanes, J. N., Suner S., and Donoghue, J. P. (1990). Dynamic organization of primary motor cortex output to target muscles in adult rats. I. Long-term patterns of reorganization following motor or mixed peripheral nerve lesions. *Exp. Brain Res.* **79**, 479–491. [312, 339]

Sapienza, S., Talbi, B., Jaquemin, J., and Albe-Fessard, D. (1981). Relationship between input and output of cells in motor and somatosensory cortices of the chronic awake rat. *Exp. Brain Res.* **43**, 47–56. [324]

Sato, K. C. and Tanji, J. (1989). Digit-muscle responses evoked from multiple intracortical foci in monkey precentral motor cortex. *J. Neurophysiol.* **62**, 959–970. [313, 315, 317]

Satomi, H., Takahashi, K., Aoki, M., and Kosaka, I. (1988). Anatomical evidence for the re-crossing of lateral corticospinal fibers via the posterior gray commissure in the cat spinal cord. *Neurosci. Letts.* **88**, 157–160. [112]

Satomi, H., Takahashi, K., Kosaka, I., and Aoki, M. (1989). Re-appraisal of projection levels of the corticospinal fibers in the cat, with special reference to the fibers descending through the dorsal funiculus: a WGA-HRP study. *Brain Res.* **492**, 255–260. [83]

Sayer, R. J., Redman, S. J., and Andersen, P. (1989). Amplitude fluctuations in small EPSPs recorded from CA1 pyramidal cells in the guinea pig hippocampal slice. *J. Neurosci.* **9**, 840–850. [56]

Schell, G. R. and Strick, P. L. (1984). The origin of thalamic inputs to the arcuate premotor and supplementary motor areas. *J. Neurosci.* **4**, 539–560. [276, 277]

Schell, G. R., Hodge, C. J., and Cacayosin, E. (1986). Transient neurological deficit after therapeutic embolization of the arteries supplying the medial wall of the hemisphere including the supplementary motor area. *Neurosurgery* **18**, 353–356. [294]

Schmidt, E. M. and McIntosh, J. S. (1979). Microstimulation of precentral cortex with chronically implanted microelectrodes. *Exp. Neurol.* **63**, 485–503. [339, 341]

Schmidt, E. M. and McIntosh, J. S. (1984). Microstimulation mapping of precentral cortex in awake behaving monkeys. *Soc. Neurosci. Abstr.* **10**, 737. [23]

Schmidt, E. M., Porter, R., and McIntosh, J. S. (1992). The effects of cooling supplementary motor area and midline cerebral cortex on neuronal responses in area 4 of monkeys. *E. E. G. clin. Neurophysiol.* **85**, 61–71. [295]

Schoen, J. H. R. (1964). Comparative aspects of the descending fibre systems in the spinal cord. *Prog. Brain Res.* **11**, 203–222. [87]

Schreiber, H., Lang, M., Lang, W., Kornhuber, A., Heise, B., Keidel, M., Deecke, L., and Kornhuber, H. H. (1983). Frontal hemispheric differences in the Bereitschaftspotential associated with writing and drawing. *Human Neurobiol.* **2**, 197–202. [290]

Schreyer, D. J. and Jones, E. G. (1983). Growing corticospinal axons by-pass lesions of neonatal rat spinal cord. *Neurosci.* **9**, 31–40. [97, 98]

Schultz, A. H. (1968). Form und Funktion der Primatenhände. In *Handgebrauche und Verständigung bei Affen und Frühmenschen* (ed. B. Rensch), pp. 9–25. Huber, Berne. [93]

Schwartzman, R. J. (1978). A behavioural analysis of complete unilateral section of the pyramid tract at the medullary level in macaca mulatta. *Ann. Neurol.* **4**, 234–244. [110, 113, 115]

Schwindt, P. C., Spain, W. J., Foehring, R. C., Chubb, M. C., and Crill, W. E. (1988a). Slow conductances in neurons from cat sensorimotor cortex in vitro and their role in slow excitability changes. *J. Neurophysiol.* **59**, 450–467. [52]

Schwindt, P. C., Spain, W. J., Foehring, R. C., Stafstrom, C. E., Chubb, M. C., and Crill, W. E. (1988b). Multiple potassium conductances and their functions in neurons from cat sensorimotor cortex in vitro. *J. Neurophysiol.* **59**, 424–449. [52]

Schwindt, P. C., Spain, W. J., and Crill, W. E. (1989). Long-lasting reduction of excitability by a sodium-dependent potassium current in cat neocortical neurons. *J. Neurophysiol.* **61**, 233–244. [52]

Sears, T. A. and Stagg, D. (1976). Short-term synchronization of intercostal motoneurone activity. *J. Physiol.* **263**, 357–381. [175]

Seitz, R. J., Roland, P. E., Bohm, C., Greitz, T., and Stone-Elander, S. (1990). Motor learning in man: a positron emission tomographic study. *NeuroReport* **1**, 17–20. [352, 360]

Seltzer, B., and Pandya, D. N. (1980). Converging visual and somatic sensory cortical input to the intraparietal sulcus of the rhesus monkey. *Brain Res.* **192**, 339–351. [297]

Sessle, B. J. and Wiesendanger, M. (1982). Structural and functional definition of the motor cortex in the monkey (macaca fascicularis). *J. Physiol.* **323**, 245–265. [73, 75, 313, 315, 322, 324, 329]

Shapovalov, A. I. (1975). Neuronal organization and synaptic mechanisms of supraspinal motor control in vertebrates. *Rev. Physiol. Biochem. Exp. Pharmacol.* **72**, 1–54. [144, 195]

Sherrington, C. S. (1885) quoted from Liddell, E. G. T. (1960) *The discovery of reflexes*. Clarendon Press, Oxford. [3]

Sherrington, C. S. (1889). On nerve-tracts degenerating secondarily to lesions of the cortex cerebri. *J. Physiol.* **10**, 429–432. [3]

Sherrington, C. S. (1893). Experiments in examination of the peripheral distribution of the fibres of the posterior roots of some spinal nerves. *Phil. Trans. R. Soc.* **184**, 641–763. [3]

Sherrington, C.S. (1898). Experiments in examination of the peripheral distribution of the fibres of the posterior roots of some spinal nerves Part II. *Phil. Trans. R. Soc.* **190**, 45 186. [3, 122, 172]

Sherrington, C. S. (1906). *The integrative action of the nervous system.* Yale University Press, New Haven. [4, 9, 348, 349]

Sherrington, C. S. (1933). *The brain and its mechanism.* Cambridge University Press. [200]

Shima, K., Aya, K., Mushiake, H. Inase, M., Aizawa, H., and Tanji, J. (1991). Two movement-related foci in the primate cingulate cortex observed in signal-triggered and self-paced forelimb movements. *J. Neurophysiol.* **65**, 188–202. [285]

Shinoda, Y. and Kakei, S. (1989). Distribution of terminals of thalamocortical fibers originating from the ventrolateral nucleus of the cat thalamus. *Neurosci. Letts.* **96**, 163–167. [49, 50]

Shinoda, Y., Arnold, A. P., and Asanuma, H. (1976). Spinal branching of corticospinal axons in the cat. *Exp. Brain Res.* **26**, 215–234. [147]

Shinoda, Y., Zarzecki, P., and Asanuma, H. (1979). Spinal branching of pyramidal tract neurons in the monkey. *Exp. Brain Res.* **34**, 59–72. [147]

Shinoda, Y., Yokota, J. I., and Futami, T. (1981). Divergent projection of individual corticospinal axons to motoneurons of multiple muscles in the monkey. *Neurosci. Letts.* **23**, 7–12. [148]

Shinoda, Y., Yokota, J. I., and Futami, T. (1982). Morphology of physiologically identified rubrospinal axons in the spinal cord of the cat. *Brain Res.* **242**, 321–325. [144]

Shinoda, Y., Kano, M., and Futami, T. (1985a). Synaptic organization of the cerebello-thalamo-cerebral pathway in the cat. I. Projection of individual cerebellar nuclei to single pyramidal tract neurones in areas 4 and 6. *Neurosci. Res.* **2**, 133–156. [310]

Shinoda, Y., Futami, T., and Kano, M. (1985b). Synaptic organization of the cerebello-thalamo-cerebral pathway in the cat. II. Input–output organization of single thalamocortical neurons in the ventrolateral thalamus. *Neurosci. Res.* **2**, 157–180. [310]

Shinoda, Y., Ohgaki, T. and Futami, T. (1986a). The morphology of single lateral vestibulospinal tract axons in the lower cervical cord of the cat. *J. Comp. Neurol.* **249**, 226–241. [144, 145]

Shinoda, Y., Yamaguchi, T., and Futami,T. (1986b). Multiple axon collaterals of single corticospinal axons in the cat spinal cord. *J. Neurophysiol.* **55**, 425–448. [147, 181]

Sholl, D. A. (1953). Dendritic organization in the neurons of the visual and motor cortices of the cat. *J. Anat. (Lond.)* **87**, 387–406. [38]

Sholl, D. A. (1956). *The organization of the cerebral cortex*. Methuen, London. [36]

Sloper, J. J. (1973). An electron microscope study of the termination of afferent connections to the primate motor cortex. *J. Neurocytol.* **2**, 361–368. [40]

Sloper, J. J. and Powell, T. P. S. (1979). An experimental electron microscopic study of afferent connections to the primate motor and somatic sensory cortices. *Phil. Trans. R. Soc. Lond.* **285**, 199–226. [49, 50]

Sloper, J. J., Hiorns, R. W., and Powell, T. P. S. (1979). A qualitative and quantitative electron microscopic study of the neurons in the primate motor and somatic sensory cortices. *Phil. Trans. R. Soc. Lond.* **285**, 141–171. [37, 45]

Sloper, J. J., Brodal, P., and Powell, T. P. S. (1983). An anatomical study of the effects of unilateral removal of sensorimotor cortex in infant monkeys on the subcortical projections of the contralateral sensorimotor cortex. *Brain* **106**, 707–716. [100]

Smith, A. M. (1979). The activity of supplementary motor area neurons during a maintained precision grip. *Brain Res.* **172**, 315–327. [281, 284]

Smith, A. M. (1981). The coactivation of antagonist muscles. *Can. J. Physiol. Pharm.* **59**, 733–747. [94, 225, 227, 346]

Smith, A. M., Hepp-Reymond, M.-C., and Wyss, U.R. (1975). Relation of activity in precentral cortical neurons to force and of force change during isometric contractions of finger muscles. *Exp. Brain Res.* **23**, 315–332. [219, 221, 226]

Smith. A. M., Bourbonnais, D., and Blanchette, G. (1981). Interaction between forced grasping and a learned precision grip after ablation of the supplementary motor area. *Brain Res.* **222**, 395–400. [284]

Smith, T. G. Jnr., Marks, W. B., Lange, G. D., Sheriff, W. H. and Neale, E. A.

(1989). A fractal analysis of cell images. *J. Neurosci. Methods* **27**, 173–180. [43]

Smith, T. G. Jnr., Behar, T. N., Lange, G. D., Marks, W. B., and Sheriff, W. H. (1991). A fractal analysis of cultered rat optic nerve glial growth. *Neurosci.* **451**, 159–169. [43]

Smith, W. S. and Fetz, E. E. (1989). Effects of synchrony between cortico-motoneuronal cells on post-spike facilitation of primate muscles and motor units. *Neurosci. Letts.* **96**, 76–81. [162, 163]

Spain, W. J., Schwindt, P.C., and Crill, W. E. (1987). Anomalous rectification in neurons from cat sensorimotor cortex in vitro. *J. Neurophysiol.* **57**, 1555–1576. [54]

Spain, W. J., Schwindt, P. C., and Crill, W. E. (1991a). Two transient potassium currents in layer V pyramidal neurones from cat sensorimotor cortex. *J. Physiol.* **434**, 591–607. [52]

Spain, W. J., Schwindt, P. C., and Crill, W. E. (1991b). Post-inhibitory excitation and inhibition in layer V pyramidal neurones from cat sensorimotor cortex. *J. Physiol.* **434**, 609–626. [52, 53]

Stafstrom, C. E., Schwindt, P. C., and Crill, W. E. (1984a). Repetitive firing in layer V neurons from cat neocortex *in vitro*. *J. Neurophysiol.* **52**, 264–289. [52]

Stafstrom, C. E., Schwindt, P. C., Flatman, J.A., and Crill, W. E. (1984b). Properties of subthreshold response and action potential recorded in layer V neurons from cat sensorimotor cortex *in vitro*. *J. Neurophysiol.* **52**, 244–263. [52]

Stanfield, B.B., and O'Leary, D. D. M. (1985). The transient corticospinal projection from the occipital cortex during the postnatal development of the rat. *J. Comp. Neurol.* **238**, 236–248. [79, 97]

Stanton, G. B., Cruce, W. L. R., Goldberg, M.E., and Robinson, D. L. (1977). Some ipsilateral projections to areas PF and PG of the inferior parietal lobule in monkeys. *Neurosci. Letts.* **6**, 243–250. [297]

Stephens, J. A., Usherwood, T.P., and Garnett, R. (1976). Technique for studying synaptic connections of single motoneurones in man. *Nature* **263**, 343–344. [31, 133]

Sterling, P. and Kuypers, H. G. J. M. (1967). Anatomical organization of the brachial spinal cord of the cat. II. The motoneuron plexus. *Brain Res.* **4**, 16–32. [122]

Stewart, M., Quirk, G. J., and Amassian, V. E. (1990). Corticospinal responses to electrical stimulation of motor cortex in the rat. *Brain Res.* **508**, 341–344. [86]

Stoney, S. D., Thompson, W. D., and Asanuma, H. (1968). Excitation of pyramidal tract cells by intracortical microstimulation: effective extent of stimulating current. *J. Neurophysiol.* **31**, 659–669. [306]

Strick, P. L. (1987). In *Motor areas in the cerebral cortex* (eds. G. Bock, M. O'Connor, and J. Marsh) Vol. 132, discussion on p. 58. CIBA Foundation Symp. Wiley, Chichester. [276]

Strick, P. L. and Preston, J. B. (1978a). Multiple representation in the primate motor cortex. *Brain Res.* **154**, 366–370. [254, 312]

Strick, P. L. and Preston, J. B. (1978b). Sorting of somatosensory afferent information in primate motor cortex. *Brain Res.* **156**, 364–369. [256, 258, 312]

Strick, P. L. and Preston, J. B. (1982a). Two representations of the hand in area

4 of a primate. I. Motor output organization. *J. Neurophysiol.* **48**, 139–149. [315, 334]

Strick, P. L. and Preston, J. B. (1982b). Two representations of the hand in area 4 of a primate. II. Somatosensory input organization. *J. Neurophysiol.* **48**, 150–159. [334]

Strick, P. L. and Sterling, P. (1974). Synaptic termination of afferents from the ventrolateral nucleus of the thalamus in the cat motor cortex. A light and electron microscope study. *J. Comp. Neurol.* **153**, 77–106. [49]

Takahashi, K. (1965). Slow and fast groups of pyramidal tract cells and their respective membrane properties. *J. Neurophysiol.* **28**, 908–924. [238]

Tan, U., Marangoz, C., and Senyuva, F. (1979). Antidromic response latency distribution of cat pyramid tract cells: three groups with respective extracellular spike properties. *Exp. Neurol.* **65**, 573–586. [82]

Tanji, J. (1975). Activity of neurons in cortical area 3a during maintenance of steady postures by the monkey. *Brain Res.* **88**, 549–553. [253, 264]

Tanji, J. and Evarts, E. V. (1976). Anticipatory activity of motor cortex neurons in relation to direction of intended movement. *J. Neurophysiol.* **39**, 1062–1068. [229, 231]

Tanji, J. and Kurata, K. (1979). Neuronal activity in the cortical supplementary motor area related with distal and proximal forelimb movements. *Neurosci. Letts.* **12**, 201–206. [278, 283, 284]

Tanji, J. and Kurata, K. (1982). Comparison of movement-related activity in two cortical motor areas of primates. *J. Neurophysiol.* **48**, 633–652. [284]

Tanji, J., and Wise, S. P. (1981). Submodality distribution in sensorimotor cortex of the unanaesthetized monkey. *J. Neurophysiol.* **45**, 467–481. [256, 258, 315, 335, 336]

Tanji, J., Taniguchi, K., and Saga, T. (1980). Supplementary motor area: Neuronal response to motor instructions. *J. Neurophysiol.* **43**, 60–68. [281, 283]

Tanji, J., Okano, K., and Sato, K. C. (1987). Relation of neurons in the nonprimary motor cortex to bilateral hand movement. *Nature* **327**(6123), 618–620. [76, 235]

Tanji, J., Okano, K., and Sato, K. C. (1988). Neuronal activity in cortical motor areas related to ipsilateral, contralateral, and bilateral digit movements of the monkey. *J. Neurophysiol.* **60**, 325–343. [280]

Tatton, W. G., Bawa, P., Bruce, I. C., and Lee, R. G. (1978). Long loop reflexes in monkeys: an interpretative base for human reflexes. *Prog. Clin. Neurophysiol.* **4**, 229–245. [255, 260]

Thach, W. T. (1975). Timing of activity in cerebellar dentate nucleus and cerebral motor cortex during prompt volitional movement. *Brain Res.* **88**, 233–241. [218]

Thach, W. T. (1978). Correlation of neuronal discharge with pattern and force of muscular activity, joint position, and direction of intended next movement in motor cortex and cerebellum. *J. Neurophysiol.* **41**, 654–676. [211, 216, 220]

Theriault, E. and Tatton, W. G. (1989). Postnatal redistribution of pericruciate motor cortical projections within the kitten spinal cord. *Devel. Brain Res.* **45**, 219–237. [98, 99]

Thilmann, A. F., Schwarz, M., Töpper, R., Fellows, S. J., and Noth, J. (1991). Different mechanisms underlie the long-latency stretch reflex response of active human muscle at different joints. *J. Physiol.* **444**, 631–643. [265]

Thomas, A., Westrum, L. E., Devito, J.L., and Biedenbach, M. A. (1984). Unmyelinated axons in the pyramidal tract of the cat. *Brain Res.* **301**, 162–165. [82]

Thomson, A. M. (1986). Comparisons of responses to transmitter candidates at an N-methyl-D-aspartate receptor mediated synapse in slices of rat cerebral cortex. *Neurosci.* **17**, 37–47. [55]

Thomson, A. M., Girdlestone, D., and West, D. C. (1989a). A local circuit neocortical synapse that operates via both NMDA and non-NMDA receptors. *Br. J. Pharmacol.* **96**, 406–408. [55]

Thomson, A. M., Walker, V. E., and Flynn, D. M. (1989b). Glycine enhances NMDA-receptor mediated synaptic potentials in neocortical slices. *Nature* **338**, 422–424. [55]

Tolbert, D. L. (1989). Absence of impulse activity in cortical neurons with transient projections to the cerebellum. *Dev. Brain Res.* **50**, 241–249. [96, 97]

Tolbert, D. L. and Der, T. (1987). Redirected growth of pyramidal tract axons following neonatal pyramidotomy in cats. *J. Comp. Neurol.* **260**, 299–311. [99]

Tomasch, J. (1969). The numerical capacity of the human cortico-ponto-cerebellar system. *Brain Res.* **13**, 476–484. [80]

Towe, A. L. (1973). Relative numbers of pyramidal tract neurons in mammals of different sizes. *Brain Behav. Evol.* **7**, 1–17. [80, 90, 91]

Towe, A. L. and Harding, G. W. (1970). Extracellular microelectrode sampling bias. *Exp. Neurol.* **29**, 366–381. [82]

Towe, A. L., Patton, H. D., and Kennedy, T. T. (1964). Response properties of neurons in the pericruciate cortex of the cat following electrical stimulation of the appendages. *Exp. Neurol.* **10**, 325–344. [249]

Tower, S. S. (1940). Pyramidal lesions in the monkey. *Brain* **63**, 36–90. [104, 109, 110, 121]

Toyoshima, K. and Sakai, H. (1982). Exact cortical extent of the origin of the corticospinal tract (CST) and the quantitative contribution to the CST in different cytoarchitectonic areas. A study with horseradish peroxidase in the monkey. *J. Hirnforsch* **23**, 257–269. [70, 73, 76]

Tracey, D. J., Asanuma, C., Jones, E.G., and Porter, R. (1980a). Thalamic relay to motor cortex: afferent pathways from brain stem, cerebellum and spinal cord in monkeys. *J. Neurophysiol.* **44**, 532–554. [261]

Tracey, D. J., Walmsley, B., and Brinkman, J. (1980b). Long-loop reflexes can be obtained in spinal monkeys. *Neurosci. Letts.* **18**, 59–65. [265]

Travis, A. M. (1955). Neurological deficiences following supplementary motor area lesions in Macaca mulatta. *Brain.* **78**, 155–173. [284, 294]

Tsukahara, N., Fuller, D. R. G., and Brooks, V. B. (1968). Collateral pyramidal influences on the corticorubrospinal system. *J. Neurophysiol.* **31**, 467–484. [62]

Tsumoto, T., Nakumura, S., and Iwama, K. (1975). Pyramidal tract control over cutaneous and kinaesthetic sensory transmission in the cat thalamus. *Exp. Brain Res.* **22**, 281–294. [270]

Ugolini, G. (1991). Anatomical evaluation of transneuronal transfer of herpes simplex virus 1 from peripheral nerves to central nervous system. PhD. Thesis, Cambridge University. [79]

Ugolini, G. and Kuypers, H. G. J. M. (1986). Collaterals of corticospinal and pyramid fibres to the pontine grey demonstrated by a new application of the fluorescent fibre labelling technique. *Brain Res.* **365**, 211–227. [65]

Ugolini, G., Kuypers, H. G. J. M., and Strick, P. L. (1989). Transneuronal transfer of herpes virus from peripheral nerves to cortex and brainstem. *Science* **243**, 89–91. [78, 79]

Vallbo, Å.B., Hagbarth, K.-E., Torebjörk, H. E., and Wallin, B. G. (1979). Somatosensory, proprioceptive, and sympathetic activity in human peripheral nerves. *Physiol. Rev.* **59**, 919–957. [206]

Valverde, F. (1966). The pyramidal tract in rodents. A study of its relations with the posterior column nuclei, dorsolateral reticular formation of the medulla oblongata, and cervical spinal cord. *Zeitschrift für Zellforschung* **71**, 297–363. [61, 86]

Verhaart, W. J. C. (1970). *Comparative anatomical aspects of the mammalian brain stem and the cord*, Vol. 1. Van Gorcum, Assen. [83]

Vicario, D. S. and Ghez, C. (1984). The control of rapid limb movement in the cat. *Exp. Brain Res.* **55**, 134–144. [219]

Vierck, C. J. (1975). Proprioceptive deficits after dorsal column lesions in monkeys. In *The somatosensory system* (ed. H. H. Kornhuber), pp. 310–317. Georg Thieme, Stuttgart. [110]

Vierck, C. J. (1978). Comparison of forelimb and hindlimb motor deficits following dorsal column section in monkeys. *Brain Res.* **146**, 279–294. [110]

Villablanca, J. R., Gémez-Pinilla, F., Sonnier, B. J. and Hovda, D. A. (1988). Bilateral pericruciate cortical innervation of the red nucleus in cats with adult or neonatal cerebral hemispherectomy. *Brain Res.* **453**, 17–31. [99]

Vogt, C. and Vogt, O. (1919). Allgemeinere Ergebnisse unserer Hirnforschung. *J. Psychol. Neurol. (Lpz)* **25**, 277–462. [13, 15, 24]

Wada, J. and Rasmussen, T. (1960). Intracarotid injection of sodium amytyal for the lateralization of cerebral speech dominance. Experimental and clinical observations. *J. Neurosurg.* **17**, 266–282. [115]

Wallace, S. A. and Weeks, D. L. (1988). Temporal constraints in the control of prehensile movements. *J. Mot. Behav.* **20**, 81–105. [356]

Walmsley, B., Wieniawa-Narkiewicz, E., and Nicol, M. J. (1985). The ultrastructural basis for synaptic transmission between primary muscle afferents and neurons in Clarke's column of the cat. *J. Neurosci.* **5**, 2095–2106. [143]

Walmsley, B., Edwards, F. R., and Tracey, D. J. (1988). Nonuniform release probabilities underlie quantal synaptic transmission at a mammalian excitatory central synapse. *J. Neurophysiol.* **60**, 889–908. [143]

Wannier, T. M.J ., Toeltl, M., and Hepp-Reymond, M.-C. (1986). On the problem of multiple hand representations in area 4 of the alert *Macaca fascicularis*. *Experientia* **42**, 711. [256, 258]

Wannier, T. M. J., Maier, M. A., and Hepp-Reymond, M.-C. (1991). Contrasting properties of monkey somatosensory and motor cortex neurons activated during the control of force in precision grip. *J. Neurophysiol.* **65**, 572–589. [216, 218, 219, 226, 227]

Ward, A. A., Peden, J. K., and Sugar, O. (1946). Cortico-cortical connections in the monkey with special reference to area 6. *J. Neurophysiol.* **9**, 453–461. [273]

Waxman, S. G. and Swadlow, H. A. (1978). The conduction properties of axons in central white matter. *Prog. Neurobiol.* **8**, 297–324. [82]

Webb-Haymaker (1953). *The founders of neurology*. Thomas, Springfield, Illinois. [11]

Weil, A. and Lassek, A. (1929). The quantitative distribution of the pyramidal tract in man. *Arch. Neurol. Psychiat.* **22**, 495–510. [83]

Weinrich, M. and Wise, S. P. (1982). The premotor cortex of the monkey. *J. Neurosci.* **2**, 1329–1345. [299, 329]

Weinrich, M., Wise, S. P., and Mauritz, K-H. (1984). A neurophysiological analysis of the premotor cortex of the monkey. *Brain* **107**, 385–414. [299]

Weisberg, J. A. and Rustioni, A. (1979). Cortical cells projecting to the dorsal column nuclei of cats. An anatomical study with the horseradish peroxidase technique. *J. Comp. Neurol.* **168**, 425–438. [61]

Welt, C., Aschoff, J. C., Kameda, K., and Brooks, V. B. (1967). Intracortical organization of cat's motorsensory neurons. In *Neurophysiological basis of normal and abnormal motor activities* (eds. M. D. Yahr and D. P. Purpura), pp. 255–288. Raven, New York. [259]

Werner, W., Bauswein, E., and Fromm, C. (1991). Static firing rates of premotor and primary motor cortical neurons associated with torque and joint position. *Exp. Brain Res.* **86**, 293–302. [219]

Westling, G., and Johansson, R. S. (1987). Responses in glabrous skin mechanoreceptors during precision grip in humans. *Exp. Brain Res.* **66**, 128–140. [260, 357]

Whitsel, B. L., Petrucelli, L. M., and Werner, G. (1969). Symmetry and connectivity in the map of the body surface in somatosensory area II of primates. *J. Neurophysiol.* **32**, 170–183. [281]

Widener, G. W. and Cheney, P. D. (1988). Effects on muscle activity from microstimuli applied to primary somatosensory cortex (SI) during voluntary movement in the monkey. *Neurosci. Abstr.* **14**, 509. [160]

Wiesendanger, M. (1969). The pyramidal tract. Recent investigations on its morphology and function. *Ergeb. Physiol.* **61**, 73–136. [67, 115]

Wiesendanger, M. (1973). Input from muscle and cutaneous nerves of the hand and forearm to neurones of the precentral gyrus of baboons and monkeys. *J. Physiol.* **228**, 203–219. [254]

Wiesendanger, M. (1981a). The pyramidal tract. Its structure and function. In *Handbook of behavioural neurobiology* (eds. A. L. Towe and E. S. Luschei) Vol. 5, pp. 401–490. Plenum, New York. [64, 65, 115]

Wiesendanger, M. (1981b). Organization of secondary motor areas of cerebral cortex. In *Handbook of physiology – The Nervous System II* (eds. J. M. Brookhart and V. B. Mountcastle), pp. 1121–1147. American Physiological Society, Bethesda, Maryland. [274, 275]

Wiesendanger, M. and Wiesendanger, R. (1984). The supplementary motor area in the light of recent investigations. *Exp. Brain Res.* suppl. 9, 382–392. [275, 276]

Wiesendanger, M., Séguin, J. J., and Künzle, H. (1973). The supplementary motor area. A control system for posture? In: *Control of posture and movement* (eds. R. B. Stein, K. B. Pearson, R. S. Smith, and J. B. Redford), pp. 331–346. Plenum, New York. [285]

Wiesendanger, M., Hummelsheim, H., Bianchetti, M., Chen, D. F., Hyland, B., Maier, V., and Wiesendanger, R. (1987). Input and output organization of the supplementary motor area. In *Motor areas of the cerebral cortex* (eds. G. Bock., M., O'Connor, and J. Marsh), vol. 132, pp. 40–53. CIBA Foundation Symp. Wiley, Chichester. [284]

Willis, W. D., Tate, G. W., Ashworth, R. D., and Willis, J. C. (1966). Monosynaptic excitation of motoneurons of individual forelimb muscles. *J. Neurophysiol.* **29**, 410–424. [128]

Wilson, S. A. K. (1914). An experimental research into the anatomy and physiology of the corpus striatum. *Brain* **36**, 427–492. [358]

Wing, A. M., Turton, A., and Fraser, C. (1986). Grasp size and accuracy of approach in reaching. *J. Mot. Behav.* **18**, 245–260. [355]

Wise, R., Chollet, R., Hadar, U., Friston, K., Hoffner, E., and Frackowiak, R. (1991a). Distribution of cortical neural networks involved in word comprehension and word retrieval. *Brain* **114**, 1803–1817. [359]

Wise, R., Hadar, U., Howard, D., and Patterson, K. (1991b). Language activation studies with positron emission tomography. In *Exploring brain functional anatomy with positron tomography* (ed. R. Porter), pp. 218–228. CIBA Foundation Symposium. Wiley, Chichester. [359]

Wise, S P. (1985). The primate premotor cortex fifty years after Fulton. *Behav. Brain Res.* **18**, 79–88. [297]

Wise, S. P. and Donoghue, J. P. (1984). Motor cortex of rodents. In *Cerebral cortex* (eds. E. G. Jones and A. Peters) Vol. 5, pp. 243–270. Plenum, New York. [79, 86]

Wise, S. P. and Mauritz, K-H. (1985). Set related neuronal activity in the premotor cortex of rhesus monkeys: effects of change in motor set. *Proc. R. Soc. Lond. Ser. B.* **223**, 331–354. [299]

Wise, S. P. and Tanji, J. (1980). Neuronal responses in sensorimotor cortex to ramp displacements and maintained positions imposed on hindlimb of the unanaesthetized monkey. *J. Neurophysiol.* **45**, 482–500. [281]

Wise, S. P. and Tanji, J. (1981). Supplementary and precentral motor cortex: contrast in responsiveness to peripheral input in the hindlimb area of the unanaesthetized monkey. *J. Comp. Neurol.* **195**, 433–451. [281]

Wise, S. P. Hendry, S. H. C., and Jones, E. G. (1977). Prenatal development of sensorimotor cortical projections in cats. *Brain Res.* **138**, 538–544. [96, 98]

Wise, S. P., Fleshman, J. W., and Jones, E. G. (1979). Maturation of pyramidal cell form in relation to developing afferent and efferent connections of rat somatic sensory cortex. *Neurosci.* **4**, 1275–1297. [97]

Wise, S. P., Weinrich, M., and Mauritz, K-H. (1983). Motor aspects of cue-related neuronal activity in premotor cortex of the rhesus monkey. *Brain Res.* **260**, 301–305. [299]

Wolpaw, J. R. (1979). Electromagnetic muscle stretch strongly excites sensorimotor cortex neurons in behaving primates. *Science* **203**, 465–467. [255]

Wolpaw, J. R. (1980). Correlations between task-related activity and responses to perturbation in primate sensorimotor cortex. *J. Neurophysiol.* **44**, 1122–1138. [255, 260, 262, 263]

Wong, Y. C., Kwan, H. C., MacKay, W. A., and Murphy, J. T. (1978). Spatial organization of precentral cortex in awake primates. I. Somatosensory inputs. *J. Neurophysiol.* **41**, 1107–1118. [254, 255, 334, 335]

Wong, Y. C., Kwan, H. C., and Murphy, J. T. (1979). Patterns of early and late discharges in somato-topically identified precentral neurons in awake monkeys in response to somatic inputs. *Can. J. Physiol. Pharmacol.* **57**, 574–577. [344]

Wood Jones, F. (1920). *The principles of anatomy as seen in the hand.* Bailliére, Tindall, and Cox, London. [96]

Woodbury, J. W. and Patton, H. D. (1952). Electrical activity of single spinal cord elements. *Cold Spr. Harb. Symp. Quant. Biol.* **17**, 185–188. [126]

Woody, C. D., Baranyi, A., Szente, M. B., Gruen, E., Holmes, W., Nenov, V., and Strecker, G. J. (1989). An aminopyridine-sensitive, early outward current recorded in vivo in neurons of the precruciate cortex of cats using single electrode voltage-clamp techniques. *Brain Res.* **480**, 72–81. [52]

Woolsey, C. N., Settlage, P. N., Meyer, D. R., Sencer, W., Hamuy, T. P., and Travis, A. M. (1952). Patterns of localization in precentral and 'supplementary' motor areas and their relation to the concept of a premotor region. *Res. Publ. Ass. Nerv. Ment. Dis.* **30**, 238–264. [276, 313, 314, 332]

Woolsey, C. N., Górska, T., Wetzel, A., Erickson, T. C., Earls, F. J., and Allman, J. M. (1972). Complete unilateral section of the pyramidal tract at the medullary level in macaca mulatta. *Brain Res.* **40**, 119–123. [114, 332]

Yakolev, P. I. and Lecours, A. R. (1967). The myelogenetic cycles of regional maturation of the brain. In *Regional development of the brain in early life* (ed. A. Minkowski), pp. 3–70. Blackwell, Oxford. [100, 107]

Yamamoto, T., Samejima, A., and Oka, H. (1990). The mode of synaptic activation of pyramidal neurons in the cat primary somatosensory cortex: an intracellular HRP study. *Exp. Brain Res.* **80**, 12–22. [38, 49]

Yumiya, H. and Ghez, C. (1984). Specalized subregions in the cat motor cortex: Anatomical demonstration of differential projections to rostral and caudal sectors. *Exp. Brain Res.* **53**, 259–276. [335]

Yumiya, H., Kubota, K., and Asanuma, H. (1974). Activities of neurons in area 3a of the cerebral cortex during voluntary movements in the monkey. *Brain Res.* **78**, 169–177. [253]

Zarzecki, P. (1991). The distribution of corticocortical, thalamocortical, and callosal inputs on identified motor cortex output neurons: mechanisms for their selective recruitment. *Somatosens. Motor Res.* **8**, 313–325. [253]

Zarzecki, P. and Wiggin, D. M. (1982). Convergence of sensory inputs upon projection neurons of somatosensory cortex. *Exp. Brain Res.* **48**, 28–42. [253]

Zarzecki, P., Shinoda, Y., and Asanuma, H. (1978). Projections from area 3a to motor cortex by neurons activated by group I muscle afferents. *Exp. Brain Res.* **33**, 269–282. [253]

Zecevic, N., Bourgeois, J.-P. and Rakic, P. (1989). Changes in synaptic density in motor cortex of rhesus monkey during fetal and postnatal life. *Dev. Brain Res.* **50**, 11–32. [97]

Index

active touch 66, 356
akinetic mutism, following SMA
    damage 294
apraxia 292
area 3a, *see* cerebral cortex

basal ganglia 49, 80, 216, 245, 348
    projections from SMA 276
    regional cerebral blood flow (rCBF) 287

cerebellum 49, 80, 216, 245, 264, 348
    activation in essential tremor 359
    adaptive functions 343
    plasticity 361
    positron emission tomography (PET)
        studies 359
    projections from SMA 276
cerebral cortex
    ablation results in
        degeneration in pyramidal tract 6
        paresis, deficits in movement
            performance 6
    afferent connections
        callosal 50
        cortico-cortical 50
        excitatory synapses on pyramidal
            cells 49
        projections from muscle afferents 249
        thalamocortical 49
    area 3a 76, 249, 261
        maintenance of steady force 264
        projections to area 4 253
        sensation of movement
            (Kinaesthesia) 271
    cingulate cortex 285
    histology of motor areas
        basket cells 45
        Campbell's description 10
        in the human brain 12
        pyramidal neurones 37
            axon collaterals 38, 40, 47
            clustering of 40, 73
            complexity revealed by fractals 43
            excitatory coupling between 47
            intracellular labelling 38, 40
            morphology 38, 54
            radial arrangement 48
            synapses, on the surface of 38
        stellate cells 45

intermediate precentral area (area 6) 15,
    20, 22, 24
intracortical connectivities 25
intrinsic connectivity 45, 49
laminar organization 56, 58
localization of function, *see also*: maps
    finger movements 17
    history
        Broca's contribution 2, 15
        Goltz and Ferrier, a battle of the
            giants 2
        Penfield, precentral and/or
            postcentral 22
        Vogts, correlation with
            cytoarchitecture 24
        Wernicke, sensory aphasia 2
    outputs activated by electrical stimuli
        25
postcentral sensory area 22, 216
precentral motor area (M1) 15
    discharges of neurones with
        conditioned responses 212
        contralateral, ipsilateral and bilateral
            movements 235
        cutaneous afferent inputs 257
        direction of movement 231
        force development 219
        joint movement 254
        joint stiffness 228
        movement performance 210, 238
        object slip 259
        onset of movement 215
        precision grip 225, 236
        prior instruction 231
        reaching 233
    flexibility of associations 235
    inputs from peripheral receptors 249
    projections from muscle spindle
        afferents 254
    regional cerebral blood flow (rCBF)
        changes 239, 244
prefrontal cortex and delayed
    responses 296
premotor cortex 24
    bilateral associations 299
    connections with motor cortex 273,
        297
    contributions to corticospinal tract 274
    cytochrome oxidase histochemistry 300
    electrical stimulation of 25
    lesions of 295